AF779624

Psychology and Buddhism

From Individual to Global Community

International and Cultural Psychology Series

Series Editor: **Anthony Marsella**, *University of Hawaii, Honolulu, Hawaii*

ASIAN AMERICAN MENTAL HEALTH
Assessment Theories and Methods
Edited by Karen S. Kurasaki, Sumie Okazaki, and Stanley Sue

THE FIVE-FACTOR MODEL OF PERSONALITY ACROSS CULTURES
Edited by Robert R. McCrae and Jüri Allik

PSYCHOLOGY AND BUDDHISM
From Individual to Global Community
Edited by Kathleen H. Dockett, G. Rita Dudley-Grant, and C. Peter Bankart

A Continuation Order Plan is available for this series. A continuation order will bring delivery of each new volume immediately upon publication. Volumes are billed only upon actual shipment. For further information please contact the publisher.

Psychology and Buddhism

From Individual to Global Community

Edited by

Kathleen H. Dockett
University of the District of Columbia
Washington, D.C.

G. Rita Dudley-Grant
Virgin Islands Behavioral Sciences
Christiansted, St. Croix, Virgin Islands

C. Peter Bankart
Wabash College
Crawfordsville, Indiana

Kluwer Academic / Plenum Publishers
New York, Boston, Dordrecht, London, Moscow

Library of Congress Cataloging-in-Publication Data

Psychology and Buddhism: from individual to global community/edited by Kathleen H. Dockett, G. Rita Dudley-Grant, C. Peter Bankart

p. cm. — (international and cultural psychology)

Includes bibliographical references and index.

ISBN 0-306-47412-3

1. Psychotherapy—Religious aspects—Buddhism. 2. Healing—Religious aspects—Buddhism. 3. Buddhism—Psychology. I. Dockett, Kathleen H., 1942- II. Dudley-Grant, G. Rita, 1951- III. Bankart, C. Peter, 1946- IV. Series.

BQ4570.P56 P78 2002
294.3′375—dc21

2002034180

ISBN 0-306-47412-3

©2003 Kluwer Academic / Plenum Publishers, New York
233 Spring Street, New York, New York 10013

http://www.wkap.nl/

10 9 8 7 6 5 4 3 2 1

A C.I.P. record for this book is available from the Library of Congress

All rights reserved

No part of this book may be reproduced, stored in a retrieval system, or transmitted in any form or by any means, electronic, mechanical, photocopying, microfilming, recording, or otherwise, without written permission from the Publisher, with the exception of any material supplied specifically for the purpose of being entered and executed on a computer system, for exclusive use by the purchaser of the work.

Printed in the United States of America

To my husband Ron Dockett and my Buddhist mentors
for their wisdom and compassion
KHD

To my husband Richard, my daughter Megan,
my parents George, Gertrude, and Ariel,
and my Sensei, Daisaku Ikeda, for their support
GRD-G

To Soong and Rog Elliott for 40 years of friendship
CPB

Contributors

C. Peter Bankart, Ph.D., is professor of psychology and director of the Student Counseling Service at Wabash College in Crawfordsville, Indiana. He is author of *Talking Cures: A History of Western and Eastern Psychotherapies* (1997), and numerous publications that explore the integration of Eastern thought with Western psychotherapeutics. He has taught on the faculty of the International Division of Waseda University in Tokyo.

David W. Chappell, Ph.D., is professor of religion at the newly established Soka University of America in Aliso Viejo, California. His publications include *Buddhist Peacework* (1999), *T'ien-t'ai Buddhism: An Outline of the Fourfold Teachings* (1983) and *Buddhist and Taoist Studies*, 2 vols. (1977, 1987). He was founding Director of the Buddhist Studies Program, and former Graduate Chair of the Department of Religion, University of Hawaii.

Kathleen H. Dockett, Ed.D., is professor of psychology and former Chairperson of the Department of Psychology and Counseling at the University of the District of Columbia. She is author of *Resources for Stress Resistance: Parallels in Psychology and Buddhism* (1993). A community psychologist, her research and presentations at APA meetings focus on Buddhism as a resource for the promotion of personal and societal well-being and its application to diversity and ethnic conflict.

G. Rita Dudley-Grant, Ph.D., MPH, ABPP, is a licensed clinical psychologist and director of Program Development at the Virgin Islands Behavioral Services in St. Croix. She is an APA Fellow, a member of the Board of Professional Affairs, past chair of the Committee on International Psychology, and past president of the Virgin Islands Psychological Association. She has presented on and been instrumental in a series of American Psychological Association programs examining the intersection of Buddhism and psychology.

Richard P. Hayes, Ph.D., is associate professor of Buddhist Studies and Sanskrit at McGill University, where he is Buddhist chaplain for the McGill Chaplaincy Service. His principal research interests are Indian Buddhist philosophy and Sanskrit poetry. A collection of his essays on Buddhism appears in *Land of No Buddha* (1998).

Leonard A. Jason, Ph.D., is a professor of psychology at DePaul University and the director of the Center for Community Research. He received the 1997 Distinguished Contributions to Theory and Research Award from the Society for Community Research and Action. He is the author of *Community Building: Values for a Sustainable Future* (1997), which integrated Eastern and Western thought and religions and the practice of community psychology.

Belinda Siew Luan Khong, LLB, Ph.D., is a lecturer in psychology at Macquarie University, Sydney, Australia, and a practicing psychologist. Her recent doctoral dissertation examined the concept of responsibility in Daseinsanalysis, Heidegger's philosophy, and Buddhist psychology. Her publications include comparative analysis of Jungian psychology and Taoist philosophy, and Existential and Buddhist psychology.

John Moritsugu, Ph.D., is professor of psychology at Pacific Lutheran University and a licensed clinical psychologist. He has co-edited texts on preventive psychology and written on minority status stress. A Fellow of the American Psychological Association, he has been co-president of the Society for the Psychological Study of Ethnic Minority Issues, Division 45 of the APA, and president of the Washington State Psychological Association.

Doris North-Schulte, M.A., is director of Educational Programming at WBEZ Chicago Public Radio where she researches and develops multicultural and humanistic curriculum for elementary, middle, and high schools. She is an independent researcher, trainer, and lecturer on Buddhism and diversity.

Edward S. Ragsdale, Ph.D., a psychotherapist in New York City for the last 16 years, recently moved his practice to the Los Angeles area. He retains interest in systematic issues in psychology (e.g., the problem of value, the mind–body relation), and has made numerous presentations on these topics at APA meetings and elsewhere.

Polly Young-Eisendrath, Ph.D., is clinical associate professor of psychiatry at the University of Vermont Medical College in Burlington, Vermont. A psychologist and Jungian psychoanalyst, she practices in central Vermont. Her most recent books include *Women and Desire* (1999), *The Cambridge Companion to Jung* (1997), and *Awakening and Insight* (2002).

Shuichi Yamamoto, Sc.D., is professor of geochemistry and environmental education at Soka University and researcher of Buddhism and environmental problems at the Institution of Oriental Philosophy in Tokyo, Japan. He is co-author of *Deep Ocean Circulation* (1993), *Dynamics and Characterization of Marine Organic Matter* (2000), *Role of Religion in Society* (1998) and author of *Environmental Ethics* (1996), and *Environmental Education* (1998).

Acknowledgments

This book is the product of many years of collaboration among a truly diverse group of scholars and professionals from around the world, each of whose contribution was essential to the task. The friendships that have resulted from this collaboration are the best rewards for all our labor we could have imagined. The book's coeditors working at vast and inconvenient distances from each other discovered that their shared commitment to the Buddha nature made working together a joyful and productive learning experience.

We want especially to express our deep appreciation for the inspiration and encouragement of our series editor, Anthony Marsella. Tony's indefatigable commitment and optimism never wavered even as we sometimes struggled with the completion of what we humorously dubbed the "elephant birth" of this volume. Our thanks too to the help and support of a large group of colleagues who helped by their careful and constructive reading of various drafts of the contents of this volume: Brenda Bankart, Steve Morillo, David Blix, Dan Fisher, George Howard, Greg Martin, Guy McCloskey, Bill Aiken, Barbara Davis, Cora Christian, and Lenard Lexier.

Thanks too to the library staffs at Dartmouth College and Wabash College for their extensive help in tracking down elusive sources, and to the Department of Psychology at Dartmouth for extending to Peter the benefits of Visiting Researcher status. Thanks too to the Faculty Development fund of Wabash College that generously supported Peter's participation in this project. Appreciation also goes to Kathleen's graduate assistants, Benjamin Siankam and Addis Berek, for editing the manuscript for APA reference citation style. Thanks to Virgin Islands Behavioral Services for the support of Rita's involvement in this book and to the University of the Virgin Islands in their assistance in various aspects of her research.

Numerous people at Kluwer International, on both sides of the Atlantic, helped with the production of this book. Thanks to you all, but especially Christiane Roll, Marianna Pascale, Susan Vorstenbosch, Sharon Panulla, Sarah Williams, and Herman Makler.

Contents

III. EMPOWERMENT, RESPONSIBILITY, AND THE CHALLENGES OF CHANGE

IV. FUTURE DIRECTIONS: GLOBAL IMPACT

Introduction

G. Rita Dudley-Grant, C. Peter Bankart, and Kathleen H. Dockett

Buddhism, one of the world's oldest religions, and psychology, one of the newest humanistic sciences, are both dedicated to the rigorous pursuit of human understanding. Both disciplines engage scholars whose primary goal is the pursuit of the deepest possible knowledge of the human capacity for growth, self-knowledge, and the transformation of human behavior and functioning. Buddhism shares with psychology an almost infinite faith in the inherent possibilities within human beings to transcend historical and immediate experience in order to fully actualize human potential. Both disciplines are ultimately profoundly optimistic about the universal human capacity to move beyond suffering, to live productive and humane lives, and to establish communities where people can live in peaceful cooperation. Moreover, psychology and Buddhism both espouse a rigorous humanistic epistemology rooted in the ideal of empowerment through the exercise of reason, intentional action, and learning about the human condition through a scrupulous empiricism.

Over the last half-century most of the scholars who have explored the interface between the two disciplines have focused primarily on the implications of Buddhist teachings and psychological theories for the development and betterment of individual lives. Psychologists from a broad range of theoretical perspectives ranging from psychoanalysis and existentialism to radical behaviorism have explored links between their practices and a wide range of Buddhism teachings on meditation practices, prescriptions for ethical living, and intricate theories of the self, to name just a few. In recent years numerous authors such as Bankart (1997), Reynolds (1997) and Molino (1998) have encouraged interested students to pursue these intellectual intersections to build a foundation for a transcultural and transpersonal psychotherapeutic revolution combining the most valuable insights and techniques from both worlds.

However, both traditions have philosophical areas of concern not just on the micro/individual level, but also on the community and even global level. Within psychology, community psychology has a long history of looking at the growth and development of healthy communities. Buddhism also has some doctrines that move beyond the individual to the communal level. Indeed some Buddhist traditions, such as the Nichiren sect, have devoted their entire mission to the establishment of world peace. There are some Buddhists, such as the Vietnamese monk Thich Nhat Hanh (1993) whose entire practice is devoted to the promotion of peace. Yet there has not been a serious consideration of how the traditions and practices of community psychology can be informed and enriched by the Buddhist traditions which transcend the individual to consider the interconnectedness of all things, or the relatedness and responsibility that we each have towards the other. This vision is in complete accord with the goals of community psychology to create healthy empowered communities where individuals can thrive and live to their fullest potential.

At the time of this writing, the heinous September 11, 2001 terrorist attack on the World Trade Center and the Pentagon had just occurred. An unprecedented 2,823 lives (McCool, 2002) were violently ended on that day. This rift in our human-ness shocked the global community and elicited immediate responses from religious and community leaders around the world. Buddhist leaders from many countries issued statements of compassion and called for a nonviolent response reflecting the most fundamental tenets of Buddhism: respect for the sanctity of human life and the dependent co-arising of all causes and conditions. The following quotes from select Buddhist social activists illustrate well the application of these principles to the "911" disaster.

Thich Nhat Hanh (2001), upon inaugurating a ten-day fast and calling for others to join him in prayer and meditation to put peace into action, stated:

> All violence is injustice. Responding to violence with violence is injustice, not only to the other person but also to oneself. Responding to violence with violence resolves nothing: it only escalates violence, anger, and hatred. It is only with compassion that we can embrace and disintegrate violence ... The violence and hatred we presently face has been created by misunderstanding, injustice, discrimination, and despair. We are all co-responsible for the making of violence and despair in the world by our way of living, of consuming, and of handling the problems of the world. ... America possesses enough wisdom and courage to perform an act of forgiveness and compassion, and I know that such an act can bring great relief to America and to the world right away. (p. 1)

Daisaku Ikeda (2001), peace activist and leader of a large international lay-Buddhist organization, made the following appeal to the global community:

> we have been reminded of the immense value of human life.... I call for a just and equitable international tribunal to be established to try those responsible for acts of terrorism and other crimes against humanity.... But the struggle against terrorism requires more than short-term international cooperation.... It is the function of evil to divide; to alienate people from each other and divide one country from another... In the end, the evil over which we must triumph is the impulse toward hatred and destruction that resides in us all. Unless we can achieve a fundamental transformation within our own lives, so that we are able to perceive our intimate connection with all our fellow human beings and feel their sufferings as our own, we will never be free of conflict and war. In this sense, I feel that a 'hard power' approach, one that relies on military might, will not lead to a long-term, fundamental resolution... dialogue holds the key to any lasting solution... (p. 2)

This book takes a bold step towards moving beyond the individual to the community and global level, furthering the Buddhism and psychology dialogues. Given the highly volatile nature of the world at the time of this writing, with ethno-political warfare being waged world wide, it is critical that psychologists be willing to become socially active, using our science and practice to assist our world in moving beyond the boundaries of delusion which lead to hatred and violence to the enlightened living which is the potential and the promise of Buddhism.

The editors of this book, who are also the authors of several of its chapters, come from distinctly different psychological-professional and Buddhist perspectives. We are all psychologists, but Peter Bankart is an example of an "elite" Buddhist interested almost exclusively in Zen. His clinical work focuses on developmental processes in young men, and proceeds from a cognitive behavioral orientation. Kathleen Dockett is a community psychologist and an example of a socially engaged Buddhist who has practiced Nichiren Buddhism with the Soka Gakkai International-USA for 17 years. She has comfortably integrated these two identities in her research on the role of religion in individual and community well-being. Rita Dudley-Grant is a psychodynamically trained clinical psychologist who has practiced Nichiren Shoshu Buddhism with the Soka Gakkai International (SGI-USA) for over 20 years. She uses her Buddhist practice to inform her clinical work.

Their separate contributions to this book clearly reflect their differing approaches to the challenge of bringing the fruits of Buddhist teachings and practices to the discipline and practice of psychology. The other authors of this book likewise bring a wide range of perspectives and scholarly interests to their work. It may end up being the task of the reader to sort out whose biases are showing, and at what points. We do hope and believe, however, that the reader will find a "big picture" here that will, if nothing else, serve as an invitation for further study, discussion, and reflection.

Overview of the Book

Part I: Foundations

The first chapter, authored by the three editors, "On the Path of the Buddha: a Psychologists' Guide to the History of Buddhism," is a brief history of Buddhism and psychology. It takes a sweeping, broad-brush approach to the extremely complex subject of Buddhism's history, emphasizing the growth of theories with shared commonalities between the two disciplines. The chapter presents Buddhist doctrine, practice, and a short review of the most well-known Buddhist systems including Theravada and Mahayana, and Vipassana, Tibetan, Zen, and Nichiren. Practices such as mindfulness meditation, Tara Ropka therapy, and chanting are also reviewed. Finally, an analysis of Buddhism as it is practiced in the West today is presented, with its implications for psychological praxis.

In the next chapter, "Five Manifestations of the Buddha in the West: A Brief History," Peter Bankart recounts the frustrations, missed opportunities, and even downright failures that psychologists have experienced over the last century in their attempts to incorporate lessons from Buddhist philosophy into psychological practice. One of the most disturbing aspects of this history is that many of those who explored non-Western traditions seem to have done so with their judgments severely clouded by European-American ethnocentrism. The distortions seen in their reports of Buddhism are so distorted, in fact, they must be judged to have been influenced by that form of racism known as Orientalism. Will the efforts being made in this book and by many other contemporary psychologists fare better when judged 25 or 50 years from now? One of the challenges is to develop sensitivity to the deep philosophical messages of Buddhism so that as those messages are translated into Western theory and practice, they will retain an essence that the Buddha would recognize as coming from the wellspring of his teachings.

Edward S. Ragsdale, in "Value and Meaning in Gestalt Psychology and Mahayana Buddhism," has accepted the challenging responsibility of reviving a much neglected phase in experimental psychology's history, Gestalt Psychology, and shows clearly how the application of Buddhist philosophy helps to carry that psychology to the next stage of clarity and utility. The problem that Ragsdale addresses is one that psychologists have struggled with for all of their history. How can one make meaningful and coherent value judgments about anything important in life, when the construction of those events is almost entirely subjective? Ragsdale's answer is that Buddhism shows us how to avoid the traps of both the mistaken absolutism of nihilism and its epistemological opposite – absolutist assertions of truth. The answer lies in the Buddha's teachings about dependent origination, a doctrine that attunes us to the irreducible value of compassion and persuades us of our absolute interdependency through the exercise of reason.

Part II: Healing and Psychotherapy: Alternatives in Psychotherapy

Rita Dudley-Grant, in "Buddhism, Psychology, and Addiction Theory in Psychotherapy," provides us with a clear and substantive exposition on the application of Buddhist principles to the extraordinary challenge of responding to the epidemic of substance abuse that has torn Western civilization apart over the past half century. She initially reviews how the two disciplines of psychology and Buddhism can be seen to have shared goals in seeking to provide a path for optimal living. Both psychodynamic and cognitive behavioral commonalities with Buddhist theories and practices are reviewed. Conceptions of the self, self-control, and addiction theory are presented for their Buddhist and psychological links. In presenting her theories on addiction, Dudley-Grant describes Buddhist conceptualizations of addiction from Tibetan and Nichiren perspectives. She then analyzes the apparent dichotomy of the 12-step program and Buddhist philosophy. The Alcoholics Anonymous approach to recovery has deep roots in Judeo-Christian beliefs of a "higher power greater than ourselves." Dudley-Grant suggests that the Buddhist commitment to community can allow Buddhists struggling with addiction to benefit from this highly successful approach to recovery. She suggests that the greatest commonality and healing comes from the commitment to community, to other rather than self, beliefs held in both Christian and Buddhist faiths.

Polly Young Eisendrath, in "Suffering from Biobabble: Searching for a Science of Objectivity," addresses the relative poverty of Western's psychology's attempts to address and come to terms with *dukkha* (suffering), the ever-present problem of human suffering. She finds the problem to be embedded within Western science's dedication to an epistemology that is better used to describe the motions of planets than the dilemmas of living beings. Can Buddhism help us to more fully develop and articulate a genuine science of human experience? Young-Eisendrath argues that it can because Buddhism does not impose a rigid Cartesian dualism on the human condition. She envisions a unique and powerful human science that will inform human services so that it can respond compassionately and comprehensively to the realities of wide spread human suffering. Moreover, Young-Eisendrath presents a cogent argument for similarities between psychodynamic formulations of the psychic compulsions that lead to repetitive dysfunctional behavior and the Buddhist conceptualizations of karma. She challenges the increasing tendency to relinquish responsibility for one's behavior attributing it to genetic maladaptation or biological determinism. Rather she suggests that analysis and Buddhist practice can be equally empowering. They hold people accountable for their actions, thus providing the possibility for change. She strongly suggests the use of Buddhist and clinical psychological methods of research to study the ultimate impact and efficacy of these two great traditions.

In "Role of Responsibility in Daseinsanalysis and Buddhism," Belinda Siew Luan Khong's background that combines her psychological training with a degree in law and an appreciation of classical European philosophy is evident. Khong's goal is to elucidate the clarifying synergy between the concept of human responsibility in Heidegger's philosophy, existential analysis, and the notion of dependent origination in Buddhism. As she reviews the fundamentals of both systems, she shows how the idea of individuals taking responsibility for their lives and experience is central to the reduction of human suffering. Buddhism, moreover, extends the notion of responsibility in a way that informs our ability as human beings to see the true nature of things – through which comes the true experience of freedom. One of the many interesting points that Khong makes is that both in Buddhism and in daseinsanalysis the individual's journey of discovery is made possible by the faithful companionship of a teacher, a teacher who may largely be a silent partner whose attentiveness supports the client's efforts towards mindfulness.

Richard Hayes, in "Classical Buddhist Model of a Healthy Mind," has contributed a chapter that clearly takes a major step in the direction of translating Buddhist philosophy into terms that are both accessible and meaningful to an audience interested in Western psychology. Hayes stresses the importance of taking from Buddhist teaching the importance of creating and preserving a healthy mind by avoiding extremes of self-denial on the one hand, and self-indulgence on the other. Buddhism's "middle way" requires us to remain actively involved in the world both as change agents and seekers of the good. But we must do so without allowing our egos either to overwhelm the natural environment, or be overwhelmed by forces that we cannot control. The path to accomplishing and maintaining this difficult balance is shown through a combination of ethics, contemplation, and wisdom; and by staying in connection with family and other members of the community.

Part III: Empowerment, Responsibility, and the Challenges of Change

Part III of the book addresses the issues of Buddhism, community psychology, and social responsibility. Western psychology's primary interest in Buddhist traditions has centered on how they can be applied in psychotherapies, stress-reduction, and other healing modalities. Yet Buddhism has considerably more to offer as a resource for community empowerment and broad-based social change. As early as the 1950's Vietnamese Buddhist monk Thich Nhat Hanh coined the term "engaged Buddhism" to capture the active involvement of Buddhist monks and laity in the problems of society. Today there are schools of socially engaged Buddhism and Buddhist-scholar activists who are deeply committed to macro level change through the application of Buddhist principles to create ethical, social, political, economic, and ecological reforms (Kraft, 1996; Rothberg, 1998). These themes resonate with community psychology and it's goals of promoting well-being, increasing empowerment, and preventing the development of problems of communities, groups, and individuals.

In what is the unique contribution of this book to the Western psychological literature, Part III addresses the intersection between socially engaged Buddhism and community psychology and other applied psychologies. The five chapters in this section discuss the contributions of Buddhism to psychological models of empowerment, foundational values to guide ecological interventions, ethical guides for the resolution of environmental problems, principles of integration for transcending difference, and principles of social action. A discussion of the application of Buddhist principles of social action to the prevention of ethnic group conflict, and to community and societal-level change are found in the chapters by Chappell (Chapter 12), by Dockett and North-Schulte (Chapter 10), and also by Dockett (Chapter 8).

Empowerment models of social and community change are concerned with methods for enhancing perceived and actual control over one's life. Community psychologist Kathleen H. Dockett adopts such a perspective in "Buddhist Empowerment: Individual, Organizational, and Societal Transformation." Using psychology's empirically derived models of stress-resistance (Kobasa, 1982) and of empowering organizations (Maton & Salem, 1995) as a framework, Dockett draws upon her 12-year case study of Nichiren Buddhism and the Soka Gakkai International-USA lay Buddhist organization to illustrate the processes and structures through which Buddhist empowerment may occur. At the level of individual empowerment, she describes Buddhist philosophies and practices that appear to promote the development of hardy stress-resistant personality traits, including a sense of personal control. This process calls for Westerners to make major paradigm shifts in worldview, the most difficult of which is the belief that we are totally responsible for and totally in control of our destiny. At the community setting level, Dockett describes how Buddhist-inspired organizational norms, structures, and processes may promote empowerment of organizational members, and lastly she describes how socially engaged Buddhism of various types may promote societal-level or political empowerment. Dockett points to the commonalities that exist in the goals, interests, and methods of social change of community psychology and socially engaged Buddhism, and suggests the potential for a collaborative partnership where each can inform the other's understanding of processes and structures for empowerment.

In "The Role of Religion and Spirituality in Community Psychology," community psychologists Leonard A. Jason and John Moritsugu propose that a synthesis of community psychology and Buddhist philosophy may provide more comprehensive solutions to the problems of human suffering. They critique major models of social and community change used in community psychology (social competence, empowerment, and ecological) and find them lacking in the foundational values needed to guide our interventions. For example, in the case of ethnic group conflicts, the questions of what values should guide our selection of groups with whom to collaborate, how resources should be redistributed and toward what ends is left unanswered. The main thesis of this chapter is that Buddhist traditions could provide guides for energizing the visions of community psychology. Jason and Moritsugu review the foundational values of Buddhist schools of thought, and show how these values might be applied in assessment and therapy, with implications drawn to broader community-level interventions. The chapter advances our thinking on the question of how it is possible to join the value basis of the spiritual traditions with the action-oriented perspective of ecological community psychology, as suggested in Spretnak's (1991) concept of "Ecological Postmodernism."

In "Transcending Self and Other: Mahayana Principles of Integration," Kathleen H. Dockett and Doris North-Schulte address the contributions of Buddhist philosophy to understanding and preventing ethnic conflict. From psychological and Buddhist analyses of the root causes of ethnic conflict, the authors conclude that a crisis of identity lies at the core of much of the ethnic violence around the globe. Observing that under conditions of group threat, people retrench into their primal cultural identities (e.g., as Muslims, Americans, Arab Palestinians, Jewish Israelis) and become alienated from their more universal or cosmic identities, the authors propose that a failure to understand the nature of our existence, our identity, and our mutually interdependent relationships with one another is at issue. Dockett and North-Schulte then discuss how Buddhist values and principles may be applied to conflict prevention and propose four Mahayana principles of integration (unity) that provide an alternative conceptualization of "self" and "other" and hold the promise of a harmonious co-existence.

The theme of an ethic of care, the idea that science can inform and be informed by compassion, and the assertion that every living person can be empowered by coming to direct terms with the essence of his or her own existence has been recognized by some psychologists as constituting the beginnings of a deep ecological commitment to preservation of the earth (see for example, Barash, 2001). In "Environmental Problems and Buddhist Ethics: From the Perspective of the Consciousness-Only Doctrine," Shuichi Yamamoto sets forth an analysis of our environmental dilemma in a way that permits us to see and understand that the only solution that will save the planet is a solution that involves a fundamental change in human consciousness. By stressing such concepts as a fundamental biospheric egalitarianism in humans, living things, and non-living things Yamamoto's analysis leads us to a recognition that the ecological movement to save the earth from destruction requires both the great compassion and the energy of the wisdom of the way of the Buddha.

David W. Chappell introduces the concept of "social mindfulness" as a dimension of Buddhist mindfulness practice in "Buddhist Social Principles." His thesis is that the same process we pursue in the inner dialogue that is mindfulness (i.e., stopping, calming, and seeing) can be extended to the nexus of our social dialogues. Growing out of a lucid engaging description of the teachings and behavior of the Buddha, Chappell derives a set of Buddhist social principles that today guide the peace work of Buddhist social activists. He cautions us, however, that neither dialogue nor Buddhist morality are enough to resolve special problems, such as structural violence, social oppression, and environmental degradation. In these instances, he calls for the "middle path" of social responsibility backed by legal safeguards to ensure the stability of social change.

A key point made in this chapter is that while dhyana and pragna (meditation and wisdom) or samatha and vipassana (calming and insight) are two legs of the Buddhist chair, social action is the third leg without which the chair cannot stand. It is important to understand that the Buddha did not remain in isolated meditation but was socially active. Most of his career was spent on the road, actively engaging others, of all walks of life, in dialogue and reform. Not only was the Buddha a social activist, pacifying a vicious mass murderer Angulimala who wore a necklace of fingers taken from his nearly 1,000 victims; repeatedly intervening to dissuade rulers from waging war on neighboring kingdoms; and teaching kings, untouchables, bandits, and Brahmins alike; but he also sent the Buddhist community into society to help others. The Buddha's sense of responsibility represents a foundational value and model for our interventions.

Part IV: Future Directions: Global Impact

Finally, in "On the Path to Peace and Wholesomeness: Conclusion to Psychology and Buddhism," the editors state their belief that the ultimate benefit of the enrichment of Western psychology by Buddhism will be in the empowerment of human beings to work together to build sustainable communities that can pursue the never-ending work of creating a more peaceful world. As much as anything this transformation of psychology will come about by helping the profession engage the real, the deep, and the universal needs of the inhabitants of the planet. The vehicle for this transformation will not be in further glorification of the scientific canon or the "final victory" of the members of any specific psychological enclave. It will come through the transformation of our understanding as psychologists of the interdependence of all life and of the immense power of human consciousness to transform the human condition.

This book is intended to inform, stimulate, and broaden the thinking of psychologists and others interested in the interface between psychology and Buddhism. As the interest in Buddhism grows within the psychological community, the need for more information on theoretical as well as practical levels becomes apparent. In this book we move from considerations of the individual, through the community to global conceptions for world peace. We attempt to further the dialogue between psychology and Buddhism at many points along the continuum. Individuals and communities, empowered and ready to engage the millennium ultimately will have global implications for the future of humankind. Given the severe challenges to peace facing our world, the editors hope that this book will provide one more resource for those who would seek to transform the way in which human beings understand and interact with each other within and across all boundaries globally.

References

Bankart, C. P. (1997). *Talking cures: A History of Western and Eastern psychotherapies*. Pacific Grove, CA: Brooks/Cole.

Barash, D. (2001, February 23). Buddhism and the 'Subversive Science.' *The Chronicle of Higher Education*. Available from http://chronicle.com/weekly/v47/i24/24b01301.htm

Ikeda, D. (2001, September 25). Renewing Our Faith in Humanity (Tentative translation, to appear in *World Tribune*, October 19, 2001). Retrieved September 25, 2001, from http://smtp:wtex-press@sgi-sa.org/thesgiusa/community/Statements/PresIkedaEssay.html

Kobasa, S. C. (1982). The hardy personality: Toward a social psychology of stress and health. In J. Suls & G. Sanders (Eds.), *Social psychology of health and illness* (pp. 3–32). Hillsdale, N.J.: Lawrence.

Kraft, K. (1996). Engaged Buddhism. In A. Kotler (Ed.) *Engaged Buddhist reader* (pp.64–69). Berkeley, CA: Parallax Press.

Maton, K. I. & Salem, D. A. (1995). Organizational characteristics of empowering community settings: A multiple case study approach. *American Journal of community psychology, 23*, 631–656.

McCool, G. (2002, May 30). Ceremony marks end of WTC Cleanup. *Reuters News Service*. Retrieved May 30, 2002, from AOL News.

Molino, A. (Ed.). (1998). *The couch and the tree: Dialogues between psychoanalysis and Buddhism*. New York: North Point Press.

Nhat Hanh, T. (1993). *Love in action: Writings on nonviolent social change*. Berkeley: Parallax Press.

Nhat Hanh, T. (2001, September 18). *Cultivating compassion to respond to violence: The way of peace*. Retrieved September 25, 2001, from Buddhist Peace Fellowship http://www.bpf.org

Reynolds, D. (1997). *A handbook for constructive living*. New York: William Morrow.

Rothberg, D. (1998). Responding to the cries of the world: Socially engaged Buddhism in North America. In C. S. Prebish, & K. K. Tanaka (Eds.), *The faces of Buddhism in America* (pp. 266–286). Berkeley: University of California Press.

Spretnak, C. (1991). *States of grace*. New York: HarperCollins.

Part I

Foundations

Chapter 1

On the Path of the Buddha

A Psychologists' Guide to the History of Buddhism

C. Peter Bankart, Kathleen H. Dockett, and G. Rita Dudley-Grant

Siddhartha Gautama was the heir of the rajah of the small republic of Saka near the southern border of today's Nepal, in the foothills of the Himalayan Mountains of northeastern India some twenty five hundred years ago. His father, Suddhodana, was a member of the Kshatriya warrior caste and therefore undisputed ruler of his kingdom. Legend has it that because of a prophecy that Suddhodana's son would grow up to be a great king only if he did not choose to become a great holy man, Siddhartha's father (his mother had died shortly after giving birth) made the decision that the boy should be raised in great luxury. This way he would ensure that the young prince would never be tempted to renounce his throne to pursue life as a homeless holy man and ascetic.

Thus Suddhodana decreed that the noble family should live in splendid isolation. And since his kingdom was both economically rich and politically stable the rajah was able to devote much of his life to giving his son a splendid and, by design, an almost entirely uneventful royal childhood. Siddhartha married at age 16 and his first son was born some ten years later.

The dominant religious practices of the time dated back at least a thousand years and focused on burnt offering sacrifices made to thirty-three gods known as *devas*. Only Braham priests were considered sufficiently pure to make these sacrifices, and they developed a wide range of esoteric practices to purify themselves before each sacrifice. These practices based on various aspects of what we know today as Yoga included intensive practice in meditation, fasting, celibacy, social isolation, and physical privation.

The ultimate purpose of these religious practices was to achieve liberation from reincarnation after death, which was to be achieved by the accumulation of *karma*, benefit derived from performing appropriate sacrifices. Many of these Brahmic beliefs and practices would eventually be codified into the religion of Hinduism, but at the time of Siddhartha's life and teaching they represented the practices of the dominant folk religion of "the people of the woods" – holy men who had withdrawn from society to live solitary ascetic lives devoted to pious ritual and practice. This was, of course, precisely the lifestyle choice that Suddhodana was most desperate to keep from his growing son.

As many famous princes have done, and continue to do, the boy Siddhartha grew to a jejune manhood untroubled by the concerns of ordinary mortals. His closest friend and constant companion was Channa, who also served as the young prince's chauffeur, charioteer, and informant about the world beyond the family cloister. The two young men conspired to have adventures, as young men will; but Siddhartha reached the age of marriage and even became a father without once experiencing the joys or sorrows of the real world just beyond his illusion of his reality.

Gradually, however, Siddhartha grew increasingly curious about life beyond the walls of the royal compound, and he prevailed upon his loyal friend to take him on a clandestine excursion around his kingdom. What he encountered on this trip and its effects on the young man's consciousness were destined to change human history.

What Siddhartha saw in the world that his father had tried to hide from him was nothing at all like the world his loving father had so carefully constructed for him in the first 25 years of his life. With his own eyes he experienced a world filled with human misery and despair. On that day, in rapid succession the young prince encountered a withered old man bent with infirmity and close to death, another man who was consumed by a disfiguring disease, and then to his ultimate dismay, he saw his first corpse – borne aloft by a large group of tearful mourners. He was struck senseless by the horror of the sorrowful world he saw all around him. Bewildered, he asked the loyal Channa if this is the world in which all men lived. Channa replied, "Yes, master, there is no escape. Old age, sickness, and death – such is the lot of all men."

This discovery of the sorrows of life had a profound effect on the young prince, and he was devastated to learn that there were no learned men who could soften or even explain the brutal truths that he had so unexpectedly learned. This new knowledge profoundly changed the young prince, who now withdrew into a period of intense introspection. He could not fathom how ordinary life could be so unrelentingly harsh. Beyond that he understood all at once that all of the pleasures of his youth had been false; that his happiness had been permitted only by his utter and complete ignorance of the sorrow of the world all around him. In his despair he entertained the idea that life was utterly futile and that there could be little justification even to bring children into the world. What meaning could anything have in life with the inevitability of disease, infirmity, and ultimately death?

At the depths of his anguish, searching everywhere for answers to questions he could barely comprehend, Siddhartha encountered the fourth great image that would shape his character and the religious faith of millions of people in the future. He observed one of the thousands of mystic ascetic men of the forest who populated India during this era.

The prince inquired of this strange man, this beggar who struck him as being both wise and untroubled, how he could learn about the meaning of life and get to the heart of the nature of all the suffering he saw all around him. Being an ascetic, the wanderer of course told the prince that the only path to finding the answers to his questions required the young man to resign his privileged place and to take up a life as a wandering seeker, to devote his life to solitude.

So, at age 25 Siddhartha left the court, his wife, and his infant son and took up the life of a religious ascetic. He became the pupil of a series of holy men who instructed him in mental and physical discipline, and spent the next six years in self-imposed exile, sustained only by what he could beg from the common people. He nearly died from this regimen of starvation and asceticism, but became a master of what we know today as the practice of hatha yoga. In six years of rigorous self-denial he learned how to master his desires and how to quiet and focus the "drunken monkey" mind of ordinary consciousness. He had conquered the desires of his body and he had tamed his mind; beyond this, he had gained a significant following of disciples. But he was still no closer to answering the great questions in his heart about life, suffering, and death that continued to demand answers.

At the end of this period in his life, and near death from starvation, he came to the realization that continuing the severe regimen of privation that he was following would almost certainly bring about his demise before it would lead to his enlightenment. He understood that the answers he was seeking required him to harness not only the energy of his mind, but the resources of his body and his heart as well. So he left the company of the ascetics and accepted food and drink from a young woman named Sujata, who had been caused by a dream to bring him a meal of rice-milk in a golden bowl.

Nourished by this worldly gift, Siddhartha now embarked on a continuous meditation under an ancient fig tree known in Buddhist legend as the Bodhi Tree, or Tree of Wisdom. He vowed to remain under the tree until he had attained the Great Enlightenment. On the 49th day of his meditation, under the full moon of May in 544 BCE Siddhartha attained the Supreme Enlightenment and became the Buddha, the enlightened one.

> No one, it is said, can possibly explain enlightenment. It does not lend itself to description or explanation in words. The man who has awakened, however, is in no doubt about the occurrence. Although unable to describe it, he knows what has happened to him, just as someone in love may not be able to describe his feelings, yet is himself in no doubt about his particular physical and emotional state, or as a man dying of thirst will know when his thirst is quenched. As a term, Enlightenment signifies a direct, dynamic spiritual experience brought about, in the Buddhist view, through the faculty of intuition, a faculty developed and sharpened by such spiritual disciplines as intensive meditation and contemplation. It is a condition beyond the power and pull of "the opposites," a full realization of the universe and the self as one. (Ross, 1981, pp. 14–15)

After he attained enlightenment, Siddhartha was called Shakyamuni, which means "sage of the Shakyas", the clan his father ruled. The Buddha would spend the rest of his life spreading the word of his Enlightenment to his disciples throughout India. These disciples in turn carried the message southward into the Southeast Asian countries of Sri Lanka, Burma, Thailand, Vietnam, and Cambodia and eastward into China, Tibet, Korea, and Japan.

The message that the Buddha's disciples carried was one of supreme compassion. Their mission was to offer humankind the opportunity to make the same discoveries about the nature of life, and of suffering, that the Buddha himself had made. There were, of course, certain central propositions that the Buddha's disciples taught, but the central message of Buddhism always was, and to this day continues to be, an experiential one.

> A perfected Buddhist might be described as a human being who has reached a state in which moral training has become so deeply a part of his nature that it would be impossible for him to be involved in violence, cupidity, insensibility, low physical passion or other "unawarenesses." (Ross, 1981, pp. 36–37)

One of the principal things that stands out about this legend is that the central teachings that inform Buddhism were not revealed to the Buddha in a divine message "received" from on high. They came to a mortal man who had spent six long years of his life in relentless search of a philosophy that would inform his existence and make the world around him sensible to him. To this day Buddhist teaching is much less about doctrine than it is a dedication to a set of mental practices, a firm mental discipline, through which Truth is revealed by the fullest awakening of the human mind. Buddhism holds out the prospect of peace, fulfillment, and ultimately release from suffering not through any sort of divine intercession, but through the exercise and control of one's own mind and senses. The release that is spoken of in Buddhism is not into a supernatural realm, but into a human zone where greed, hate, and delusion are turned aside – simply by the disciplined act of systematically letting go of attachment and desire. Reduced to its core, Buddhism is about developing a form of universal wisdom rooted in compassion for all living things.

The great power of Buddhism for many psychologists is that it is so completely and powerfully true. Day after day we encounter clients who work single mindedly and furiously against their own best interests. They seek to impose their will upon the world in order to secure love, respect, or devotion. Yet the harder they rail against reality, the more isolated, alienated, and alone they become. We want to say to them: Be still! Give your kids a chance to come to you; risk not controlling every human interaction; trust that your heart can lead you where you want to go. Calm your monkey-mind! Listen to the wisdom of your body. See that there are no closed doors; feel the release that comes with every breath.

The wisdom of the Buddha's revelation is that the answers to life's most perplexing and persistent dilemmas are not outside ourselves. The therapist cannot cure; God is unlikely to rescue you. Love is a gift that is offered – it can no more be seized, contained, controlled, or consumed than air. There is no meaningful distinction between you and me. Age, gender, skin color, infirmity, flags of nations – none of these constructs are for you a different world than the one I inhabit. Our tears are the same; our children are the same; our fears, our hopes, and our minds are the same. Every atom that divides us is an illusion. Every perception, attitude, sensory impression is arbitrary; every distinction, every category, every drawn line in the sand is meaningless. There is no fixed trait that is the center of a human being, any more than there is a fixed point that is the center of the universe. Life is a never static. All life is *process*; it is not in any way, shape or form a fixed entity. Life is an ever-moving stream of atoms, molecules, energy fields, beings, becomings and, yes, even extinctions.

The one great idea that defines Buddhism, and that informs every chapter in this book, is that the universe is a system of interrelated parts – a seamless, beginingless, endless flow of energy and appearances. You try to explain to your client that she can't coerce her spouse into loving her; you try to help him to see that whatever power he achieves will only deepen the insecurities that haunt him. Joy is not in the substance – be it gold or crack cocaine. You try through your work with families, schools, communities, and legislative bodies to increase motivation to end the violence in human society; to end the greedy destruction of our trees, rivers, and oceans; and to cultivate moral responsiveness to other beings and to the life of Earth itself. Yet the false gods all require us to suspend our rational powers – to discredit what we have known intuitively since infancy; that the possibility of human happiness can only be realized by embracing our humanity and recognizing that it exists only in connection with others and the rest of creation. The greatest and most powerful human faculty is empathy. The most profound and transformative human motive is compassion.

The central problem addressed by Buddhism is: How can we overcome the universal illusion of our unique, separate, bounded individuality? How do we get beyond the false notion that I am "I" and you are "other"? How do we strike through the masks, the pretensions, and the cowardice of the illusion of our own immortality? For the central irony of our existence is that our life long quest for union, for oneness with the universe, and for transcendence, in reality, ultimately requires us to develop an extraordinary sense of our own being and non-being. The key to solving this problem lies in the development of our consciousness; for if we do not preserve and deepen our natural consciousness, how can we ever see the truth? True, I am just a subatomic speck in the universe, but I am a subatomic speck with mind! I possess potential awareness not only of my own "speckness," but also of the thousands, and even millions of other specks all around me. The faculty of comprehension that I need to understand this awareness is the defining characteristic of "I" – but not a separate, separated, and independent I. This comprehension is what Buddhism refers to as the "compassionate oneness" of the self.

Roger Walsh, a psychiatrist who has spent many years focusing on the ways in which Buddhist practice and modern psychology inform each other about the nature of reality, has developed a special interest in how Buddhism casts a light on the experience of the self. Walsh (1998) has written:

> The extent to which consciousness is normally occupied by fantasy is enormous. That this gross encroachment on awareness has gone largely unnoticed, for example, by behavioral scientists, represents a significant hiatus in Western psychology. Meditation tends to reduce the amount of this fantasy, and initial fantasy-free episodes may elicit feelings of strangeness, unreality, and discomfort. Reduction in the amount of fantasy, therefore, may reduce the sense of separation from others. It may be impossible to think or work one's way out of these fantasies and, in fact, such attempts may even exacerbate them. However, withdrawing attention from them and continually fixing the mind on a neutral object may collapse them. (Walsh, p. 19)

The Basic Teachings of the Buddha

After attaining enlightenment the Buddha spent the rest of his years teaching the truths that he had realized. He was never doctrinaire in his teaching, and always instructed his followers to "Work with diligence. Be lamps unto yourselves. Betake yourselves to no external refuge. Look not for refuge to anyone beside yourself. Hold fast to the Truth as to a lamp." Indeed he taught the ideal that his followers should "just sit" and engage their practice, so that others might join them in their own practice. No salesmanship, no proselytizing; in the Buddhism of the Buddha there is no dogma, no hierarchy, and no idea of an elect group of keepers of a received Truth.

The Buddha died after eating a meal of poison mushrooms in the forest. He instructed his followers to burn his body, and asked that his relics be placed in a Stupa, or burial mound, at a place where four roads meet. He then said, "And whoever shall put flowers or scents on it, or whitewash, or shall express devotion or feel confidence in his heart here, that will be long for his welfare and happiness" (Harvey, 1990, p. 27). And that was the end.

The Core Teachings of the Buddha

So the ultimate Truth of the Buddha is that the answers to life's most pressing and vexing questions lie entirely within us. These Truths, however, will not become clear to us so long as we lead lives that are disruptive and full of the contamination of the "three consuming fires" of greed, hate, and delusion. We must, therefore, adopt habitual practices to center our attention and cultivate our consciousness. We must come to understand our lives, ourselves, as ever changing and infinite yet universal and part of the totality of the universe. At the heart of the teaching lies the idea that everything matters, everything is connected, and that we are vulnerable to suffering because suffering is part of being a living thing.

Dukkha, or suffering, is the principle focus of the core of the Buddha's teaching. Indeed, almost everyone who has had any passing acquaintance with Buddhism knows that among the Four Noble Truths identified by the Buddha, the first and most profound truth is that "All life is suffering." For Buddhists, however, this dukkha, this suffering, is a sort of universal sickness, not unlike in its nature the Christian concept of original sin. To be human, to have awareness, and to participate fully in life one must encounter the inescapable facts of sickness, death, and decay. Because we are human we are vulnerable to sorrow, pain, grief, and despair, to separation from what we love, what we want, and what we need. Life is never precisely as we would have it, and thus life is always to some degree unsatisfactory. The problem is that we become attached to our desires, and when they cannot be fully met, we feel discouraged, abandoned, and resentful. Every happiness eventually passes into regret for its unsustainability, and we become greedy, fearful that we haven't had our fair share, that life has cheated us.

This doctrine is not just a rephrasing of the wisdom of the ascetic forest dwellers, however. The Buddha had experienced the extremes of deprivation, and knew that extreme hardship was not the route to enlightenment or self-discovery. It is not the experience of pleasure that Buddhism sees at the heart of the human dilemma. It is attachment – dependency – on the things that bring those pleasures that must be overcome.

> Giving up attachments does not mean giving up enjoyments of life's pleasures. It means rather, never being *dependent* on the pleasures. It means being ready to forgo the pleasures without frustration. If a splendid meal is available, enjoy it; if not, be content with a humble meal. You've gotten tickets to this special concert?

Wonderful! If not, find some other useful way to spend the evening. If you have nice clothes, enjoy them; if you have shabby clothes, ignore them. (Levine, 2000, p. 44)

The Second Noble Truth therefore explains that the suffering that is so central to and so much a part of our lives, is something that we create out of our ignorant greed and grasping. Our suffering is rooted in our desires; and our desires are rooted in our selfish self-centeredness. We are too attached to a world that, in reality, is completely transitory. But we both console and fool ourselves into believing that if we can just possess "just one more" person or thing, that we can escape the sorrows associated with being alive. We crave pleasures – that are never just exactly what we crave them to be because the world is constantly changing and is never perfectly as we desire it to be. We seek pleasures, and even beliefs, to enhance our own being, but we are blindly and perhaps deliberately ignorant of the cost of those pleasures and beliefs to other beings.

At the heart of the Buddha's teachings about these desires were his teachings about the nature of the self. Especially in the West we tend to see ourselves as detached, independent, autonomous actors – "This is the basic attitude of 'I am': deep-rooted self-assertion or egoism, which is concerned about how 'I' measure up to 'others'" (Harvey, 1990, p. 54). Buddhism replaces this egoism with the unifying concept of *Conditioned Arising*, or *Dependent Origination.* Almost every chapter that follows in this volume is directly or indirectly concerned with this concept. The Buddha himself and his closest disciples considered this specific doctrine to be so clearly at the heart of the teaching that it was said that until the Truth of Conditioned Arising is comprehended there is no possibility for enlightenment.

The essence of this doctrine is the idea that every aspect of creation originates from every other aspect of creation; no part stands alone or outside the whole. This principle, called the *principle of conditionality*, states that all things, mental and physical, arise and exist due to the presence of certain conditions, and cease once their conditions are removed. Nothing is independent. The most obvious, but in some ways most obscure lesson to be learned is the absolute interdependence of everything in creation. This is the teaching of Buddhism that demonstrates that concern for the environment, for other species, and for all other organisms isn't just anthropomorphic sentimentality, but is actually a profound spiritual concern. This doctrine of Conditioned Arising is the source of the deep ecology that many Buddhists practice in their politics and in their daily lives (Barash, 2001).

Buddhism directly applies these principles to the whole concept of suffering, *dukkha*; and this is where many psychologists find the most relevance of the teachings to their personal and professional lives. The conditions that give rise to suffering, which can be thought of as constituting spiritual ignorance, can be changed through education. Thus suffering can be eliminated by the destruction of the ignorance that gives rise to it. Ignorance is abolished through the development of conscious compassionate awareness.

Thus is derived the Third Noble Truth, that suffering is not permanent or eternal; that the roots of suffering – egoism, greed, selfishness and the like, can be known, understood, and rooted out. When craving comes to an end, it brings about the end of *dukkha*. This is the teaching that comes closest to the Buddha addressing the process of renunciation. But what is critical in this doctrine is that it is not the prospect of happiness, harmony, or enlightenment that is renounced – Buddhism is most definitely not an iteration of nihilism or of any sort of radical relativism. The renunciation one focuses on in Buddhism is the renunciation of craving – the usual Buddhist metaphor is the quenching of fire.

> This [the Buddha's "fire sermon"] teaches that everything internal and external to a person is "burning" with the "fires" of attachment, hatred, and delusion, and of birth, ageing and death. Here the "fires" refer both to the causes of *dukkha* and to *dukkha* itself. Attachment and hatred are closely related to craving for things and craving to be rid of things, and delusion is synonymous with spiritual ignorance. *Nibbana* [Nirvana] during life is frequently defined as the destruction of these three "fires" or defilements. When one who has destroyed these dies, he cannot be reborn and so is totally beyond the remaining "fires" of birth, ageing and death, having attained final *Nibbana*. (Harvey, 1990, p. 61)

The ability to vanquish desire is developed, according to the Fourth Noble Truth, by living one's life in accord with a set of eight highly refined principles, widely known in the Western world as the Noble Eightfold Path. These are the so-called eight "rights" – right understanding, purpose, speech, conduct, livelihood, effort, mindfulness, and concentration. Nancy Wilson Ross (1980) presented these as they were reconceptualized rather gracefully by the Anglo-Irish historian and philosopher, Gerald Heard (1971):

> 1. First you must see clearly what is wrong.
> 2. Next you must decide that you want to be cured.
> 3. You must act and
> 4. Speak so as to aim at being cured.
> 5. Your livelihood must not conflict with your therapy.
> 6. That therapy must go forward at the "staying speed," that is, the critical velocity that can be sustained.
> 7. You must think about it incessantly and
> 8. Learn how to contemplate with the *deep mind*.
>
> These were the basic precepts of the Way of Life which the Buddha undertook to preach in forty-five years of active ministry after he had made the initial great decision to "beat the drum of Dharma [truth] in the darkness of the world." (Ross, 1981, pp. 24–25)

Thus the Buddha's message is that we can control and even extinguish our suffering if we dedicate ourselves to a drastic change in our consciousness through a deliberate recharting of the way we think, perceive, and relate to others (karmic tendencies). This is more than just following Alfred Adler's admonition to ask each day what you can do today to make life better for someone else [though that is surely a good start!]. It is a change in our moral reasoning, a transformation in the way we live – carried out in order to increase our understanding of own nature, and our place in creation.

The problem of course is, that as the famous Buddhist prayer recognizes, "though the number of my passions is infinite; I vow to conquer them all." The struggle to live life on the correct path, to take charge of one's passions, and to recognize the futility of trying to escape from taking responsibility for one's thoughts, motives, and deeds is indeed difficult. But it has one powerful ally deep within one's own consciousness. For the Buddhist prayer quoted above has a second verse; it goes something like this: "Though the number of feeling, thinking beings is infinite; I vow to help them all." This is how the actions of ordinary men and women create and maintain *karma*, the Buddhist term for deeply engrained patterns of thoughts, words, and deeds that constitute our style of relating in the world.

Compassion is the priceless jewel in the center of the granite carving of the Buddha at his most serene. As Ross (1981) has noted, Buddhism goes beyond the doctrine that you should be your brother's keeper or that you should treat everyone as your brother; it states that you *are* your brother. Compassion is a sort of compass that keeps one clear about the course of the Noble Eight-fold path. Compassion subverts my devotion to preserving a separate and isolated "I." It is the heartfelt aspiration that all living beings will know relief from the harshness of the world.

Compassion connects me to all living things. In an ancient Buddhist chant, followers are told to "conquer anger by loving kindness; conquer evil by good; conquer the stingy by giving; conquer the liar by truth."

> May all beings be happy and secure, may they be happy-minded! Whatever living beings there are – feeble or strong, stout or medium, short, small or large, seen or unseen, those dwelling far or near, those who are born or those who await rebirth – may all beings, without exception, be happy-minded! Let none deceive another nor despise any person whatever in any place; in anger or ill-will let them not wish any suffering to each other. Just as a mother would protect her only child at the risk of her own life, even so, let him cultivate a boundless heart towards all beings. Let his thoughts of boundless loving kindness pervade the whole world: above, below and across, without obstruction, without any hatred, without any enmity. Whether he stands, walks, sits or lies down, as long as he is awake, he should develop his mindfulness. This, they say, is divine abiding here. Not falling into wrong views, virtuous and endowed with insight, he gives up attachment for sense-desires. He will surely not come again to any womb. (quoted by Harvey, 1990, pp. 209–210)

Buddhist Practice

The practice of Buddhism can be seen to have three basic components. These include, the development of a moral lifestyle informed by a strong ethical code; membership in a community, or *Sangha*, where one fulfills one's responsibilities to society; and developing mindfulness, or meditation, chanting or enlightenment.

As should be clear, the cornerstone of Buddhist ethics is the eradication of sorrow and suffering from the world. Thus one's thoughts, speech, and behavior should all be attuned to creating the greatest amount of happiness for one's self and others. This is not an ethics that is described by rituals and duties; it is a natural ethics that evolves out one's awareness of the suffering of others.

> I get the impression that when people are not much interested in religion they also neglect values like compassion, a sense of sharing, a sense of caring – all the things that people consider to be a religious message and reject. That's a mistake. These are secular ethics, not a religious message, and they are for everyone. Everyone can understand that being human, you want a happy life, a happy family, and to be a happy individual. But material things will not provide you with genuine inner peace or inner happiness. Human values are essential. We must find a way to present basic human values to everyone – and present them not as religious matters but as secular ethics that are essential whether you are religious or not. (Dalai Lama, 2001, p. 57)

As we have seen, the doctrine of Conditioned Arising clearly defines the self as existing only in relation to all other beings. If I behave in a way that causes another pain, it cannot have any effect except to increase my own pain and alienation as well. As one sutra says: "Since the self of others is dear to each one, let him who loves himself not harm another." When I help you I am, in fact, helping myself; and by helping myself I further my potential to help others. Beyond this general principle, there are five ethical precepts that constitute the core of Buddhist ethical teaching (Harvey, 1990).

The first precept here is to avoid taking or injuring another life. The second is to foreswear any act of theft or thievery, fraud, or cheating. The third is to refrain from any inappropriate sexual acts, although Buddhism does not provide any universal definitions of what is or is not appropriate sexual interaction. The fourth precept prohibits any form of lying or intentional deception. Lying is bad when it manipulates others for one's own gain, of course; but it is also a bad practice because it removes one from the course of finding the Truth – in other words lying increases delusion and self-deception. The fifth precept warns against the use of intoxicants or engaging in any practice that clouds the judgment or disturbs mental clarity.

At the heart of all Buddhist ethical systems is a clear concern for compassion and developing loving kindness towards all beings. And this generalizes into one's actions towards and responsibilities to the other members of one's community, the *Sangha*. In the ancient texts the writings about the *Sangha* were intended to set out the rules by which monks and nuns should live and practice with each other in closed religious communities. In modern usage the *Sangha* refers more broadly to all of the members of one's religious community. Beyond that, in this book, the editors and several of the authors would like to extend the notion of the *Sangha* to include all of the members of one's professional and residential community, and ultimately to extend that concept to all the people of the world. Thus Buddhists around the world are increasingly concerned with issues such as social justice, human rights, the protection of the environment, the rights of women, the development of strong community structures, the plight of refugees, and world peace.

An exemplar of this tradition, the current Dalai Lama, his Holiness Tenzin Gyatso, whose writings are widely distributed around the world, is widely regarded as one of the leaders of the modern era who is most clearly identified with the promotion of world peace and the resolution of global conflicts. Other major Buddhist figures promoting world peace are Thich Nhat Hanh, the Vietnamese Buddhist priest whose writings for peace are also known world wide, and who has been nominated for the Nobel Peace Prize; and Daisaku Ikeda, the President of the Soka Gakkai International whose peace proposals have been made to the United Nations since 1978 and whose mission for *Kosen Rofu* or World Peace is practiced by his 12 million followers in 177 countries and territories around the world.

The third domain of practice refers to the activities undertaken by individuals, whether or not they call themselves "Buddhist" to engage in certain practices with the aim of developing wisdom or *prajna*. The collective name we give to all of these practices is "meditation" but as we will see, the scope of various meditative practices ranges far beyond the common notion of sitting silently in the lotus position while repeating a mantra in one's mind to include chanting a mantra, reciting the Buddha's teachings, mandala meditation and many other highly disciplined practices.

The sort of meditation one learns to practice depends as much upon geography as anything else. As Buddhism spread across Asia in the centuries after the Buddha's death, it took on the distinctive characteristics of the cultures where it took root. These regional and cultural variations differ more in form than in substance (although important differences in teachings do exist), and we can expect that as Buddhism gains increasing numbers of adherents in the Western world, the practices employed by Western Buddhists will take on a flavor and character of their own.

Theravada or Hinayana Buddhism. This is the oldest of the Buddhist branches. The Theravada branch has been defined as "The Way of the Elders," a term for the Buddhist community in Sri Lanka and Southeast Asia based on the Buddhist scriptures preserved in the Pali language (Chappell, 1999). It traces its roots to the time of the Indian Emperor Ashoka (264–226 BCE) who was responsible for the spread of Buddhism into Southeast Asia and Sri Lanka. According to legend Ashoka converted to Buddhism after encountering a Buddhist monk who refused to be physically or emotionally disturbed by the process of being boiled in a cauldron of water in the emperor's torture chamber. The emperor witnessed the monk chatting affably with the men who were stoking the fire under the caldron, and was so impressed that he converted to Buddhism on the spot. The monk went on to become the king's religious teacher (Levine, 2000), and Ashoka's daughter, Sanghamitta, went on to bring Theravada Buddhism to the people of Sri Lanka.

The Theravada Buddhists eventually created a vast, powerful, and enlightened empire throughout Southeast Asia over the ensuing centuries. The vast temple complexes in Cambodia, Thailand, Burma, and Sri Lanka are testimony to the extraordinary technical and aesthetic heights achieved by these communities.

Vipassana or Insight Meditation. Vipassana or Insight meditation has as its primary goal the development of a calm centered comprehension of the self and the world. Practitioners of this form of meditation are concerned with developing "mindfulness" – a heightened state of awareness of all of the sensations associated with ordinary acts such as breathing, walking, digesting, and experiencing moods and emotions. It is said that the skilled practitioner of Vipassana meditation can find Truth in every dimension of his/her being – s/he knows no such thing as a "distraction." The progress of the student of Vipassana meditation is first to achieve the ability to experience a global Calming [sic] of the body and mind "to temporarily suspend, and thus weaken, attachment, hatred and delusion" (Harvey, 1990, p. 253); and then to deepen that practice to move beyond calm into an experience of Insight, the product of a higher level of mindfulness while the physical body is in a near state of suspended animation. When Calm and Insight can be achieved effortlessly and spontaneously the practitioner is said to have experienced *Nibbana*.

The quest of the practitioner of mindfulness meditation is to break through the illusions of ordinary consciousness to become aware of the "fundamental three marks" of all experienced phenomena. This includes comprehension of impermanence, of the pervasiveness of frustration, unsatisfactoriness and suffering, and of *anatta*, the principle of not-self. Of these the doctrine of *anatta* is probably the most difficult for Westerners to grasp. The key to understanding this teaching is the realization that the world exists independent of my self's relation to it. It will not die when I die, it will not change as I change, and it is void or empty of any "extra" meaning that I impart to it.

> The teaching [on *anatta*] is not only intended to undermine the Brahmanical or Jain concept of self, but also much more commonly held conceptions and deep-rooted feelings of I-ness. To feel that however much one changes in life from childhood

> onwards, some part remains of the "real me", is to have a belief in a permanent self. To act as if only *other* people die, and to ignore the inevitability of one's own death, is to act as if one had a permanent self. To relate changing mental phenomena to a substantial self which "owns" them: "I am worried ... happy ... angry", is to have such a self-concept. To identify with one's body, ideas, or actions, etc. is to take them as part of an "I". (Harvey, 1990, p. 51)

The doctrine of *anatta* has a strongly psychological flavor to it. The observation that my life is continuous, and that I have various personality traits and characteristic ways of perceiving and behaving, is in Buddhism simply a reflection of the empirical self – a pattern of conditioned responses to the events of life – recurring patterns of responses to patterned stimuli. Moreover, while some Buddhist teachings assert that many such patterns are nearly automatic and difficult if not impossible to alter with the will, other teachings hold that precisely because one's life is continuous and constantly changing, the tendency to respond in a certain way (an aspect of one's karma) is subject to behavior modification through developing new conditioned responses. But this does not make relatively fixed behavioral patterns absolute or essential. The existence of distinctive patterns of thought and behavior does not demonstrate some sort of super-human attachment to the world. Rather it simply calls on us to examine such phenomena with interest – to see these patterns as clearly and as objectively as we see anything else. "Buddhism sees no need to postulate a permanent self, and accounts for the functioning of personality, in life and from life to life, [is understood] in terms of a stream of changing, conditioned processes" (Harvey, 1990, p. 53).

These are truths that can be confirmed in the practice of meditation. As Harvey (1990) has observed, these truths are there for anyone to see who pursues mindfulness. They are not conceptual, or intellectually abstract; in fact as some Buddhist teachers have pointed out, they are as evident and irreducible as mathematics. They are the key observations that a human being makes in the process of gaining understanding of the self and the universe – of attaining wisdom.

Mahayana Buddhism. Mahayana Buddhism has been defined as "a term for the Buddhist community in East Asia based on a new scriptural collection that appeared after the death of Gotama Buddha which survives in Chinese and Tibetan and encourages the use of new methods of practice based on the emptiness and interdependency of all things, the compassion of the Buddha, and the equality of practitioners as fellow bodhisattvas" (Chappell, 1999, p. 245). Mahayana Buddhism arose more than a thousand years after the Buddha's death, and has developed over the ensuing millennium almost completely independently of any "alien" influences from Western culture. It was initially a social reform movement and Bodhisattvic practice of helping others, embodying the Bodhisattva ideal as the epitome of Mahayana ethics. The great Indian philosopher Nagarjuna (1st Century CE) is credited as being the father of the Mahayana movement, having established the dominance of the Mahayana teachings over both Hinayana and Brahman teachings. The central core of Mahayana teaching recognizes the supremacy of the Lotus Sutra and the primacy of the doctrine of the emptiness of all phenomena, non-self (*sunyata*).

Northern Buddhism or Tibetan Buddhism (also known as Vajrayana Buddhism). This form of Buddhism developed through interaction with a very different set of local cultures, traditions and religious practices. One of the major practices following the Mahayana Buddhist teachings is a much more exotic and colorful practice with less emphasis on the early teachings of the Buddha as in Theravada, and more emphasis on a wide range of deities, spirits, and tantric practices. Many scholars of Buddhism believe that as a result of its many centuries of sociopolitical and geographical isolation, Tibetan Buddhism is a manifestation of ancient Mahayana Buddhism in its purest form.

The central teachings of Tibetan Buddhism replace the notion of the sorrow and pain of life with the observation that, as befits the ancient experience of a nomadic people, life is in a constant state of flux. In addition to their transmission by scriptural text, the core of the teachings of Tibetan Buddhism have historically been passed along through successive generations of the nomadic population as a central part of their oral tradition – scripture is more likely to be recalled than to be read. The great teachers of Tibetan Buddhism are revered as those who possessed great wisdom, and their lineage is believed to be passed down through successive generations of holy Lamas through the process of reincarnation.

With the incursion of China into Tibet in 1959, the Tibetan way of life changed dramatically. In order to preserve the tenets and practices of Tibetan Buddhism the Dalai Lama was forced to flee the country, residing in India and traveling extensively throughout the world. One consequence of this Diaspora is that Tibetan Buddhism has become widely accessible to the Western World for virtually the first time in its thousand plus year existence. Many Lamas have come to America and have set up major centers for prayer and study further expanding the availability of the practice to the West. American Vajrayana has modified many traditional practices, most notably reducing the traditional separation between monastic and lay communities. Thus Tibetan Lamas in the Kagypa and Nyingmapa orders have taught their senior American disciples ancient tantric practices and their accompanying rituals, that were rarely if ever practiced in Tibetan households (Lavine, 1998).

Robert Thurman, a Buddhist scholar and holder of the first endowed chair in Indo-Tibetan Buddhist Studies in America, was the first Western Tibetan Buddhist monk. Thurman studied under the Dalai Lama and has been a major force in bringing Tibetan Buddhism to the west. He expounds the ancient Mahayana doctrines of the eight-fold path, the four noble truths, karma, personal and community responsibility, and the enlightenment movement. Thurman (1998) teaches that appropriate awareness of these truths, along with proper meditation and other practices will produce the "inner revolution" that will ultimately lead to peace in the world. His writing offers the Western reader a vision of the enlightened community by way of the example of Tibet as a model for how religious beliefs and practices can move a society to the full achievement of peace.

Tibetan beliefs and practices have also been incorporated into therapeutic institutions. One example of this is in the Tara Rokpa Therapy (www.tararokpa.org/article.htm). Rokpa is the humanitarian, medical, and spiritual teaching of Dr. Akong Tulku Rinpoche. It utilizes techniques such as relaxation massage, and art therapy training to aid in physical and emotional healing. It challenges the familiar notions of western psychopathology by suggesting that the "Buddhist notions of the mind open the possibility that we could experience the world without this defensiveness, without emotional cloud between us and reality, without the suffering created by this defensiveness. That we could even find within ourselves joy, and the ability to open to further caring, and to a very full life" (Sweeney, 1996). Rinpoche's writings explain that Tara is a method of freeing or creating spaciousness – which holds everything through love and compassion. Rokpa means help, the creation or harmony or coordination between inner and outer environment. Tara Ropka therapy allows one to encounter the raw experience of life directly so that it can manifest the understanding that is already within us; indeed revealing our highest self is a key concept in Mahayana Buddhism.

It is important to note that Tibetan Buddhism is a philosophy, but it is also a political and social movement that has a strong following in the West in the struggle for Tibetans to regain their freedom and autonomy from China. Significantly, many scholars have pointed out that the traditional Tibetan society historically demonstrated the most advanced form of the integration of religion, politics, and society that has ever been seen. This is, of course, completely consistent with the living tradition of Buddhism throughout the ages, but it is largely contrary to strongly held belief in North America in the separation of "church and state."

Distinction between Theravada and Mahayana: Engagement with the World. As we have seen, there are many types of Buddhism; and Buddhist-derived practices that vary in goals, philosophy, and practice. Their goals may range from personal enlightenment to human revolution, social reform, and world peace.

The traditional Theravada branch was a monastic order based in Sri Lanka and Southeast Asia. Its practitioners removed themselves from society to engage in rigorous practice in pursuit of their spiritual development. Thus Theravada was absent of a proselytizing spirit, remained aloof from politics, and largely inaccessible to the masses of working people.

Mahayanans on the other hand have been described as social and political activists. They are said to have viewed Buddhism as a faith to be vigorously disseminated throughout society; not merely practiced by monks confined in a cloister but spread to the masses who lived in poverty and misery. Mahayanans were more likely to make political statements based on Buddhist ideals embodied in the Dharma, and to actively challenge the social order. However, as Ikeda (1977) pointed out, "Though dissatisfaction with the apolitical attitude of the early Hinayanaists was among the factors leading to the rise of the Mahayana school, the problem of the proper relationship between politics and religion is a highly complex one and cannot be settled in haste" (p. 82–83).

These early distinctions between Theravada and Mahayana are beginning to fade in the modern era with the emergence of Socially Engaged Buddhism. For example in Southeast Asia, the Zen Buddhist monk Thich Nhat Hanh who coined the phrase is quoted as saying:

> When I was in Vietnam, so many of our villages were being bombed. Along with my monastic brothers and sisters, I had to decide what to do. Should we continue to practice in our monasteries, or should we leave the meditation halls in order to help the people who were suffering under the bombs? After careful reflection, we decided to do both – to go out and help people and to do so in mindfulness. We called it engaged Buddhism. Mindfulness must be engaged. Once there is seeing, there must be acting.... We must be aware of the real problems of the world. Then, with mindfulness, we will know what to do and what not to do to be of help. (as cited in Rothberg, 1998, p. 268)

Currently Socially Engaged Buddhism is a modern movement of Buddhists committed to social reform, and guided by liberal and progressive values. It includes a broad range of approaches which collectively involve the direct application of Buddhist teachings and practices to the social, economic, political, and environmental concerns that have not been traditionally associated with Buddhist practice" (Rothberg, 1998, p. 268). These concerns include human rights, social justice, ecological sustainability, community development and empowerment, and prevention of nuclear warfare.

Internationally, a number of Buddhists have entered the political process to affect social reforms including for example, English Vipassana teacher Christopher Titmuss who ran twice as Green party Candidate for parliament, and Soka Gakkai members in Japan who maintain a powerful, albeit controversial, elected presence in the Japanese government's Komeito Party. Many North American Buddhist organizations are presently involved in socially engaged Buddhism, organized under the Buddhist Peace Fellowship, which has a national and international advisory board of members of prominent socially engaged organizations; the International Network of Engaged Buddhists; and the Soka Gakkai International-USA.

The question of the legitimacy of religion's involvement in social reform and public policy is reminiscent of an analogous concern in the history of Western psychology. Not unlike the emergence of engaged Buddhism, community psychology emerged out of clinical psychology as a social change movement within the mental health field. Its emphases have some interesting parallels to those of engaged Buddhism: leaving the clinics and going out into the community; collaborating with the people as equals to solve the social problems of the masses; emphasizing prevention through individual competency building, empowerment, and ecological interventions; community capacity building; and reforming policy to protect the welfare of human society. These parallels are further discussed in Dockett's chapter on community empowerment in this book. On the question of whether scientists should be involved in public policy, Reiff (1971) took the position, common among members of the Critical Psychology movement, that all scientific activity is a political statement, either for or against the status quo (see Fox & Prilleltensky, 1997). Thus the question is not whether one should be involved but rather to be conscious of one's involvement and the values that involvement supports. The same may apply in the case of religion but the jury is still out on that point. Jason and Moritsugu address the issue of values to guide our interventions in a later chapter in this volume.

Zen Buddhism. Zen Buddhism is a form of Mahayana Buddhism introduced into Japan from China in the 12th Century BCE. The earliest traces of Buddhism in China trace to around the year 50 CE, brought there by traders who were practicing Buddhists. As Buddhism spread through China in the first two centuries of the current era it was influenced by both Confucianism, with its emphasis on filial piety, duty, and harmonious social relationships, and Taoism. Taoism was a religious and philosophical tradition that encouraged meditation, contemplation, alchemy, and spiritual immortality. Perhaps more profoundly, however, Chinese Buddhism encountered two distinctly Chinese philosophical traditions: a deep and pervasive humanism and down to earth pragmatism (Chan, 1967a). Chinese humanism resisted seeing the Buddha as a god or a divine; instead he was viewed as a man of extraordinary and wonderful moral achievements. What was enshrined about the Buddha was that he was a man of supreme virtue; indeed Chinese Buddhist temples were called *jen-tz'u*, "temples of goodness."

Chinese humanism didn't depict the Buddha as sitting on a heavenly throne; instead it shows him sitting in a bamboo grove, carrying a baby, or holding a fish basket (Chan, 1967a). Moreover what the Chinese valued in the life of the Buddha was the Buddha's dedication to the human world, the world of responsibilities, relationships, and duty. As Chan (1967a) pointed out, the Chinese Buddha was also a very good Confucian.

Chinese pragmatism is seen most clearly in the practices that emerged in the centuries following the Buddha's death. Chinese Buddhists focused on a doctrine that held that human beings were responsible for their own salvation, and as Chan wrote, "What is more interesting, salvation is to be achieved here and now.

And most interestingly of all, it is to be achieved 'in this very body'" (1967a, p. 21). In emphasizing the importance of seeing, clarifying, and strengthening one's own nature Chinese Buddhists incorporated both the moral rigor of Confucianism and the ideal of an everlasting life on earth from Taoism.

By the 5th Century CE Chinese Buddhism had divided into two branches. The larger and more successful branch became known as Pure Land Buddhism. Pure Land Buddhism was and continues to be a religious sect whose followers are concerned almost exclusively with issues related to spiritual salvation. It has a creed of faith, religious practices, and is primarily concerned with salvation of souls; until the 10th Century it was headed by a group of patriarchs who controlled and issued the faith's doctrines. It is called Pure Land Buddhism because it has interpreted Enlightenment as arrival in the land of the Buddha of Infinite Light – a concept analogous to the Christian teaching about heaven. Because it is almost devoid of philosophical implications, it does not seem to have much direct relevance to the work of psychologists.

The other branch of Chinese Buddhism, Ch'an Buddhism, however, is all about philosophy and psychology. It is, almost supremely, about *practice*. In fact one of its legendary founders spent nine years in meditation gazing at a wall, until his legs fell off! (Harvey, 1990). Ch'an has really only one aim, and that is to enable a person to come to a full and even serene knowledge of his or her innermost nature.

> Ch'an is basically a method, not a method of writing or words, which the school rejects, but a method of "direct intuition into the heart to find *Buddha*-nature." Nevertheless, this method is based, on the one hand, on the assumption of the eightfold negation of production and extinction, annihilation and permanence, unity and diversity, and coming and departing, and, on the other hand, on the affiliation of the reality of *Buddha*-nature in all things. The Ch'an method of "direct intuition," together with its "sudden enlightenment," gave the Chinese mind a way of ready and complete release, and for this reason had a peculiar charm. Above all, its sole reliance on meditation imposed on the Chinese mind a severe mental and spiritual discipline which was invigorating and quickened the Chinese imagination.... (Chan, 1967b, p. 56)

Under the T'ang dynasty (618–907) both China and Buddhism flourished. Much to the displeasure of the Taoists, Buddhist monasteries became rich and powerful by becoming a sort of court religion, until it fell out of court favor and onto hard times both politically and economically.

During the period of its greatest power, however, Ch'an Buddhism spread into both Korea and Japan. By sometime in the late 6th Century under the Emperor Shotoku, Buddhism became the official court religion of Japan (and Confucianism became the official court philosophy – even then showing the Japanese genius at incorporating diverse foreign elements into their culture and life). During the height of the Heian period (794–1185) the royal court was moved from Nara to Kyoto, and Buddhism essentially subsumed the native Japanese religion of Shinto – by the clever expedient of naming the spirit *kami*, the central component of Shinto, as *Bodhisattvas*.

Tensions between Pure Land Buddhism and Ch'an Buddhism followed the movement across East Asia and into Japan. Ch'an Buddhism was the Buddhism of court and of the elite. It was the practice of the warrior class, but it had little impact on the masses, whose allegiance was to the Pure Land Sect. By the beginning of the 12th century this schism was so great, and the varieties of Ch'an practice so diffuse that a new practice was begun that did not carry with it the baggage of centuries of theological debate and division over practice. This new Buddhism was Zen.

> The monk Eisai (1141–1215) first introduced [Zen] from China ... and experienced opposition from [other] monks when he said that Zen was the best form of practice. ... He argued that [Zen] would strengthen [the people] and protect the land. Indeed, Zen's meditational and ethical discipline, and indifference to death, appealed to the samurai, who were thereby better able to resist two attempted Mongolian invasions in 1274 and 1281. Eisai gained the protection of the Shogun at the capital Kamakura, and established the long-lasting alliance between [Zen] and the samurai. This can be seen as an example of "skillful means", in the form of adaptation of Buddhism to the way of life of a group of people. (Harvey, 1990, p. 165)

Zen thus became the Buddhism of the samurai warrior and the hard working farmer. It is vastly less verbal, less scriptural, and less spiritual than all other forms of Buddhist practice. It is a form of Buddhism with austere temples, a strict and disciplined life, and practice that can be reduced to its essence of "just sitting."

There is at times a clearly stated anti-intellectualism in Zen, and there are hundreds if not thousands of Zen stories that focus on the moral superiority of the well disciplined student of Zen who makes a fool out of the visiting Southeast Asian Buddhist monk whose life is full of religious teaching, but who does not know how to separate his practice from his devotion to the sutras. The jokes, tricks, and pointed lessons aimed at followers of Pure Land Buddhism are even more numerous. Here is just one such story:

> A monk came to Master Ma Tsu for help in solving the *koan* (a sort of riddle that cannot be solved with logic) he had been given "What is the meaning of Bodhidharma's coming to China?" The Master suggested that before preceding with the problem the monk should make him a low bow. As he was dutifully prostrating himself, Ma Tsu, the great Master, applied his foot to the monk's posterior. The unexpected kick resolved the murky irresolution in which the monk was floundering for some time. When he felt the impact of his teacher's foot, he is said

> to have "attained enlightenment." Subsequently he said to everyone he met, "Since I received the kick from Ma Tsu I haven't been able to stop laughing". (Ross, 1981, p. 170)

Zen can be seen as a deliberate reaction to both the scholarly Buddhism of Southeast Asia and the "bells and whistles" of Tibetan Buddhism. Zazen, the practice of Zen meditation is not seen as a route to some higher order of being, a path to enlightenment strewn with golden lotus flowers – the practice of zazen is understood *as* Enlightenment. As Shunryo Suzuki (1970) always reminded his students, everything else is "extra" and must be gotten out of one's practice.

> A person must sit in *zazen* with constant awareness [as befits a warrior] and with faith that he is already a Buddha. The process is one of self-forgetting in which the Buddha-nature gradually unfolds its infinite potential throughout one's life. As an aid to this, physical, mental, moral, and intellectual discipline provides a fitting framework for the life of selfless action. (Harvey, 1990, p. 166)

Zen practice involves a wide range of disciplined activities including flower arranging, calligraphy, writing haiku poetry, arrowless archery, ink painting, drinking tea, solving mental puzzles, and above all – telling stories. Zen stories are all about the destruction of ego, and the foolishness of hollow pride. They generally focus on the wisdom of the body, and of the uselessness of the over-educated intellectual rule keeper. In Zen monks die standing on their heads – just to prove it can be done. They break all the rules, forget the sacred lines, and deflate the pompous with the turn of a quick-witted phrase. Zen is the only form of Buddhism where enlightenment can come on a person who is engulfed in laughter, after a truly satisfying meal, while viewing cherry blossoms, or while watching a cascade of autumn leaves falling from a thousand-year-old oak.

> In summation, what can one finally say about Zen? It is not easy; in fact it may be impossible. One can only try. First, perhaps, it should be reaffirmed that there is in truth no goal to be attained. Even *satori*, enlightenment, is not to be imagined as something achieved after arduous effort. Arduous effort may be involved, to be sure, but it is not the real meaning. The real meaning, the real enlightenment, happens in the way a ripe fruit falls from a tree. All the effort of the seed struggling up through the soil, the tree putting down roots and putting out branches, leaves, blossoms, its patient endurance of the many opposing natural forces – all in the end produce the fruit which, when fully ripe, silently, easily falls. Yet, this whole process of fruition was a *process*, not a goal and the seed itself was as much the goal, the *reality* as the fruit itself. The seed as seed is eternal; an apple seed is eternally an apple seed, and given the chance it will become an apple tree producing more apple seed. As Dogen said, wood is wood and ashes are ashes. Enlightenment is, then, to live in accordance with one's true nature. That is what the Buddha did. That is how he was "Enlightened". (Ross, 1981, pp. 172–173)

The role of the teacher is supremely important in Zen practice, and this is probably one of the main reasons why so many Western psychotherapists and counselors have been attracted to its application in the consulting room. This is also, of course, one of the main potential drawbacks to the application of Zen in therapeutic settings. The teacher/therapist/Master/sensei is so important and so powerful in the life of the student that the danger of abuse and exploitation is always present. Reading first-hand accounts of encounters of somewhat naïve Westerners with unscrupulous "Buddhist" gurus (Bankart, 1997; Singer & Lalich, 1996) will fill any ethical therapist with anger and disappointment.

As a great many other writers have noted, individuals encounter great risk in the process of finding either a therapist or a teacher. It is sadly unlikely that many people in the West will ever encounter a *sensei* with the skill, moral fortitude, personal openness, and human compassion that is required to guide a student/client through the labyrinth of self discovery that is involved in wisdom practices. The possibilities for personal, financial, and sexual exploitation are too numerous, and the screening/training of Western therapists is too superficial for us to imagine otherwise. It has taken our profession altogether too long to recognize the vulnerability of women and girls in this process; and we still don't have any deep awareness of how often boys and men are also exploited by others in positions of trust (Bankart, 2000).

Nichiren Buddhism. This Buddhism is a socially engaged form of Mahayana Buddhism. It emerged in 13th-century Japan at a time of considerable confusion in the religious community about which of a conflicting array of teachings and practices represented the definitive teachings of the Buddha. It was also a time of unprecedented natural disasters, man-made conflicts, and great suffering among the people. Remonstrations, propagation, and conversions among different sects were the order of the day as they debated which of the Buddha's sutras was correct and therefore had the power to alleviate the sufferings of the people and the disasters befalling the nation.

Nichiren (1222–1282), the only son of a poor fisherman's family, was dissatisfied with the contradictory teachings of the eight Buddhist sects of his day. Deeply motivated to discover the wisdom of Buddhism and the correct practice to alleviate the people's suffering, he entered the priesthood at age 16 and devoted the remainder of his life to study and propagation. Exhaustive study of all the sutras of the Buddha and the eight sects of Japan led Nichiren to conclude that the correct teaching for the time was the Lotus Sutra. This sutra is "a core Mahayana Buddhist scripture that emphasizes the worth of all people as possessing the Buddha nature and the mission of Buddhists to be socially active to help others based on compassion and the sustaining power of eternal Buddhahood" (Chappell, 1999, p. 245).

At age 32, Nichiren proclaimed that chanting the phrase Nam-myoho-renge-kyo, the title and essence of the Lotus Sutra, would lead one to perceive the essential, enlightened nature of their life and thereby attain Buddhahood. Believing the practice of propagating the Lotus Sutra to be *shakubuku*[1], the refutation of competing doctrines, Nichiren assumed the role of a religious reformer (similar to Martin Luther in the Protestant Reformation [Hurst, 2000]) and sharply criticized the Pure Land, Zen, and other schools for not adhering to the highest teaching of the Buddha – the Lotus Sutra. His proclamations and remonstrations with the government and other Buddhist sects had severe repercussions, marking the beginning of a series of persecutions, exiles, and attempted assassinations that persisted throughout the remainder of Nichiren's life until his death at age 61. Yet he was never dissuaded from his vision of propagation throughout the world and took his persecutions as proof of the power of his teachings. Nichiren's early forms of "social engagement" aimed at securing the peace of the land were to continue albeit in different forms throughout the history of this school as practiced by the Soka Gakkai lay Buddhist organization, and today represent a world-wide movement for peace.

Nichiren Buddhism holds that all living beings possess the potential for enlightenment. The Lotus Sutra teaches that this state of freedom is accessible to us in this lifetime and through our own efforts. It teaches that life is eternal; that the accumulated effects of our thoughts, words, and deeds determine our current life circumstances; and that by taking control of our cognitions in a single moment of life, we can change each of the moments that follow. As stated by Nichiren in 1222, *On Attaining Buddhahood* (*Writings of Nichiren Daishonin*, 1999):

> If you wish to free yourself from the sufferings of birth and death you have endured since time without beginning and to attain without fail unsurpassed enlightenment in this lifetime, you must perceive the mystic truth that is originally inherent in all living beings. This truth is Myoho-renge-kyo. Chanting Myoho-renge-kyo will therefore enable you to grasp the mystic truth innate in all life.
>
> The Lotus Sutra is the king of sutras, … it reveals the principle of the mutually inclusive relationship of a single moment of life and all phenomena. That is why this sutra is the wisdom of all Buddhas.
>
> Life at each moment encompasses the body and mind and the self and environment of all sentient beings in the Ten Worlds as well as all insentient beings in the three thousand realms, including plants, sky, earth, and even the minutest particles of dust. Life at each moment permeates the entire realm of phenomena. To be

[1] As Hurst states, "Although one possible translation of shakubuku is 'break and subdue,' this has been most often used by critics of the method. One Soka Gakkai leader told me, 'The *break and subdue* translation of shakubuku is misleading perpetuating the unsubstantiated accusations of violent proselytization which affected Nichiren himself and the Soka Gakkai centuries later. Even the word *forceful* suggests physical, rather than moral strength. Shakubuku does mean to refute (break) another's attachment to provisional Buddhist views and to remove (subdue) the suffering, which accompanies such attachments.' " (Hurst, 2000, p. 72)

> awakened to this principle is itself the mutually inclusive relationship of life at each moment and all phenomena. (p. 3)

Nichiren's teachings of the theories of the "ten realms" (i.e., the Ten Worlds) of existence and the "nine consciousnesses" are key concepts for understanding how and why the transformation of the self is possible (SGI-USA, 1997):

> The expression of the "ten realms" describes the ten basic states of life, or life-conditions that comprise the life potential of every human being. Everyone possesses and intermittently experiences each of these life states, which range from the lowest–Hell, Hunger, Animality, and Belligerence–through Tranquility, Rapture, Learning, and Realization to Bodhisattva and, ultimately, Buddhahood or Enlightenment. These states should not be mistaken for moods we pass through. They are patterns into which one's entire existence falls, and although each person tends toward one particular state more than any other, whatever one's life-condition at a given moment, in the next it can readily fall into a lower state or be raised to a higher one. The aim of Nichiren's Buddhism is to establish and maintain the predominance of the state of Buddhahood. (p. 10)

The theory of the nine consciousnesses[2] presents a construct for understanding the layers of the mind. The first five correspond to the five senses; the sixth integrates information from the five senses and allows us to make judgments and function in our daily lives. The seventh, or *mano* consciousness, allows for abstract thought, thereby fostering an awareness of and attachment to our sense of self (ego) as a unique, separate entity, isolated from other things. The eighth consciousness is our "karma storehouse" or *alaya* consciousness, which contains memories of all our experiences in the current lifetime and in the remote past. Due to the "karmic seeds" or latent causes stored there, the *alaya* consciousness imperceptibly influences everything we experience, including the functioning of all lower levels of awareness. The ninth consciousness is our pure or *amala* consciousness. Unaffected by karma, it allows us to purify all other functions and manifest our Buddhahood. It is the ninth level of consciousness that "manifests the wisdom to understand that we are one with the cosmic life force.... that, at the most profound level, we are all interconnected and interdependent (Kawada, 2001, p. 22). Nichiren taught that chanting Nam-myoho-renge-kyo allows us to access this level, thus transforming all layers of consciousness to bring forth our enlightened nature in the present moment. The correspondence between the theory of the nine consciousnesses and concepts elaborated by Sigmund Freud and Carl Jung (ego-consciousness, personal unconsciousness, and collective unconsciousness) is of interest to scholars of psychology and Buddhism

[2] Contributions of the Consciousness-Only School that the brothers Vasubandu and Asanga of the Yogacara School (the second main school of the Mahayana Branch along with Nagarjuna's Madhyamika School) introduced from India to China.

(cf., Kawada, 2001; Stacks, 1996; Yamamoto's chapter on the consciousness-only theory in this book).

At its core, Nichiren Buddhism is a teaching of psychological empowerment. Practitioners learn self-control, self-responsibility, and self-change. Through an empowering philosophy and practice, members learn that they can achieve enlightenment in this lifetime just as they are; that they have within themselves the power to transform everyday sufferings into happiness. As practiced through the lay organization of the Soka Gakkai International, Nichiren Buddhism has two aims. One is to teach individuals how to uncover their highest potential, which is the Buddha nature inherent within their life. The second aim, which is inextricably linked to the first, is to promote peace through the collective "happiness" of enlightened individuals who act in harmony with others and with the universe. As articulated in the Soka Gakkai International Charter (SGI-USA, 1995), members "embrace the fundamental aim and mission of contributing to peace, culture and education based on the philosophy and ideals of the Buddhism of Nichiren Daishonin."

The core philosophy of Nichiren Buddhism (SGI-USA, 2001)

> is expressed in the concept of human revolution, a process of inner transformation that centers on the idea that the causes we make through our thoughts, words, and actions have influence that extends beyond their immediate context to affect the vast and complex web of life. Through undergoing our individual human revolution, we awaken to the responsibility we each have for our own circumstances and for our environment. Our inner transformation will lead us to take the actions that bring about personal fulfillment and help us contribute to the harmony and healthy development of society. These ideals are based on the Buddhist worldview of dependent origination, a concept of interrelation where all things in the realms of humanity and nature are dependent upon each other for their existence and nothing can exist in isolation. (p. 1)

Among the various schools of Buddhism in America, Soka Gakkai Nichiren Buddhism is unique in several ways. First, it has the largest, most ethnically and racially diverse membership of all forms of North American Buddhism. It "is the only North American Buddhist group with a large number of African Americans and Hispanics (who represent over 20 percent of local leadership). This contrasts sharply with the Zen and Tibetan communities in North America which are largely educated, middle class, European Americans and have virtually no African Americans, Latin Americans, or Asian Americans from other Asian countries" (Chappell, 2000, pp. 302–303).

In the 41 years since 1960 when Soka Gakkai International President Daisaku Ikeda first visited the United States for the purpose of spreading Nichiren Shoshu Buddhism in America, the Soka Gakkai-USA has grown to a reported membership of 300,000 members and 77 community centers (SGI-USA, 1997).

Internationally its membership of 12 million people from 177 countries and territories throughout the world including 8 million in Japan (McCloskey, 2001) attests to the successful efforts of Ikeda and his predecessors. What began in 1930 Japan as a society influenced by Nichiren's teachings and dedicated to educational reform under the leadership of Tsunesaburo Makiguchi and Josei Toda, the first and second presidents of the Soka Kyoiku Gakkai (Value-Creating Education Society), has become a vehicle for societal reform based on the values of Nichiren Buddhism. Under Ikeda's leadership the movement's goals have shifted from the worldwide propagation of Nichiren Buddhism to the establishment of world peace through cultural, educational, religious, global outreach, and diplomatic activities as a Non-Governmental Organization of the United Nations. It's values as articulated in the Soka Gakkai International Charter (SGI-USA, 1995) include respect for life, human rights, religious tolerance and interfaith collaboration, cultural diversity, environmental protection, and humanistic education.

The board-based appeal of Soka Gakkai in America is consistent with the desire of the Buddha to alleviate the suffering of the masses. Several factors may explain the attraction of this form of Buddhism. (a) The simplicity of its practice, which involves chanting Nam-myoho-renge-kyo at a shrine in one's own home without necessarily understanding complicated theories, renders it readily accessibility to all socio-economic classes and language groups. (b) Its ability to foster a sense of personal control over one's life is appealing to all people and especially to disenfranchised groups such as African Americans, Latin Americans, and people who are poor. (c) Its method of propagation, which in the past involved assertive proselytizing to people of all walks of life, reaches out to diverse segments of the population.

Second, as Chappell's (2000) research shows:

> Among all Buddhist groups in America, Soka Gakkai excels in its organizational capacities. The social solidarity in Soka Gakkai is not an accidental feature or a byproduct of its teaching, but is at the core of its understanding and practice. One of the reasons why the Soka Gakkai was so attractive to those without social stability in the 1960's and 1970's was its capacity to welcome them into the organization and to develop their abilities. Homeless youth in the drug culture in the 1960s discovered that Soka Gakkai did not discriminate against them… Everyone was accepted and encouraged to chant for whatever they wanted, lofty or mundane – for world peace or for money… (p. 323)

The social organization of the Soka Gakkai provides a network of constant personal support and a host of public events that provide a training ground for honing interpersonal, social, and leadership skills. Against this backdrop and combined with the practice of chanting, members undergo a transformation. They learn to accept responsibility for their lives, experience the control they have producing positive outcomes (internal locus of control), and become confident, optimistic, and empowered. According to Chappell (2000) "This social development is not a major part of Zen, or Tibetan Buddhism, or Vipassana, but it is at the heart of Soka Gakkai, which is not just socially active, but is socially transforming at the very core" (p. 324) "... The organizational strength of Soka Gakkai is not a method to control membership as critics might claim, but an expression of social connectedness and social responsibility, which Soka Gakkai regards as the life of a bodhisattva and as their highest mission" (p. 325). Compared to other popular forms of American Buddhism, the Soka Gakkai probably provides the best example of an active sangha, which is one of the three basic practices of the Buddha.

Lastly, "The secret at the heart of Soka Gakkai is the discovery that, through practice, individuals participate in a universal reality that unleashes their personal creativity to transform life's problems into blessings, to 'change poison into medicine' (*hendoku iyaku*). This is the fuel that feeds the life of Soka Gakkai" (Chappell, 2000, p. 303).

As an organization that intentionally blurs the distinction between the public and the private, the personal and the political, and the spiritual and the secular, SGI has always been at the center of considerable controversy. The following excerpts from Professor of Religion Jane Hurst (1992; 2000) provide a view of some of the controversies surrounding the SGI.

> The Soka Gakkai movement has not been without controversy, both in America and elsewhere.... Reaction to the Soka Gakkai movement in Japan has been highly emotional and steeped in controversy from the start.... From the beginning people distrusted the Soka Gakkai because it promoted a passionate belief in the truth of its own cause (Hurst, 1992, pp. 107–108). To outsiders, there is much to criticize in the wealth and power of the Soka Gakkai and its dedication to its leaders, especially President Ikeda. The Komeito Party's unofficial affiliation with Soka Gakkai is suspect and troubling in a nation that formally separates church and state...
>
> [The split in 1991 when] the Nichiren Shoshu priesthood excommunicated all 11 million Soka Gakkai members, [brought] to an end the more than fifty-year cooperation between the largest of the Nichiren sects and its lay organization. The causes of this split are complex, but largely have to do with disagreement over matters of Nichiren Shoshu Buddhist teachings, the function and power of the leadership in each of the two groups, and certain financial issues. (Hurst, 2000, p. 77)
>
> It is probable that some of the criticisms of Soka Gakkai in the early phases of the movement have some basis in the facts of the behavior of an overzealous young organization [e.g., aggressive proselytizing]. What is disturbing is that these negative treatments of Soka Gakkai all discount the validity of Nichiren Shoshu Buddhism as a legitimate religion.... To research a new religious movement without taking seriously its religious aspects is an unacceptable approach. It has been used all too often with regard to Soka Gakkai. (Hurst, 1992, p. 112)
>
> In simple functional terms, Soka Gakkai helped members organize their lives by encouraging personal hard work and participation in group activities.

> Furthermore, Nichiren's Buddhism, with its absolute insistence on the ability of the individual to change his or her own destiny by chanting to the Gohonzon, gives Nichiren … believers a sense of personal power. In the modern world, such a sense of power is not often experienced by individuals, and in fact its opposite, anomie, seems to be a fixed feature of modern life. One might in this sense see Soka Gakkai as a socializing agent, creating group identity and personal strength in its members. (Hurst, 1992, pp. 113–114)
>
> What is most impressive is the spiritual work for self and society that these SGI members are doing in an era in which materialism and greed are so easily rewarded. The members of this group have high ideals for themselves and for the future. Whether or not one agrees with their method for achieving them, the fact that these ideals are held and worked for is admirable. (Hurst, 1992, p. 195)

The interested reader should see Dockett's chapter on empowerment in this volume for a more detailed explication of the SGI's activities for world peace.

Buddhism and the West Today

Buddhism first came to North America with the Chinese immigrants who began coming to California in the middle of the 19th century. By the time of the great California gold rush, 10 percent of the population of California was Chinese, and Buddhist temples had been erected all along the coast and throughout the San Francisco Bay area. They were joined a half-century later by a surge of immigrants from Japan, so that by the turn of the century there was a large thriving community of Buddhists on the west coast, most of whom were practitioners of Zen (Prebish, 1998).

In the United states today there are active Buddhist organizations representing the various Buddhist traditions of immigrants from all over the world; in addition there are a number of Westernized secular Buddhist organizations whose emphasis is on personal development. Interestingly enough, however, the same tensions that broke the Buddhist legacy into dozens of competing schools in ancient times are still very much at work today. We can suggest that most of these concepts and divisions can be understood within the framework of three primary competing forces that even the Buddha's immediate followers faced.

The first force is the impact of what the noted scholar Charles Prebish (1998) has called "ethnic Buddhism." Originally this referred to the problem of exporting the Buddha's teachings from the foothills of the Himalayas in Northeast India to the various kingdoms in Southeast Asia, Sri Lanka, Tibet, China, Korea, Japan, and a thousand places and principalities in between. In North America however it refers to the types of Buddhism practiced by immigrants who came to the United States for various reasons and brought their religion with them (also referred to as "baggage Buddhism.") These Buddhist communities are deliberately and primarily mono-ethnic and use their religion in part to preserve their sense of cultural identity as well as for the spiritual benefits. Ethnicity is a primary defining characteristic of these communities (Nattier, 1998). One of the brilliant aspects of Buddhism is that it is easily adapted to the mores, customs, values, and existing belief structures of people all around the world; "Sit and practice; and some will sit and practice with you." However, as Prebish has noted, the task of reconciling the differences between these various doctrinal schools is truly formidable.

Buddhism in northern California probably doesn't look much like Buddhism in Southern California, Buddhism in the Green Mountains of Vermont, Buddhism in the inner city of Washington DC, or Buddhism among the diverse people who live in the Virgin Islands. So is there a consistent practice that is "truly" Buddhism? Prebish (1999) tells us that the Buddhism that is practiced by many Americans doesn't look a thing like the Buddhism practiced by Vietnamese or Lao immigrants to the United States. Pure Land Buddhists and Zen Buddhists have little to say to each other after a thousand or so years of doctrinal disputes. Prebish has wisely observed that we run the danger of so westernizing our practice that it becomes "Buddhism without the Buddha" (Prebish, 1999).

At the other end of the continuum is "socially inclusive" Buddhism. According to Buddhist scholar David Chappell (2000), the primary characteristic of these Buddhist communities is the ethnic, racial, and social class diversity of their membership. The Soka Gakkai International-USA is the "single most prominent example of socially inclusive Buddhism;" it is "more culturally diverse and multiracial than any other form of Buddhism either in Japan or in America" (Chappell, 2000, p. 302).

A competing characterization of the Soka Gakkai by some writers is that of "Evangelical Buddhism" (Nattier, 1998; Tweed & Prothero, 1999). Evangelical Buddhism is spread by missionary activity, by Buddhists who seek to engage their practice for spiritual enlightenment and the attainment of world peace. The Soka Gakkai International, the largest Buddhist organization operating in North America, is a prime example of this force.

The SGI-USA aims to empower its members to take control and responsibility for transforming the suffering in their lives into happiness. It also embraces the mission of contributing to peace, culture and education based on the philosophy and ideals of Nichiren Buddhism (SGI-USA, 1995). Through active proselytizing of these "missions" in a wide range of settings, it has become the largest and most diverse Buddhist organization since setting foot on American soil in 1960. The mid-1990's split with its exclusivistic Japanese priesthood and the establishment of participatory lay leadership methods changed the Soka Gakkai from a charismatic cult to a denomination (SGI-USA) (Chappell, 2000, p. 300).

Meanwhile another group of Western "Buddhists," those identified by Tweed and Prothero as "Elite Buddhists," seek only the transcendental benefits of Buddhist practice. They eschew its spiritualist connections, seeking empowerment of individuals, groups, and communities in roughly the same way that the long-ago Samurai sought empowerment by their adherence to Zen and zazen practice. This group is so labeled because its defining characteristic, even though most members are of European ancestry, is social class background. Most are middle to upper class Americans who have the leisure time and economic opportunity to engage in travel to sometimes expensive training sites and pursue strenuous meditation training. Tibetan, Vipassana, and Zen sects of Buddhism tend to attract those of privileged class background (Nattier, 1998) and thus have been labeled "Elite Buddhism." The divisions between the Elite Buddhists and the Evangelical Buddhists at some level also obscure the fact that these two movements hold vastly different attractions to racial and ethnic minorities, women, homosexuals, intellectuals, radical humanists, and those with a missionary zeal.

The use of these classification systems – "elite," "ethnic," "evangelical," etc. – is problematic. They use non-parallel bases of classification, specifically member characteristics for "elite" and "ethnic" and propagation method for the "evangelical." A consistent application of the dominant characteristic or the membership criterion would result in a reclassification of "elite,", "ethnic," and "socially inclusive." Moreover, the labels probably exaggerate the differences in the actual practices between different groups of modern Buddhists, especially those who live (and practice) in the West. Yet it is important to recognize that Buddhism is not a monolithic enterprise, and further to recognize that there are a wide variety of motivations, practices, and belief systems subsumed by the term "Buddhist."

In the midst of all this diversity, Western psychology has also "discovered" Buddhism, and Western psychologists and psychotherapists have been intrigued by the evident power of Buddhist practice to transform individual lives as the following passage, composed more than a quarter century ago, shows.

> Perhaps more than any other areas of cultural life in the West, modern psychology, psychotherapy, and psychiatry have felt the impact of Buddhism. The great discovery of the unconscious by Freud, Adler, and Jung paved the way into hitherto unexplored regions: the drives underlying human behavior, the sources of artistic and intellectual images and ideas, and the causes of mental disturbance and physical illness. This breakthrough to the level of the unconscious caused European thinkers to realize the import of various forms of Eastern meditation, above all of Buddhist meditation. Not only did this centuries-old discipline lead to a deep knowledge of the unconscious; it also served as a means to exercise voluntary control over images, moods, passions, and intuitions of the unconscious mind. The psychology of the unconscious noted in amazement that the Eastern religions, especially Buddhism, had developed a methodical mental discipline in regions that had largely been hidden to European science. And thus a novel attempt was made to incorporate Eastern meditation into European psychotherapy. (Benz, 1974, p. 320)

That "the Buddha was also a social activist" (Chappell, 1999, p. 202; Chappell, Chapter 12 in this volume) is another important "discovery" of Western psychology, especially among psychologists concerned with issues of social justice, ethnic conflict, peace, environmental concerns, and community empowerment. These psychologists have discovered the applicability of Buddhist principles of ecology, compassion, non-violence, and empowerment, to social and community change. Thus an earnest effort is now underway to study models of socially engaged Buddhism that could inform our interventions to create healthy communities.

As can be seen from the preceding brief review, the interface between psychology and Buddhism has a long and rich history. There is much psychology can learn from Buddhist philosophy and practices. Most important, as psychologists take their place on the world wide stage, it is hoped that the Buddhist principles aimed towards peace and mutual understanding can be an important component of the work on all levels including research and intervention.

References

Bankart, C. P. (2000). Qigong in the West: Challenges, hazards and opportunities. In W. Weidong, Y. Sasaki, & Y. Hauruki (Eds) *Bodywork and psychotherapy in the East* (pp. 133–142). Delft, The Netherlands: Eburon.

Bankart, C. P. (1997). *Talking cures: A history of Western and Eastern psychotherapies*. Pacific Grove, CA: Brooks/Cole.

Barash, D. (2001). Buddhism and the "Subversive Science." *The Chronicle of Higher Education*, February 23, 2001.Available: *http://chronicle.com/weekly/v47/i24/24b01301.htm.*

Benz, E. (1974). Buddhism in the Western world. In H. Domoulin & J. C. Maraldo, (Eds.) *Buddhism in the modern world* (pp. 305–322). New York: Collier Books.

Chan, W. (1967a). Chinese theory and practice, with special reference to humanism. In C. A. Moore (Ed.) *The Chinese mind: Essentials of Chinese philosophy and culture* (pp. 11–30). Honolulu: East-West Center Press and The University of Hawaii Press.

Chan, W. (1967b). The story of Chinese philosophy. In C. A. Moore (Ed.) *The Chinese mind: Essentials of Chinese philosophy and culture* (pp. 31–76). Honolulu: East-West Center Press and The University of Hawaii Press.

Chappell, D. W. (1999). *Buddhist peacework: Creating cultures of peace*. Somerville, MA: Wisdom.

Chappell, D. W. (2000). Socially inclusive Buddhists in America. In D. Machacek & B. Wilson (Eds.), *Global citizens: The Soka Gakkai movement in the world* (pp. 299–325). Oxford, UK: Oxford University Press.

Dalai Lama (2001, Fall). Ethics for a secular millennium. *Tricycle, 41*, pp. 55–57.

Dockett, K. H. (1993). *Resources for stress resistance: Parallels in psychology and Buddhism*. The Philosophy and Practice of the SGI. Santa Monica, CA: Soka Gakkai International-USA.

Fox, D. & Prilleltensky, I. (1997). *Critical psychology: An introduction*. London: Sage.

Harvey, P. (1990). *An introduction to Buddhism: Teachings, history and practices*. Cambridge, UK: Cambridge University Press.

Hurst, J. (1992). *Nichiren Shoshu Buddhism and the Soka Gakkai in America: The ethos of a new religious movement*. New York: Garland.

Hurst, J. (2000). A Buddhist reformation in the Twentieth Century: Causes and implications of the conflict between the Soka Gakkai and the Nichiren Shoshu priesthood. In D. Machacek &

B. Wilson (Eds.) *Global Citizens: The Soka Gakkai Buddhist movement in the world* (pp. 67–96). Oxford, UK: Oxford University Press.

Ikeda, D. (1977). *Buddhism, the first millennium.* (B. Watson, Traner). Tokyo: Kodarsha International.

Kawada, Y. (2001, September). Nichiren Buddhism and empowerment. *Living Buddhism*, pp. 18–23.

Lavine, A. (1998). *Tibetan Buddhism in America: The development of American Vajrayana.* In C. S. Prebish & K. K. Tanaka (Eds.) *The faces of Buddhism in America* (pp. 99–115). Berkeley: University of California Press.

Levine, M. (2000). *The positive psychology of Buddhism and Yoga.* Mahwah, NJ: Lawrence Erlbaum.

McCloskey, G. (2001). Personal communication.

Nattier, J. (1998). Landscape of Buddhist America. In C. S. Prebish & K. K. Tanaka (Eds.) *The faces of Buddhism in America* (pp. 183–195). Berkeley: University of California Press.

Prebish, C. S. (1998). Introduction. In C. S. Prebish & K. K. Tanaka (Eds.) *The faces of Buddhism in America* (pp. 1–10). Berkeley: University of California Press.

Prebish, C. S. (1999). *Luminous passage: The practice and study of Buddhism in America.* Berkeley: University of California Press.

Reiff, R. (1971). Community psychology and public policy. In G. Roseblum (Ed.) *Issues in community psychology and preventive mental health* (pp. 33–54). New York: Behavioral Publications.

Ross, N. W. (1981). *Buddhism a way of life and thought.* New York: Vintage.

Rothberg, D. (1998). Responding to the cries of the world: Socially engaged Buddhism in North America. In C. S. Prebish & K. K. Tanaka (Eds.), *The faces of Buddhism in America* (pp. 266–286). Berkeley: University of California Press.

SGI-USA (1995). Charter of the Soka Gakkai International. Available from http://www.sgi-usa.org/thesgiusa/aboutsig/sgicharter.html

SGI-USA (1997). The Soka Gakkai International: Religious roots, early history, and contemporary development. Available from Soka Gakkai International-USA Website, http://www.sgi-usa.org/

Singer, M. T. & Lalich, J. (1996). *"Crazy" therapies.* San Francisco: Jossey-Bass.

Stacks, T. N. (1996, December). The nine consciousnesses and Jung's theory of the collective unconscious. *Seikyo Times*, 6–13.

Suzuki, S. (1970). *Zen mind, beginner's mind.* New York: Weatherhill.

Sweeney, B. (1996). The relevance of Buddhist methods for Western psychotherapy. From a public talk given in Berlin, August, 1996. Available from http://www.tararokpa.org./article.htm

Tara Rokpa Therapy (Internet search 9/21/01). Available from http://www.tararokpa.org./article.htm

Thurman, R. (1998). *Inner Revolution: Life, liberty, and the pursuit of real happiness.* New York: Riverhead Books.

Tweed, T. A. & Prothero, S. (Eds.) (1999). *Asian religions in America: A documentary history.* New York: Oxford University Press.

Walsh, R. N. (1978). Initial meditative experiences: Part II. *Journal of Transpersonal Psychology, 10*, 1–28.

Writings of Nichiren Daishonin (1999). Available from http://www.sgi-usa.org/thesgiusa/aboutsgi/

Chapter 2

Five Manifestations of the Buddha in the West

A Brief History

C. Peter Bankart

The purpose of this essay is to offer a brief history of the influence of Buddhist teachings on the theory and practice of Western psychotherapy. In doing so the greatest challenge has been to impose some meaningful and instructive order on a literature that is as richly diverse and eclectic as any set of writings in modern psychology. The ordering of the five-part scheme I am proposing is roughly chronological, but I don't mean to suggest that later developments are more sophisticated or synthetic than earlier ones. For one thing the five have only minimally built on or even influenced each other. To a great extent they mainly reflect five competing mostly Western interpretations of the nature of human suffering and growth.

The Five Manifestations of the Buddha in the title of this essay, then, should be understood to reflect a diversity of epistemological connections between the core of Buddhist teachings and several major paradigms of Western psychology and psychotherapy. These include: Freudian Psychodynamics; Jungian Analytical Psychology; NeoFreudian Eclecticism; Behavioral Pragmatism; and New Age Consciousness. As we explore each of these I will offer a limited commentary on the relative success and primary limitations resulting from each encounter. Our goal throughout is to examine both the ability of Western psychologists to incorporate and learn from traditional Buddhist teachings, as well as to observe what their efforts contributed to Western understanding [and sometimes misunderstanding] of the Dharma.

Phase I: Psychodynamic Orientalism

I have argued elsewhere (Bankart, 1997) that psychoanalysis, in many respects, reflects the highest flowering of the humanistic ideals of the Western Enlightenment. Its fundamental assertion is that the only valid solutions to mankind's emotional suffering are the products of Western rationalism, and in particular, Newtonian science. Indeed, as Ehrenwald (1976) observed, there is no room in Freud's detached, uncompromisingly scientific attitude toward human suffering for compromise with any doctrine that is not thoroughly objective, impersonal, value-free, and absolutely unencumbered by any religious overtones or influences. In *Civilization and Its Discontents*, for example, Freud (1930) summarily dismissed all human experience resembling oceanic feeling or religious bliss as an unfortunate consequence of a fixation at the narcissistic stage of infancy. Freud viewed such occurrences as evidence of regression to the infant's innate wish for union with the mother.

Although the metaphysical wellspring of Freud's theory is clearly traceable to the teachings of St. Augustine who, in the fourth century described human beings as "empty, desiring, deceptive, hungry, lustful, and at bottom inadequate," Freud has clearly filtered these teachings through the Enlightenment doctrines of John Locke. Locke argued that human beings have the ability to engage a pure, independent, and empowered self to transform their consciousness "into the final arbiter of truth [through the exercise of] initiative and individualism." Thus the clearly articulated ideal in Freud's metaphysics was the empowering of an autonomous individual, free from any religious or political control, who has the capacity to determine his or her own destiny. Psychoanalysis propounds a doctrine of secular salvation that celebrates, and even constructs, a "masterful, bounded, and empty self" (Cushman, 1995, pp. 361, 378, 287).

In Freud's view the greatest enemy of human freedom was mankind's ancient reliance on mysticism, superstition and religion – external sources of authority that maintain and enforce every individual's ignorance of their full human potential for personal liberation. It became the mission of psychoanalysis to liberate the "interiorized, rational, secular, hardworking, self-disciplined, fugal, [gendered], and secretly sexual and aggressive" (Cushman, 1995, p. 384) self by bringing to it a cold, clear, and thoroughly objective self-awareness.

Freud's ultimate legacy, then, was the enshrinement of individualism, intellect and reason as the ultimate sources of human liberation. Anything else was not only suspect, it was anathema to genuine psychic growth and development. In fact, alternatives ways of knowing, alternative traditions which located a central spiritual component of the psyche, *anything* that diverged from the rigorous antivitalism of 19th century physics was not only foolish, it was psychically dangerous and pathological. As the Group for the Advancement of Psychiatry put it in 1976:

> The psychiatrist will [only] find mystical phenomena of interest because they can demonstrate forms of behaviour intermediate between normality and frank

> psychosis; a form of ego regression in the service of defense against internal or external stress; and a paradox of the return of repressed regression in unconventional expression of love. (as quoted in Deikman, 1977, p. 215)

Nevertheless as psychoanalysis became the international gold standard of psychotherapy in the 1940s and 1950s in the West it seems that in the East many practitioners of Buddhist psychiatry sought to form a sort of intellectual alliance with their Western colleagues. In 1953, Kondo, a founder of Morita therapy, wrote in the American Journal of Psychoanalysis that in Eastern psychiatry, as in psychoanalysis, "all neurotic symptoms are understood as the expression of the total process constituting the inner conflicts or the sufferings from them due to the unsuccessful efforts of patients to stop, deny, or to escape from their anxiety" (Kondo, 1953, p. 31). Sato (1958) offered a systematic accounting of the similarities and differences between Eastern and Western approaches to psychotherapy, proposing strong similarities, for example, between the Buddhist doctrine of "no mind" and the psychoanalytic doctrine of free association. In a related vein in 1976, Takeo Doi, probably Japan's most noted psychiatrist, wrote an article that drew a delightful parallel between psychotherapy and the children's game of Hide and Seek. He proposed that both Western and Eastern psychotherapies seek to rescue human beings from the modern predicament by uncovering the personal secrets that always lie at the heart of neurotic misery (Doi, 1976).

There remained, however, powerful resistances within psychoanalytic circles to recognizing any kinship with non-Western modes of psychotherapy. In part, this resistance was rooted in deep philosophical differences between the two traditions. Consider, for example, Doi's observation that "individualism can be defined as contentment at being in hiding" (Doi, 1976, p. 276), or Sato's (1958) observation that Eastern psychiatrists' practices were substantially less verbal than those of Western psychiatrists, and substantially more concerned with the physical well being of their patients. Perhaps, however, differences in epistemology between Eastern and Western psychiatry lay at the heart of the divide:

> Self-knowledge is possible only when the identification of subject and object takes place; that is, when scientific studies come to an end, and lay down all their gadgets of experimentation, and confess that they cannot continue their researches any further unless they can transcend themselves by performing a miraculous leap over into the realm of absolute subjectivity. (Suzuki, 1960, p. 25)

However, it seems clear to me that there was a more profound and culturally pervasive reason for the more or less wholesale psychoanalytic rejection of traditional Eastern theory and practice. I believe Western psychiatry's response was rooted in that form of cultural bias that Said (1979) has called "Orientalism":

> Orientalism can be discussed and analyzed as the corporate institution for dealing with the Orient – dealing with it by making statements about it, authorizing views of it, discrediting it, by teaching it, settling it, ruling over it: in short Orientalism [is] a Western style for dominating, restructuring, and having authority over the Orient. (p. 3)

How else could one interpret the voluminous highly critical psychoanalytic critique of psychological phenomena inherent in Eastern traditions? Take as both seminal and illustrative a paper published in 1931 by Franz Alexander with the strident title, "Buddhistic Training as an Artificial Catatonia" (Alexander, 1931). In his paper, based on a lecture delivered in Berlin in 1922, Alexander asserted that Buddhist practices induce a profoundly deep regression into an autistic asocial abandonment of the world:

> Buddhistic self-absorption is a libidinal, narcissistic turning of the urge for knowing inward, a sort of artificial schizophrenia with complete withdrawal of libidinal interest from the outside world. [This is] a narcissistic-masochistic affair [that] leads to asceticism, [a] systematic suppression of all emotional life. (pp. 130, 131,132)

Alexander concluded his lecture/essay with a psychoanalytic interpretation of the historic Buddha's personality, concluding that the Buddha's teachings reflect the neurotic strivings of a man who had not resolved, because he had not analyzed [!], his "repressed object transference" (p. 144) with his followers.*

The assumption in the West that psychoanalysis provided the only legitimate perspective for evaluating non-Western psychotherapy prevailed throughout the middle years of the century. In 1952 two United States Navy medics visited a psychiatric hospital on the island of Kyushu (then and now a region of Japan that is rich in traditional Japanese customs and practices) to assess the current status of Japanese psychiatry and psychotherapy. It appears the two Americans had little knowledge of Buddhism or other Eastern traditions, but they described a treatment milieu where, they were told, a patient's recovery requires a "calm and well-regulated mind." Applying an implicit psychodynamic template to what they observed, Jacobson and Berenberg noted with disapproval the complete lack of Japanese interest in the roots and meanings of specific delusions. They were also concerned that no attention was paid to transference phenomena of any kind; and noted a complete lack of interest in patients' dreams. In fact, as far as they could see, the contents of the unconscious were completely ignored by post-war Japanese psychiatrists. The Americans came to the conclusion that "suppression is the dominant theme in therapy; conformity the goal"! (Jacobson & Berenberg, 1952, p. 328).

Many of these themes were still in currency in the mid 1960s when Alexander and Selesnick published their canonical History of Psychotherapy. In that volume they often appear to be trying to explain Buddhism objectively and dispassionately to an uninformed Western audience. But a more careful reading reveals the very essence of Orientalism as their intellectual frame of reference. They observe, for example, that while psychoanalysis has as its aim "the grasping of one's true nature to achieve rational understanding" such an

* Interestingly, Rubin (1996) makes a far more reasoned case for the interpersonal dangers of Buddhist teachers' lack of understanding of transference phenomena.

understanding is "inimical to the Zen Buddhist's thinking" (p. 371); and they go to some pains to advise the reader that *satori* [enlightenment] is at its heart "a regression to a state of total narcissism" (p. 372). Their argument is highly developed:

> [The Buddha] developed a psychological technique of meditation for the purpose of arriving eventually at the ultimate stage of nirvana – a tranquil state devoid of all striving and passion. This was to be achieved through a succession of four stages of meditation (jhana), leading back to the nullification of birth, which is the beginning and cause of man's troubles. The goal, therefore, is a psychological and physiological regression to the prenatal state of oblivion, of pure being, in which the difference between subject and object vanishes. In the first stage of jhana the world is renounced as a symbol of evil; contempt for the world results in renunciation of all worldly desires, and the meditating monk is beset with sorrow. This is analogous to a state of experimentally induced melancholia. These feelings of sorrow are replaced in the second stage by self-love, a drawing upon the self for all spiritual sustenance. This condition represents a still further regression and resembles psychotic states in which interest is completely centered upon the self. In the third stage the feeling of pleasure induced by self-love diminishes into apathy, which is then transformed – in the fourth stage – into complete mental emptiness and uniformity. Here the ascetic meditator is exalted above pleasure and pain, is free from love and hate, is indifferent to joy and sorrow, is indifferent indeed toward the whole world, toward gods and men, even towards himself. He emerges free from all emotion. At this point he can remember with ever-increasing clarity all the circumstances of his life down to the least detail. Significantly, recollection of one's whole development has been described by Freud as the aim of psychoanalytic treatment for mental disturbance. However, in Buddhist training the unwinding of the film of life in a reverse direction goes even further, beyond birth, back through all the previous reincarnations to the very beginning of life, reversing the developments through all previous existences. This is nirvana, the end of the regressive journey through the four stages of jhana, during which all forms of one's previous lives are reexperienced in a clairvoyant fashion. That these memories are in fact true may be open to doubt, for it is understandable that a person intent upon flight from the world and the self may, in his spiritual fervor, accept his visions as memories of previous incarnations.
>
> It is difficult to reconcile the goal of absorption, nirvana, which is a completely asocial condition, with Buddhist ethical precepts, healing and devotion to the "welfare and succor of gods and men." Absorption with oneself – withdrawal from the world and society – is an unbridgeable gap between Buddhism and Western psychiatric thought. Psychoanalysis, for example, strives to conquer the self without losing the outside world. A complete withdrawal is a goal alien to the Western cultural tradition, in which man is imbued with a drive toward achievement. This fundamental opposition of ideals explains why the influence of Eastern thought upon the development of psychiatry has been only sporadic. As the extroverted interest of European culture reached its peak in the modern era of science, eventually even psychology assumed the goals and principles of empiricism and experimentation ...
>
> It is difficult for the Western mind to understand how the satori experience leads to the achievement of humility, love, and compassion, the end goals of Zen Buddhist

> doctrines. The obvious similarities between schizophrenic regressions and the practices of Yoga and Zen merely indicate that the general trend in Oriental cultures is to withdraw into the self from an overbearingly difficult physical and social reality. Only the future can tell how much Western psychiatry will learn from this Oriental bent of thought, which for centuries coexisted with the more outward-directed Western mentality, without the two influencing each other to any appreciable degree. (Alexander & Selesnick, 1966, pp. 25–26, 372)

Support for the allegations of psychological immaturity, pathological regression, and perhaps even decadence by practitioners of Buddhism are sprinkled through the Western psychiatric literature of this era. A classic example of this sort of orientalism was reported by Abel, Metraux, and Roll (1987). It is based on data collected in 1965 by a cultural anthropologist named Spiro who was invited to visit a Buddhist monastery in an isolated village in Burma. He administered Rorschach tests to the monks, and sent the protocols to an analyst colleague for interpretation. According to Abel et al. (1987), the responses of the monks revealed to the analyst: "Definite psychopathology among the monks. Among other characteristics, they showed marked regression in manifestations of aggressive and oral needs, hypochondriasis, 'erotic self-cathexis', greater fear of female or mother figures, greater defensiveness, and latent homosexuality" (p. 62).

It was also noted that the monks' responses were indiscriminable from the responses of other males in the same village. The results put Abel et al. in mind of another study using Rorschach responses from 1944 that described the entire population of Atimelang villagers on an island in the East Indies as "brain damaged."

Various Western scholars have tried to reconcile the split between Western and Eastern theories and practices, but until relatively recently their work has carried little weight in psychoanalytic circles. Fingarette (1963) asserted that Buddhism was an antidote to the Western tendency to disregard the psychic experiences of patients by dismissing these experiences as "pale, alien, merely verbal, or 'theoretical' " (p. 208). He tried to show how psychoanalytic transformation of the self has many of the same goals as the "mystic" tradition, concluding: "In the last analysis, then, the mystic way is a 'simple' and 'obvious' way – for those who will open their eyes .... It is the liberation from neurotic fixation and dogma of all kinds" (Fingarette, 1963, p. 323).

In a more spirited, if perhaps strident, tone, Deikman (1977) described the writings of psychoanalytic critics of Eastern teachings as displaying "extreme parochialism, a lack of discrimination, and a naïve arrogance in its approach to its subject" (p. 213). He accused them of failing to discriminate between lower (sensate) and higher (transcendent) states of consciousness reported by meditators. Deikman held that this was a motivated blindness, a reaction to Eastern psychology's challenges to basic tenets of Western culture – the primacy of reason and intellect, the separate, individual nature of man, and the linear organization of time. He concluded: "Real gold exists, even though false coin abounds. Perhaps the greatest teaching of the mystics is the need for humility" (p. 217).

The Buddha once wrote: "It is better to live one single day in the pursuit of understanding and meditation than to live a hundred years in ignorance and unrestraint." It seems evident that the loss, in this case, is very much our own. Between the nearly comic misunderstanding of the nature of Buddhist theory and practice and the arrogance of nearly a century of psychiatric orientalism, much opportunity has been lost. As Imamura (1998) has written: "The goal of Buddhist psychotherapy is enlightenment – seeing things-as-they-are, the perfection of the emotions into compassion, and of cognition into wisdom" (p. 234). The potential affinity between Buddhist and psychoanalytic doctrine is unmistakable; both link salvation to an "unending examination and reevaluation of a person's assumptions in all areas of life" (Imamura, 1998, p. 234). Both teach that "the search for the real meaning in life and for the attempt to comprehend oneself, one's mind and the nature of one's experience [can be achieved] through fearless introspection." The whole purpose of Buddhism is "to apply mental therapy to a condition which, accepted as the norm, is in truth nothing but a universal delusion" (Clifford, 1984, pp. 215, 216) for:

> The entire thrust of the Buddha's teaching and the Buddha's path is to encounter the mind, become aware of how it works, and how it controls us, and then to bring it under control and through this to cure suffering. For according to Buddhism, the source of all suffering is the lack of control of mind. (Clifford, 1984, p. 215)

Phase II: Analytical Mysticism

At first reading, Carl Jung's embrace of Eastern teachings appears to be in stark contrast to its wholesale rejection by Freud and his followers. Where the psychoanalysts condemned Buddhist meditation as a regression to infantile levels of development, a much regressed state of autism, and an extreme form of autosuggestion (Ben-Avi, 1959), in 1934 Jung (1964) wrote of it: "One has the feeling of touching upon a true secret, not something that has been imagined or pretended; this is not a case of mystifying secrecy, but rather an experience that baffles all language" (pp. 11–12).

At the same time, however, Jung has strong reservations about the ability of Westerners to benefit in significant ways from Eastern teachings. As Ray (1986) pointed out, Jung expressed serious "concern about the transposition of Eastern ideas to the West... not only [because of] what he sees as the Westerner's underdeveloped awareness of the unconscious [but also because] he maintains that the West errs in its exclusive emphasis on the intellectual, the rational and the scientific." In fact as Jung himself wrote in 1962:

> ... it is sad indeed when the European departs from his own nature and imitates the East or "affects" it in any way. The possibilities open to him would be so much

> greater if he would remain true to himself and evolve out of his own nature all that the East has brought forth in the course of the millennia. (pp. 85–86)

Throughout Jung's writing on Buddhism and related Eastern teachings he adopted the orientalist convention of referring to Eastern teaching and practices as "mysticism". What is most peculiar about this convention is that Jung clearly should have known better. In concluding the very book for which Jung had written his impressive Foreword, Suzuki (1964) had emphatically claimed:

> Taking it all in all, Zen is emphatically a matter of personal experience; if anything can be called radically empirical, it is Zen. No amount of reading, no amount of teaching, no amount of contemplation will ever make one a Zen master. (p. 132)

One can argue, as Ben-Avi (1959) does, that Zen represents a radical departure from the assumptions about human nature and human suffering that are common to most forms of Western psychotherapy, but there is almost nothing "mystical" about it. In fact, in Buddhist teaching, "the essence of change, illumination, or growth, must be rooted in the immediate, the concrete experience of the individual rather than based on an intellectual or abstract formulation" (Ben-Avi, 1959, p. 1818).

Why, then, does Jung fall into this orientalist semantic convention? The answer is probably rooted in Jung's intense desire to use the teachings of the East not as universal tools of human liberation but as evidence to support the structural framework of his own theory of the topography of consciousness and unconsciousness. He argues, for example, that East and West are essentially unknowable to each other because they are predicated on different styles of consciousness, the East representing one-sided Introversion, the West one-sided Extraversion:

> As Kierkegaard says, "before God man is always wrong." By fear, repentance, promises, submission, self-abasement, good deeds, and praise he propitiates the great power, which is not himself but *totaliter aliter*, the Wholly Other, altogether perfect and "outside", the only reality. If you shift the formula a bit and substitute for God some other power, for instance the world or money, you get a complete picture of Western man – assiduous, fearful, devout, self-abasing, enterprising, greedy, and violent in his pursuit of the goods of this world: possessions, health, knowledge, technical mastery, public welfare, political power, conquest, and so on…he mind is chiefly employed in devising suitable "isms" to hide the real motives or to get more loot…. I cannot help raising the question of whether it is possible, or indeed advisable, for either to imitate the other's standpoint. The difference between them [Eastern and Western man] is so vast that one can see no reasonable possibility of this, much less its advisability. You cannot mix fire and water. The Eastern attitude stultifies the Western, and vices versa. You cannot be

> a good Christian and redeem yourself; nor can you be a Buddha and worship God. (Jung, 1954, p. xxxvii)

Jung went on in this essay to equate enlightenment to an awareness of the collective unconscious, and consistent with his theory draws a direct connection between enlightenment, introversion and insanity:

> The introverted attitude is characterized in general by an emphasis on the a priori data of apperception. [In this context] the extraordinary feeling of oneness is a common experience in all forms of "mysticism" and probably derives from the general contamination of contents, which increases as consciousness dims. The almost limitless contamination of images in dreams, and particularly in the products of insanity, testifies to their unconscious origins. (pp. xl, xivi)

Jung saw the extraverted attitude of the West struggling for greater insight into the nature of consciousness and awareness of being, and he saw the introverted East as struggling to become more rational and relational:

> I think it is becoming clear from my argument that the two standpoints, however contradictory, each have their psychological justification. Both are one-sided in that they fail to see and take account of those factors which do not fit in with their typical attitude. The one underrates the world of consciousness, the other of One Mind. The result is that, in their extremism, both lose half of the universe, their life is shut off from total reality, and is apt to become artificial and inhuman. (p. xlvii–xlix)

And he concluded with a warning to both camps:

> There is a difference, and a big one [between Christian striving for Truth and yoga]. To jump straight ... into Eastern yoga is no more advisable than the sudden transformation of Asian peoples into half-baked Europeans. I have serious doubts as to the blessings of Western civilization, and I have similar misgivings as to the adoption of Eastern spirituality by the West. Yet the two contradictory worlds have met. The East is in full transformation; it is thoroughly and fatally disturbed. (p. xlii)

Jung did see Western psychotherapy as offering a sort of metaphysical bridge between East and West, and recognized that the difference is largely an apperceptive one. He advises us, in fact, that in Zen: "It is not that something different is seen, but that one sees differently" (Jung, 1964, p. 17). From his perspective meditation practice "reverts energy needed for conscious processes to the unconscious ... and reinforces its natural supply up to a certain maximum [that] increases the readiness of the unconscious contents to break through to the consciousness" (p. 22). However, he concluded his remarks on a curious note. He wrote that since Zen is oriented toward those "ready to make any sacrifice for the sake of truth" it is fundamentally dissimilar to psychotherapy which is oriented toward "the most stubborn of all Europeans," who lack "the intelligence and will-power" that Zen demands (pp. 25, 29).

Phase III: Neofreudian Eclecticism

The writings of the neo-Freudians, Erich Fromm, Karen Horney, and Harold Kelman, constitute the core of what I am calling the Third Manifestation. These were the first sources that many Western psychotherapists encountered in their training that expressed professional interest in the ideas and principles of Buddhist psychotherapy. What they all have in common, of course, is that they were influenced and taught by the great Daisetz T. Suzuki, who introduced Zen to Western scholars in the middle years of the 20th century.

The beginnings of this movement can be more or less precisely dated to August, 1957 when Erich Fromm invited Suzuki and a group of colleagues to his home in Cuernavaca, Mexico for a one-week intensive seminar on the applicability of Zen Buddhism to psychology and psychotherapy. Wolf (1957) attended the seminar and published his summary of what was transpired in a short article in the American Journal of Psychotherapy:

> [Zen's] appeal is in its directness of approach and insistence on direct experience. Verbalization as well as organization as a school system is in a way discouraged since "He who knows does not speak and he who speaks does not know." Words can have meaning only when the speaker or writer has had the same experience as the hearer or reader. Since *satori* is a unique experience which most people have never had before, no words can convey a truly meaningful concept. (p. 868)

Here, at last, was Western psychology receiving Buddhist teaching without either the stigma of Freudian psychopathologizing, or the imposition of an overlay of Jungian mysticism. Fromm and his colleagues were open to the *idea* of consciousness, and were eager to explore the implications of what they were learning for therapeutic work with their patients.

One of the fascinating things that this generation of therapists began to discover was that the teachings and practices of Buddhism had a great power to transform them, as well as their patients. A typical example of this comes from Welwood (1983) who wrote:

> When I studied Rogerian therapy in graduate school, I felt frustrated because I was never taught how to develop "unconditional positive regard" for the client. I was told that it was essential, and it sounded good to me, but it was assumed that I should be able to feel this way toward anyone who walked into my office. What I discovered many years later was that meditation provided a concrete operational method for developing just those ingredients of acceptance and unconditional friendliness that are most essential for successful therapy. A therapist who sits through the subtle, complex twists and turns of his own thoughts and feelings is unlikely to find many of his client's problems all that alien, shocking or unfamiliar. The more a threatened therapist trusts his own basic goodness underneath his confusion, the more he can help clients find their way between those two aspects of

themselves. And the more he can face his own fear, the more fearlessly he can approach his clients' problems as well. (as cited in Claxton, 1986, p. 320)

In short, the introduction of Buddhist teachings in to mid-century Western psychotherapy offered an alternative to the rigid boundaries between self and other that were the hallmark of traditional forms of psychoanalysis. In 1985, for example, Rubin argued in the prestigious *Psychoanalytic Review* that the practice of meditation by psychoanalysts would cultivate maximum listening and refined attentiveness by training the analyst's power of attention, improving his perceptual acuity, and providing an optimal internal environment by systematically enhancing mental tranquility.

In a similar vein, Claxton (1986) argued that Buddhist teachings "provide a mirror that reflects the insights of perceptual psychologists back into our selves, and it teaches us to apply those insights reflexively" (p. 313). For the practicing therapist the product of this reflection is a newly discovered clarity of perception and knowledge of the other. It yielded, as Claxton noted, a new level of awareness that at the same time is extraordinarily intense, but also completely choiceless. It offered a treatment milieu that was essentially human and rational, and based in the healer's morality and kindness.

For Fromm, who had proclaimed psychoanalysis to be a cure for the soul, Buddhism also provided a link between psychoanalysis and humanistic religion by stressing man's innate power to seek freedom and independence through the existential search for truth (Fromm, 1950). As Fromm (1960) emphasized throughout his landmark essay that grew out of the meetings in his home, psychoanalysis and Zen Buddhism shared the dream of liberating human beings by freeing the contents of their unconscious minds into full and unfettered consciousness.

If, as Clifford (1984) noted, the central teaching of Buddhism was that "all worldlings are deranged," (p. 216) then it followed that the whole purpose of Buddhism is to apply a sort of spiritual and mental therapy to a condition that masquerades as bourgeois normalcy and "mental health" but is, in truth, nothing but a universal delusion. In short, the dissemination of the teachings of Buddhism to psychotherapy practitioners in the West provided a deeply satisfying theoretical soapbox for a generation of mid-century existential philosopher-therapists. In 1958 the existential psychotherapist Wilson van Dusen published a paper in the inaugural volume of *Psychologia* proclaiming that from reading and practicing Zen he had found "a real readiness to finally see the tree in the courtyard that has delighted adepts in Zen for centuries" (p. 229). This was highly similar to a theme sounded by the Japanese Morita therapist, Kondo (1953), who had described the plight of neurotic patients as being "so much absorbed in their egocentric demands that they forget all about [the] kind of happiness, contentment, and inspirations which everyone shares" (p. 33). Kondo called on psychotherapists to embrace the work of restoring their patients' "natural feelings" of being fully awake and alive.

Clifford (1984) articulated the vision of a great many neo-analysts of his time when he wrote:

> The entire thrust of the Buddha's teaching and the Buddha's path is to encounter the mind, become aware of how it works and how it controls us, and then to bring it under control and through this to cure suffering. For according to Buddhism, the source of all physical and mental disease and suffering is the lack of control of mind. Buddhism's means of mental therapy is a transformation of self through the development of morality, meditation, and wisdom. Through meditation one can become aware of unconscious motivations, mental habits and inner conflicts, and free oneself of bondage to them. (pp. 215, 216)

Karen Horney's interest in Buddhism resulted in her visit to Japan to meet with D. T. Suzuki in 1952. Horney died from cancer a few weeks later, so the actual record of her engagement with Buddhist teachings is necessarily rather limited. If we look at the core of her ideas, however, it is clear where her interest in Buddhism originated. In 1945 Horney wrote Our Inner conflicts: A Constructive Theory of Neurosis, a book that references the writings of D. T. Suzuki. In this work Horney stressed the central importance of whole heartedness, a quality that Horney considered to lie at the heart of human sincerity. Nobody, Horney observed, divided within himself can be wholly sincere; and she quoted Suzuki to the effect that "Sincerity, that is, not deceiving, means putting forth one's whole being, in which nothing is kept in reserve, nothing is expressed under disguise, nothing goes to waste" (as cited in Horney, 1945, pp. 162–163).

For Horney this quality of sincerity was a reflection of a person's moral integrity, and she was one of the few Western readers of Zen in those days that clearly understood the necessary connection between Zen and moral character. Strength of character, Horney argued, is reflected in "spontaneity of feeling, an awareness and aliveness of feeling, whether in respect to love or hate, happiness or sadness, fear or desire. This would include a capacity for expression as well as for voluntary control marked by the capacity for love and friendship" (pp. 241–242).

By the end of 1952 Horney had made a more definitive link between sincerity, wholeheartedness, spontaneity of feeling, and emotional awareness and the practice of Zen. In a lecture she wrote a short time prior to her death she called on her fellow analysts to listen to their patients with Zen-like concentration and non-attachment. She encouraged them to develop the ability to learn from the Zen masters that the essence of living is "being with all one's faculties," and she called on them to bring these qualities with them into the analytic session. What was demanded, she wrote, was "Wholeheartedness of concentration [where] all our faculties come into play: conscious reasoning, intuition, feelings, perception, curiosity, liking, sympathy, wanting to help, or whatever" (Horney, 1987, p. 19).

Horney's student, Harold Kelman, brought these themes together in a comprehensive essay written in 1960, and reprinted in 1976. Enlightenment, Kelman argued, is the "ultimate" goal of therapy; and it is characterized by the dissolving of all intellectual barriers between experiencing, understanding, and knowing. He even quoted Menninger to the effect that a well-trained analyst must possess "the will-power of desirelessness; he must free himself from the desire to cure" (Kelman, 1960, p. 331). He called on psychoanalysis to turn away from individualism, and to turn instead towards the interpersonal, holistic, and the unitary. Instead of man being posed as an object that must change or forever be in conflict against a society that will not, Kelman's vision was that man could become a true participant-observer in his world, engaged in life as a unitary process, as one with his environment. He continued:

> The emergence of and interest in Existentialism, the work of Buber and Zen, to me are evidence that Western man is aware that his philosophic roots are inadequate. I feel these interests are a current phenomenon of the West and a phase on the way toward something different which will unify the contributions of East and West in ways heretofore not consistent or envisioned. Existentialism is the formulated awareness of the emptiness, meaninglessness and nothingness of our previous ways of being on the basis of the subject-object dualism and the tragedy of it. It points at the experienced despair and hopelessness of hanging on to an outmoded way of being. It defines the fear of the responsibility of choosing to let go into freedom, a freedom with which the West has little experience .... The Occidental is being pushed off the precipice into the unknown, into formlessness, against his will, in terror, dread and despair. The Easterner makes this leap into formlessness through choice, in the natural course of his discipleship.
>
> The analyst will have to be aware that the only place we can ever be and experience is here; that the only time we can ever be and experience is now; and that the only feelings we can ever be, not have, are present feelings. This means that the only time and place we live is the moment. This being the moment, being it totally, is vastly different from the Western experience of urgency and emergency that demands relief and release and in which each moment is experienced as a matter of life and death but on a quite different plane. Total acceptance of the Western notion that we have to die to be reborn is more possible and widespread in the East. Each moment we die and are reborn. Each moment is new. This notion is not alien to us. Goldstein says, "If the organism is 'to be,' it always has to pass again from moments of catastrophe to states of ordered behavior." And in quantum physics energy exchange is discontinuous.
>
> I feel vaster and deeper possibilities are now open to what is now called psychoanalysis which can and does move more in the direction of the Eastern master-disciple relation. (Kelman, 1960, pp. 332, 333)

The leader of current efforts to integrate Buddhism with dynamic psychiatry is Jeffrey Rubin who has championed the idea of what he calls "contemplative psychoanalysis." In a book-length extension of his thesis that psychoanalysts can benefit dramatically in their powers of attention and concentration by practicing meditation, Rubin (1996) argues that Buddhist teachers also have much to learn from psychoanalysis. The heart of his thesis is that "Psychoanalysis and Buddhism can both enormously benefit from an egalitarian dialogue characterized by mutual respect, the recognition of differences, and a genuine interest in what they could offer each other" (p. 7).

Phase IV: Behavioral Pragmatism

Although Fromm, Horney, and Kelman published their ideas within a generation of the current day I wonder what, if any, role their contributions play in the training of contemporary psychotherapists. The behavioral revolution rolled through the graduate programs of the 1960s and 1970s and spawned the managed care revolution evident in today's treatment centers. It swept aside most of the psychodynamic, analytic, and neo-analytic training programs, but it was not altogether uninfluenced by the Eastern psychologies in the process. This is the period that I refer to as the Fourth Manifestation of the Buddha in the West.

Mikulas (1978, 1981) seems to have been among the first to take on the task of developing a systematic integration of Buddhist teachings with the literature of behavioral psychotherapy. He emphasized several key areas of overlap including:

- Overriding emphasis on self-control
- Minimal use of theoretical constructs
- Focus on real problems in daily living
- Concern with objective study of observable behaviors
- Focus on the contents of conscious experience
- Symptom-specific application of relaxation and biofeedback
- Ahistorical, here-and-now focus
- Concern for the common people
- Discrimination between behavior and personality
- Increase awareness of subtle cues from the body
- Focus on behavior change, especially through guided practice
- Meditation as an adjunct for all forms of therapy
- Focus on helping the practitioner to be more fluid and empathic, less dogmatic
- Work to clarify the vantage point of the client
- Emphasis on peace of mind and happiness achieved through systematic self observation

Mikulas also credits Lesh (1970) for demonstrating the salutary effects of Zen meditation practice in increasing a variety of measures of empathy in counselors in training.

In 1985 de Silva published a follow-up paper to Mikulas's reviews by describing five "striking parallels" between traditional "early" Buddhist approaches to suffering and "modern" behavioral interventions. These included covert sensitization, thought stopping, exposure, distraction, and thought-substitution. He also described several other interventions common to both schools of thought including: forceful restraint, various ways for dominating the mind, and the use of interpersonal influence by a "strong man" to control the actions of a "weaker man" [where "strong" and "weak" refer to the strength of each person's character].

In the mid to late 1970s hundreds of thousands of Americans became practitioners of Transcendental Meditation (TM). Included in this number were at least ten thousand licensed "trainers" (Zilbergeld, 1983) who essentially operated franchises that offered instruction in the practice of TM. Through most of the 1970s TM was the popular standard of Eastern practice, and most of the behavioral research that investigated the effects of meditation focused on TM practitioners. Wallace, Benson, & Wilson (1971), for example, recruited 36 experienced meditators through the Student's International Meditation Society, an organization officially sponsored by the TM international organization. Wallace et al. documented decreased oxygen consumption, carbon dioxide elimination, respiration rate, blood pH, blood lactate, and markedly increased skin resistance along with increases in alpha and theta wave activity during periods of meditation. They argued that TM induced a "wakeful hypometabolic physiologic state," (p. 795) distinctly different from sleep, autohypnosis, and autosuggestion. They concluded by noting that their subjects demonstrated "finer or more creative levels of thinking in an easy and natural manner" (p. 795).

In 1975 Woolfolk, writing in the Archives of General Psychiatry, reviewed forty-three recently published papers on the effects of TM, and concluded that TM was effective in inducing relaxation for global desensitization, lowered trait anxiety, decreased drug abuse, increased self-actualization, improved breathing in asthma patients, decrease systolic blood pressure in hypertensive patients, and lowered cortical and autonomic arousal. Woolfolk concluded that practitioners of TM had physiological outcomes equivalent to those observed in long-term practitioners of Zen.

Woolfolk, Carr-Kaffashan, McNulty, and Lehrer (1976) documented that meditation was an effective treatment for chronic insomnia, equivalent to other available treatments, but also resulting in inner calmness and tranquility, reduced cortical excitation, and lower metabolic rates. Benson and a group of eleven colleagues (Benson et al., 1978) reported no differences in a variety of outcome measures for treatment of anxiety disorders between meditation and self-hypnosis. With meditation they found a 34% improvement in psychiatric assessment, mixed results in terms of psychophysiological arousal reduction, and a 63% improvement in self-assessed feelings of anxiety.

Shapiro and Zifferblatt (1976a, 1976b) reported that a combination of meditation and self-management training reduced methadone dosage among heroin addicts (a reliable indicator of craving); and they pointed to similar efficacy of the combination of Zen and self-control training in reducing fear, curbing drug abuse, increasing empathy in counselors, decreasing generalized anxiety and test anxiety, reducing blood pressure and improving coronary activity among coronary rehabilitation patients.

By 1985 Jarrell could document over 1,000 published scientific papers on the beneficial effects of meditation, including some that claimed that meditators were less depressed, less anxious, less irritable, more self actualized, and significantly happier. This was in line with the conclusions published by de Silva (1986) who included much of what has just been listed, and added headaches, general tension, fatigue, excessive self-blame, pathological bereavement reactions, separation anxiety, and low frustration tolerance. As he had in his 1985 paper, de Silva paid particular attention to describing the wide range of modern behavior therapy techniques that can be extracted from traditional Buddhist practices.

Of course, there was a problem lurking behind most of these reports of the phenomenal effectiveness of TM and related practices. That problem was that most of the studies reported data from experienced TM participants, few of whom manifested any evident psychopathology. Where were the control groups, the double blinds, and all the other apparatus of carefully controlled Western science? An answer was provided by Holmes (1984) who analyzed the data from 20 well-controlled experimental studies published between 1976 and 1980 of the effects of meditation on somatic arousal. The following is excerpted from Holmes' abstract:

> A summary of the research in which the somatic arousal of meditating subjects was compared with the somatic arousal of resting subjects did not reveal any consistent differences between meditating and resting subjects on measures of heart rate, electrodermal activity, respiration rate, systolic blood pressure, diastolic blood pressure, skin temperature, oxygen consumption, EMG activity, blood flow, or various biochemical factors. (p. 1)

Holmes reviewed a further four experimental studies that investigated the effects of meditation on the anticipation of stress. These studies included diverse control groups, including one that was called anti-meditation that had subject exercise vigorously and think actively about their problems. Holmes' conclusion: "There is no evidence whatsoever that meditation facilitates the control of arousal in threatening situations" (p. 8). He further concluded that there was no reason to believe that there was any difference between the effectiveness of TM and any other forms of meditation.

As one reviews the history of these studies several things become relatively clear. There were (and probably are) real and substantial psychophysiological and psychological benefits to be derived from a regular practice of meditation. These benefits, however, are not really of a different kind or of a different magnitude than those benefits that can be shown from a wide variety of similarly aimed interventions, including distraction. Buddhism stripped of its philosophy, and reduced to a set of techniques is probably of some value compared to a no-treatment control, but it is probably not likely to be more effective than an active placebo. Meditation, particularly for the beginner, is difficult, time consuming, and requires focused attention. Further, as my colleague, Mark Blows, has repeatedly observed, much of the time, nothing happens! Metaphysically, 20 minutes of meditation a day is probably at the other end of the client use spectrum from, let's say, taking 20 mg of Prozac every day.

It would be a serious mistake, however, to dismiss the potential contribution of Buddhist philosophy and practice to behavior therapy. The overlap is, as de Silva has shown in his writing, actually quite remarkable. In fact, as a practicing cognitive therapist, virtually all of what I teach my clients can be derived from Buddhist teachings. Take, for example, the following passage from the Dhammapada, cited by Parry and Jones (1986, p. 180):

> We are what we think
> All that we are arises with our thoughts
> With our thoughts, we make the world
> Speak or act with an impure mind
> And trouble will follow you

The real problem is, as Ponce (1982) pointed out, that the Buddhist vision of psychotherapy aims at a complete transformation of the individual's paradigms or worldviews. It demands recognition that the world is in constant flux, that there is no permanent self, and that the things we believe we know about the world and our selves are nothing but delusions. It demands that we shatter our habitual ways of looking and knowing. It demands that we adopt a rigorously moral and ethical way of speech, action, effort, and occupation. The solution to our suffering requires the transformation of our limited view of reality, in an existentially authentic way, applied to the totality of our experience (Ponce, 1982). None of this is apt to be reflected in patterns of anticipatory psychophysiological reactions to stress (Bankart & Elliott, 1974). As George Kelly reminded us a generation ago: "What we think we know is anchored only in our own assumptions, not in the bedrock of truth itself, and that world we seek to understand remains always on the horizons of our thoughts" (as cited in Ray, 1986, p. 28).

Phase V: New Age Consciousness

I would like to suggest that there were three foundational events in the emergence of the Fifth Manifestation of the Buddha in Western psychology. The first was the publication in 1961 of Alan Watts' Psychotherapy East and West.

The second was the publication in 1969 of an important new source for scholarly exchange about the psychology of consciousness, the Journal of Transpersonal Psychology. The third was the integration of theory and practice of Eastern psychology into a Western developmental perspective in a book edited by Ken Wilber, Jack Engler, and Daniel P. Brown in 1986, Transformations of Consciousness: Conventional and Contemplative Perspectives on Development. Taken together these three primary sources created legitimate space for a serious extended academic discussion of consciousness, and its role in physical and psychological well-being.

As early as 1953 Alan Watts was writing in scholarly journals about the correspondence of ideals between Western psychotherapies and traditional Buddhist teachings. Watts was unhappy with the standard focus on the analysis of the unconscious that was the mainstay of psychotherapy at mid-century. He argued that consciousness could be explored without adopting the goals of diagnosis and social control; and rejected the assumption that psychotherapy was designed to produce "happy adjustment" of sick individuals to the conventions of society. He saw society populated by unhappy people, and wondered how fitting in better into such a social milieu could constitute a therapeutically desirable goal.

For Watts, the critical philosophical idea from the East was that of *mushin*, or "no mind"; a state of consciousness which is not analyzed but rather informs all life. Watts championed "the therapeutic value of the subjective abandonment of any psychological goals, in the future, coupled with the gentle but persistent focusing of attention on the immediately present totality of feeling-sensation – without any attempt to explain, diagnose, judge, or change it" (Watts, 1953, p. 28). He ended his essay with a quote from Chuang-tzu that read: "He who knows that he is a fool is not a great fool."

In his 1961 Psychotherapy East and West Watts refined his message, arguing that both Eastern teachings and Western psychotherapy seek to bring about "changes in consciousness and our ways of feeling our own existence and our relation to human society and the natural world" (Watts, 1961, pp. 15–16). But he now went on to claim that ordinary Western style consciousness was in fact a "breeding ground of mental disease" (p. 16). He argued that Eastern philosophy, and especially Buddhism, offered a powerful critique of Western culture, and he wondered out loud if traditional models of Western psychotherapy were even capable of bringing about a reconciliation between individual feeling and social norms without sacrificing the integrity of the individual.

Psychotherapy East and West was a far-reaching call for psychology and psychotherapy to facilitate the liberation of individual souls from the suffering resulting from the suffocating conformity of a joyless, sexless, over-analyzed and vastly over-controlling society. He rejected the Freudian call for what he called the domination of Eros by reason, and called, in its place, for Eros expressing itself with reason. The book was, for all extents and purposes, a vivid and heartfelt rejoinder to Freud's (1930) Civilization and Its Discontents.

The transformations of consciousness envisioned by Watts became, eventually, the subject matter of a journal that began publication in 1969. The web homepage of the Journal of Transpersonal Psychology [see References for address] provides excerpts from the writings in the journal from everyone from Abraham Maslow to Baba Ram Dass to the Dalai Lama. The focus of the journal from its inception has been on transpersonal experiences – that is, "experiences in which the sense of identity of self extends beyond (trans) the individual or personal to encompass wider aspects of humankind, life, psyche or cosmos" (Walsh & Vaughan, 1993).

The steady stream of articles published in JTP had a powerful influence on a resurgence of interest not only in studies of consciousness and "higher" mental processes, but also in a systematic rethinking of the concept of self in Western psychology. This new field of inquiry seriously challenged the psychoanalytic assumption that the "masterful, bounded, empty self... characterized by a pervasive sense of personal emptiness" (Cushman, 1995, pp. 6, 287) was the only self Western minds could experience; with psychotherapy its only solace.

In 1980 Roger Walsh asserted the currency of a way of thinking about consciousness that had lain dormant in American psychology since William James. He quoted James' famous dictum about consciousness:

> Our normal waking consciousness is but one special type of consciousness whilst all about it, parted from it by the filmiest of screens, there lie potential forms of consciousness entirely different. We may go through life without suspecting their existence, but apply the requisite stimulus, and at a touch they are there in all their completeness, definite types of mentality which probably somewhere have their field of application and adoption.
>
> No account of the universe in its totality can be final which leaves these other forms of consciousness quite disregarded. How to regard them is the question ... At any rate, they forbid our premature closing of accounts with reality. (as cited in Walsh, 1980, p. 665)

Walsh argued that the study of consciousness was a 4th Force in Western psychology, and called for the inclusion of serious inquiry into states of consciousness, meditation, modes of psychological health, peak experiences, mystical experience, and the interconnections between these studies and modern physics.

For the purposes of this essay, however, the most interesting aspect of Walsh's argument came at the end of his essay. He concluded his paper with a plea; and that plea was that behavioral scientists examine both the literature and the practices under study, and that these studies be conducted by persons with "personal experiences of these practices" (Walsh, 1980, p. 671). In short, he was calling for a new research paradigm, conducted by what he called Yogi-Scientists, trained in both Eastern and Western psychology. Without this new paradigm,

Walsh feared, the emergent study of consciousness would be forever confused with and contaminated by what he called "degenerate populisms," and subject to the systematic errors of our own Western scientific resistances as our most fundamental beliefs and worldviews were called into question.

The publication of Wilber, Engler, and Brown's *Transformations of Consciousness* in 1986 was precisely the sort of scholarship and inquiry that Walsh had urged. It developed an explicitly developmental focus that took into consideration not only failures of normal conscious development (disorders of the self-system, etc.) but also the upper reaches of the development of human consciousness. They took the challenge of understanding the voyage of the self head on, and explored with intellectual acuity the essential dilemma confronting all humans, but especially Westerners, the "bewildering experience of being both subject and object and its resultant dualism (Ben-Avi, 1959, p. 1818). Eastern teachings remind Western scholars that a robust and true science of human behavior; in Michael West's (1986) words, "needs to engage in exploration of people's most profound experiences." Further, it must retain a clear appreciation for "the importance of recognizing the individuality of such experience and its place within the person's life" (p. 267).

The success of this enterprise has the potential to transform all of Western psychology, in every one of its fields of inquiry. Take for example, the discussion of self that appeared in a recent book on the development of self in Western adolescents:

> From a Buddhist perspective, one must go beyond this form of self-observation; one must remove the watcher and the complicated bureaucracy that it creates to preserve the permanence of the self.... Once we take away the watcher, there is a tremendous amount of space, since the watcher and the bureaucracy take up so much room. Thus if one eliminates the role of the watcher, the space becomes sharp, precise, and intelligent. In fact one does not really need the watcher or observer of the self at all. (Harter, 1999, p. 189)

Concluding Thoughts

Recall that Walsh (1980) urged a new epistemology for the study of consciousness for *two* reasons. We seem to have the scholarly/experiential/new paradigm end of things well covered today. But how are we doing with the problem of what Walsh called "degenerate populisms"? As New Age bookstores have flourished and the number of neighborhood bookstores' shelves devoted to angels, crystals, and reincarnation have grown exponentially, how has this 4th Force, this Fifth Manifestation, faired as a serious field of inquiry? I will not attempt to answer that question directly – my charge as a historian of science is only to point to it, perhaps with some alarm.

At any rate, even as long ago as 1983, Bernie Zilbergeld lamented, "the problem is not that so many are constantly looking for enlightenment these days, but that so many have found it" (Zilbergeld, 1983, p. 3). The reader is urged to take a close look at Singer and Lalich (1996) for a current, and relatively independent assessment of the plethora of New Age cures, many of them sounding vaguely Eastern, that have become part of the popular cultural scene in recent years.

As therapists we must also be mindful of the potential hazards of applying Eastern practices outside of their cultural and spiritual contexts. Numerous sources have warned of the dangers of applying Eastern techniques in the West without great care. All of these sources agree it is crucial that Western psychotherapy patients explore Eastern approaches to the transformation of consciousness in the company of an experienced and trusted guide. There is substantial literature on this point in Western psychology, which we have commented on in two publications addressing integration of Eastern techniques into Western psychotherapies (Bankart, 1992; Bankart, Koshikawa, Nedate, & Haruki, 1992).

Fishman (1992), in recounting the case of a man who became deeply disturbed while practicing relaxation, deep abdominal breathing, and visualization concluded that these techniques are especially counterindicated in "individuals who have maintained rigid control over their thoughts and feelings to defend against a disruptive childhood and chronic insecurity" (p. 585). Similarly, Reynolds (1980) has advised serious caution that the "quiet therapies" may be dangerous for psychotic and depressive patients. Indeed, Transcendental Meditation and even deep relaxation have been noted to have a powerful potential for adverse psychiatric effects in some types of patients (Lazarus, 1976; Lazarus & Mayne, 1990).

Shapiro (1982) has called on Western therapists to use *extreme caution* when applying Eastern techniques with Western psychotherapy patients. In a carefully designed, systematic study Shapiro (1992) assessed the adverse effects of meditation among a group of long-term meditators (average length of meditation, 4.27 years). Sixty three percent of his participants had experienced at least mildly aversive affects, and two of his subjects (out of 27 in the sample) suffered profound adverse effects resulting in psychiatric hospitalization.

A review of this literature leads me to propose two separate but related obstacles of central concern to Western practitioners and teachers who become involved with introducing their Western clients/students to traditional Eastern techniques. The first is the general tendency in the West to look at all self-discovery regimens as essentially psychotherapeutic. The second, and more pressing problem, relates to the potential for disruptive psychological and emotional disregulation and/or regression in the wake of Eastern practices from too powerful an encounter with the self. In such cases it appears that the power of Eastern techniques overwhelms the self-structure of some psychotherapy patients, precipitating what are known in the literature as psychiatric casualties. For a more careful review of this literature see Bankart (2000).

So I want to end by coming full-circle back to the specter of orientalism that has overshadowed most of the contents of this essay. There is a great deal of evidence that in the phenomenal growth of interest in Buddhist practices and teachings in America, especially by psychologists and other therapists, Buddhism is colliding with a modern world that 2500 years of Buddhist philosophers could not have imagined. As Prebish (1999) has pointed out, the Dharma has become so disguised, it could never be proved in court. Prebish further notes that it is already pretty much unrecognizable to the three to four million practicing Buddhist Americans of Asian descent, for whom it is a traditional faith – not a recently adopted therapeutic practice.

In fact Prebish (1999) quotes Robert Thurman to the effect that Buddhism will not actually be able to succeed in its mission in America unless it is able to perform that mission without in any real sense being Buddhism! This "Buddhism without the Buddha" may become the ultimate expression of transcendental American optimism; but it will bear little resemblance to the teachings of the Buddha. Prebish sees the future of Buddhism in America as a social revolution directed toward increasing human happiness. He has a vision of a social-psycho-therapeutic movement: "increasingly lay, feminist, practice-oriented, psychological, socially concerned, [and gay-friendly, see Corless, 1998], democratic, self-critical, ... and grounded in social engagement interconnectedness, conflict resolution, environmental awareness, and right livelihood" (Prebish, 1999, pp. 253–4, 259).

Like Rubin (1996) and Prebish (1999) I wonder out loud what sort of Buddhism exists that it is all practice and action oriented, and seems to be unable to come to terms with day-to-day ethical dilemmas, and an overriding concern with ethical conduct, wisdom and compassion. Prebish and Rubin both expresses strong concern over widespread and well-documented ethical breaches, sexual abuses, and abuse of power by various American Buddhist teachers. [See Gross (1998) for a vivid and somewhat chilling glimpse into the never-never world of the sexual politics of gurus, feminists, and "postpatriarchal Buddhism" in America.]. Western Buddhists may, in fact, be in danger of the greatest act of orientalism yet committed against the ancient teachings; turning it into a massive carnival of self-glorifying power-seeking materialistic narcissism. At any rate it is difficult to argue with the observation of one Shin practitioner who wryly observed: "White practitioners practice intensive psychotherapy on their cushions in a life-or-death struggle with ego, whereas Asian Buddhists just seem to smile and eat together" [cited by Prebish, 1999, p. 65).

Perhaps, then, it is appropriate for this chapter to conclude with a reminder from Robert Thurman about the true nature of Buddhist thought and practice:

> This is the messianic drive of the Bodhisattva; the spirit of love and compassion called the enlightening soul. It is not merely the wish that all be well with all beings – it is the determination that you yourself will assume responsibility for others. (Thurman, 1998, p. 159)

References

Abel, T. M., Metraux, R., & Roll, S. (1987). *Psychotherapy and culture*. Albuquerque: University of New Mexico Press.

Alexander, F. (1931). Buddhistic training as an artificial catatonia. *Psychoanalytic Review, 18*, 129–145.

Alexander, F. G. & Selesnick, S. T. (1966). *The history of psychiatry: An evaluation of psychiatric thought*. New York: Harper & Row.

Bankart, C. P. (2000). *Qigong* in the West: Challenges, hazards, and opportunities. In W. Weidong, Y. Sasaki, & Y. Haruki (Eds.), *Bodywork and psychotherapy in the East* (pp. 133–142). Delft, the Netherlands: Eburon.

Bankart, C. P. (1997). *Talking cures: A history of Western and Eastern psychotherapies*. Pacific Grove, CA: Brooks/Cole.

Bankart, C. P. (1992). Some Western questions for an Eastern psychology. *Japanese Health Psychology, 1*, 103–112.

Bankart, C. P. & Elliott, R. (1974). Heart rate and skin conductance in anticipation of shocks with varying probabilities of occurrence. *Psychophysiology, 11*, 160–174.

Bankart, C. P., Koshikawa, F., Nedate, K., & Haruki, Y. (1992). When West meets East: Contributions of Eastern traditions to the future of psychotherapy. *Psychotherapy, 29*, 141–149.

Ben-Avi, A. (1959). Zen Buddhism. In S. Arieti (Ed.), *American handbook of psychiatry, Volume Two* (pp. 1816–1820). New York: Basic Books.

Benson, H., Frankel, F. H., Apfel, R., Daniels, M. D., Schnielwind, H. E., Nemiah, J. C., Sifneos, P. E., et al. (1978). Treatment of anxiety: A comparison of the usefulness of self-hypnosis and a meditational relaxation technique. *Psychotherapy and Psychosomatics, 30*, 229–242.

Claxton G. (1986). Therapy and beyond: Concluding thoughts. In G. Claxton (Ed.), *Beyond therapy: The impact of Eastern traditions on psychological theory and practice* (pp. 311–325). London: Wisdom Press.

Clifford, T. (1984). *Tibetan Buddhist medicine and psychiatry: The diamond healing*. York Beach, Maine: S. Weiser.

Corless, R. (1998). Coming out in the *sangha*: Queer community in American Buddhism. In C. S. Prebish & K. K. Tanaka (Eds), *The faces of Buddhism in America* (pp. 253–265). Berkeley: University of California Press.

Cushman, P. (1995). *Constructing the self, constructing America: A cultural history of psychotherapy*. Reading, MA: Addison-Wesley.

De Silva, P. (1986). Buddhism and behavior change: Implications therapy. In G. Claxton (Ed.), *Beyond therapy: The impact of Eastern traditions on psychological theory and practice* (pp. 217–231) London: Wisdom Press.

Deikman, A. (1977). Comments on the GAP report on mysticism. *Journal of Nervous and Mental Disease, 165*, 213–217.

Doi, T. (1976). Psychotherapy as "Hide and Seek." In W. P. Lebra (Ed.), *Culture bound syndromes, ethnopsychiatry and alternate therapies* (pp. 273–277). Honolulu: University Press of Hawaii.

Ehrenwald, J. (1976). *The history of psychotherapy: From healing magic to encounter*. New York: Jason Aronson.

Fingarette, H. (1963). *The self in transformation: Psychoanalysis, philosophy, and the life of the spirit*. New York: Basic Books.

Fishman, B. (1992). Therapy for an anxious patient who believes his symptoms are caused by a medical problem. *Hospital and Community Psychiatry, 43*, 583–85.

Freud, S. (1930). *Civilization and its discontents*. London: Hogarth.

Fromm, E. (1950). *Psychoanalysis and religion*. New Haven, CT: Yale University Press.

Fromm, E. (1960). Psychoanalysis and Zen Buddhism. In E. Fromm, D. T. Suzuki, & R. De Martino (Eds.). *Zen Buddhism and psychoanalysis* (pp. 77–141). New York: Harper and Row.

Gross, R. M. (1998). Helping the iron bird fly: Western Buddhist women and issues of authority in the late 1990s. In C. S. Prebish & K. K. Tanaka (Eds.), *The faces of Buddhism in America* (pp. 238–252). Berkeley: University of California Press.

Harter, S. (1999). *The construction of the self: A developmental perspective*. New York: Guilford.

Holmes, D. S. (1984). Meditation and somatic arousal reduction: A review of the experimental evidence. *American Psychologist, 39*, 1–10.

Horney, K. (1945). *Our inner conflicts: A constructive theory of neurosis*. New York: Norton.

Horney, K. (1987). Final lectures. In D. H. Ingram (Ed.), *Final lectures*. New York: Norton.

Imamura, R. (1998). Buddhist and Western Psychotherapies: An Asian American perspective. In C. S. Prebish & K. K. Tanaka (Eds.), *The faces of Buddhism in America* (pp. 228–237). Berkeley: University of California Press.

James, W. (1958). *Varieties of religious experience*. New York: New American Library.

Jacobson, A. & Berenberg, A. N. (1952). Japanese psychiatry and psychotherapy. *American Journal of Psychiatry, 109*, 321–329.

Jarrell, H. R. (1985). Meditation and psychotherapeutic effects. *Archives of General Psychiatry, 35*, 294–302. *Journal of Transpersonal Psychology* World Wide Web homepage available: *http://www.igc.apc.org/atp/perspective/quotes.html*

Journal of Transpersonal Psychology World Wide Web homepage available at: http://www.igc.apc.org/atp/perspective/quotes/html.

Jung, C. G. (1954). The development of personality. New York: Pantheon Books.

Jung, C. G. (1957). Psychological commentary. In W. Y. E. Wents (Ed.), *The Tibetan book of great liberation; or the method of realizing nirvana through knowing the mind* (pp. xxix–lxiv). New York: Oxford University Press.

Jung, C. G. (1962). Commentary on *The Secret of the Golden Flower*, R. Wilhelm (trans.). London: Routledge & Kegan Paul.

Jung, C. G. (1964). Foreword. In D. T. Suzuki, *An introduction to Zen Buddhism*. New York: Grove, pp. 9–29.

Kelly, G. A. (1977). The psychology of the unknown. In D. Barrister (Ed.), *New perspectives in personal construct theory* (pp. 1–19). New York: Academic Press.

Kelman, H. (1960). Psychoanalytic thought and Eastern wisdom. In J. Ehrenwald (1976), (Ed.), *The history of psychotherapy: From healing magic to encounter* (pp. 328–333). New York: Jason Aronson.

Kondo, K. (1953). Morita therapy: A Japanese therapy for neurosis. *American Journal of Psychoanalysis, 13*, 31–37.

Lazarus, A. A. (1976). Psychiatric problems precipitated by transcendental meditation. *Psychological Reports, 39*, 601–602.

Lazarus, A. A. & Mayne, T. J. (1990). Relaxation: Some limitations, side effects, and proposed solutions. *Psychotherapy, 27*, 261–266.

Lesh, T. (1970). Zen meditation and the development of empathy in counselors. *Journal of Humanistic Psychology, 10*, 39–74.

Mikulas, W. L. (1978). Four noble truths of Buddhism related to behavior therapy. *Psychological Record, 28*, 59–67.

Mikulas, W. L. (1981). Buddhism and behavior modification. *Psychological Record, 31*, 331–342.

Parry, S. J. & Jones, G. A. (1986). Beyond illusion in the psychotherapeutic enterprise. In G. Claxton (Ed.), *Beyond therapy: The impact of Eastern traditions on psychological theory and practice*. (pp. 173–192). London: Wisdom Press.

Ponce, D. E. (1982). Buddhist constructs and psychotherapy. *International Journal of Social Psychiatry, 28*, 83–90.

Prebish, C. S. (1999). *Luminous passage: The practice and study of Buddhism in America*. Berkeley: University of California Press.

Ray, C. (1986). Western psychology and Buddhist teachings: Convergences and Divergences. In G. Claxton (Ed.), *Beyond therapy: The impact of Eastern religions on psychological theory and practice* (pp. 17–29). London: Wisdom Press.

Reynolds, D. (1980). *The quiet therapies: Japanese pathways to personal growth*. Honolulu: University Press of Hawaii.

Rubin, J. B. (1985). Meditation and psychoanalytic listening. *Psychoanalytic Review, 72*, 599–613.

Rubin, J. B. (1996). *Psychotherapy and Buddhism: Toward an integration*. New York: Plenum Press.

Said, E. W. (1979). *Orientalism*. New York: Vintage Books.

Sato, K. (1958). Psychotherapeutic implications of Zen. *Psychologia, 1*, 213–218.

Shapiro, D. H. (1982). Overview: Clinical and physiological comparison of meditation and other self-control strategies. *American Journal of Psychiatry, 139*, 267–274.

Shapiro, D. H. (1992). Adverse effects of meditation: A preliminary investigation of long term meditators. *International Journal of Psychosomatics, 39*, (Special Issue Nos. 1–4), 62–67.

Shapiro, D. H. & Zifferblatt, S. M. (1976a). An applied clinical combination of Zen meditation and behavioral self-management techniques: Reducing methadone dosage in drug addiction. *Behavior Therapy, 7*, 694–695.

Shapiro, D. H. & Zifferblatt, S. M. (1976b). Zen meditation and behavioral self-control: Similarities, differences, and clinical applications. *American Psychologist, 31*, 519–532.

Singer, M. T. & Lalich, J. (1996). *Crazy therapies: What are they? Do they work?* San Francisco: Josey-Bass.

Suzuki, D. T. (1960). Lectures on Zen Buddhism. In E. Fromm, D. T. Suzuki, & R. DeMartino, (Eds.) *Zen Buddhism and psychoanalysis* (pp. 1–76). New York: Harper & Row.

Thurman, R. (1998). *Inner revolution: Life, liberty, and the pursuit of real happiness*. New York: Riverhead Books.

Van Dusen, W. (1958). Zen and Western psychotherapy. *Psychologia, 1*, 229–230.

Wallace, R. K., Benson, H., & Wilson, A. F. (1971). A wakeful hypometabolic state. *American Journal of Physiology, 221*, 795–799.

Walsh, R. (1980). The consciousness disciplines and the behavioral sciences: Questions of comparison and assessment. *American Journal of Psychiatry, 137*, 663–673.

Walsh, R. & Vaughan, F. (1993). On transpersonal definitions. *Journal of Transpersonal Psychology, 25*. Retrieved from *http://www.igc.apc.org/atp/perspective/quotes.html*

Watts, A. W. (1953). Asian psychology and modern psychiatry. *American Journal of Psychoanalysis, 13*, 25–30.

Watts, A. W. (1961). *Psychotherapy East and West*. New York: Pantheon.

Welwood, J. (1983). Befriending emotion. In J. Welwood (Ed.), *Awakening the Heart* (pp. 79–90). Boulder, CO: Shambala.

West, M. A. (1986). Meditation: Psychology and human experience. In G. Claxton (Ed.), *Beyond therapy: The impact of Eastern traditions on psychological theory and practice* (pp. 311–325). London: Wisdom Press.

Wilber, K., Engler, J., & Brown, D. P. (1986). *Transformations of consciousness: Conventional and contemplative perspectives on development*. Boston: New Science Library/Shambala.

Wolf, W. (1957). Reflections on Zen Buddhism, psychology, and psychotherapy. *American Journal of Psychotherapy, 11*, 866–869.

Woolfolk, R. L. (1975). Psychophysiological correlates of meditation. *Archives of General Psychiatry, 32*, 1326–1333.

Woolfolk, R. L., Carr-Kaffashan, L., McNulty, T. F., & Lehrer, P. M. (1976). Meditation training as a treatment for insomnia. *Behavior Therapy, 7*, 359–365.

Zilbergeld, B. (1983). *The shrinking of America*. Boston: Little, Brown.

Chapter 3

Value and Meaning in Gestalt Psychology and Mahayana Buddhism

Edward S. Ragsdale

This chapter seeks to build a bridge between Western psychology and Mahayana Buddhism regarding some basic questions in ethics and the psychology of values. A major problem in the West concerns our struggle to come to terms with the considerable extent to which values differ and change over place and time, and to determine what kind of validity ethics might yet rightly claim in the midst of such diversity. Clearly this is not merely an academic problem. Value conflict, in both inner and outer worlds, seems part of the fundamental human condition. Internally it arises in what Jung (1964/1970, p. 444) calls "conflicts of duty," where competing demands may pull us in opposite directions and divide us from ourselves. Externally, in our confrontation with persons and groups whose values conflict with our own, the challenge is redoubled, as we face the immense and critical challenges of cooperative living on a fast-shrinking planet.

Attempts to address the problem of value and value conflict are often formulated within the framework of the absolutism–relativism distinction. Absolutism clings tight to assumptions of validity, but at the price of rigid and rule bound exclusivity. Relativism relinquishes that exclusivity, but in so doing sacrifices any claims to validity or universality. It is questionable whether problems of ethics and value can be resolved within this duality. I believe the insights of Gestalt psychology – long neglected and often misunderstood – may provide a more viable alternative. Gestalt psychology rejects both absolutism and relativism in favor of a *relational* view as a middle way between those polar extremes. Its principle of relational determination of meaning and value respects value diversity without conceding validity or universality in value experience.

This relational approach has echoes of Mahayana Buddhism, in particular the Madhyamika, or "Middle Way" school founded by Nagarjuna near the beginning of the Common Era. Madhyamika's central teaching is the relational interdependence of all phenomena. This principle serves as an antidote to the habitual tendency to impute independent existence to persons and things. Both Gestalt theory and Buddhism view reality and experience as relational facts, and both view absolutism and relativism (cf. nihilism) as mistaken departures from relational understanding. Buddhism may be further helpful in revealing the full measure of this relationality, and in clarifying the moral significance relational understanding may hold. I hope that the benefits of mutual illumination of one viewpoint in light of the other might offset the obvious risks of comparing traditions so widely separated by time, culture, and institutional nature.

Gestalt Psychology

Let us first consider Gestalt psychology. Gestalt psychology was founded in Germany in 1912 by Max Wertheimer, who joined with Kurt Koffka and Wolfgang Köhler to build a scientific psychology relevant to human experience and respectful of the human capacity for insight and value. Gestalt theorists maintained faith in the unity of science, seeking to reveal the ultimate compatibility of mental and physical realms. They rejected the standard model – common to both introspectionism and behaviorism – of reducing mental events to atomistic and mechanistic processes in mind or body, which entails a relativism of thought and value. Rejecting traditional assumptions of elementarism, mechanism, and reductionism, Gestalt psychologists developed a field approach for psychology, to address problems in perception, cognition, interpersonal relations, and value.

A few words should be said about Köhler's (1938/1966, 1944/1971, 1947, 1959, 1969) work on the psychophysical foundations of value, and the role – in mind and body – of invariant dynamics as a third principle of causation beyond heredity and learning. Köhler expanded psychology's common view of value as a subjectively imposed, ego-driven product of the exigencies of mutation or conditioning, to reveal it as a fact of nature that is neither ego-bound nor utterly dependent on the contingencies of genetics or learning (see also Köhler, 1950/1961). Value experience may depend substantially upon processes of invariant dynamics found throughout nature (see also Henle, 1977, 1985; Ragsdale, 1999). If so, reductive and relativistic explanations will not suffice. While this view invites comparison to Buddhist teachings concerning the uncreated mind, that is not a goal of the present work.

Let us narrow our focus to one aspect of the wider view: that of the relational determination of meaning and value. Gestalt psychology's relational viewpoint is reflected in Köhler's famous statement "the whole is different from the sum of its parts." A whole – be it percept or concept, value or belief – is not a mere summation of component parts. The organization and internal structure of those parts is crucial in constituting the whole. Likewise, parts should not be viewed as independent units, since their nature or role is shaped by the function they play in completing the whole.

The Gestalt psychologists Karl Duncker and Solomon Asch applied this thinking to better understand value experience and value diversity. The valuation of a particular practice cannot be understood without reference to the context of the whole situation within which it acquires its particular meaning. Neither absolutism nor relativism may be sufficiently mindful of the role of situational context in shaping meaning and value. The Gestalt view of relational determination provides an alternative to some basic assumptions common to both.

Let us review traditional Western thinking about values and consider the contrasting Gestalt viewpoint. As far as ethics and values go, societies have traditionally embraced some form of absolutism. In the West, the Judeo-Christian ethic has predominated. Such (deontological) approaches lay out moral absolutes – laws, rules, or commandments with which to decide categorically whether a given act is good or bad. Their moral dualism depicts those categories as ultimate and unconditional. Such views may predispose their adherents to attitudes of condescension toward those with conflicting views, who may be seen as ethically immature, or less than fully human, or evil.

Our increasing exposure to diverse and conflicting moral codes, and a growing scientific skepticism concerning the possibility of objective value generally, has raised doubts about absolutism, and has produced a reaction against it, in the form of ethical relativism. Relativism denies "that there are any fixed principles of value in human relations and [asserts] that these are historically conditioned or relative to the society" (Asch, 1952, p. 367). This view has come to dominate psychology and the social sciences, including the new postmodern theories.

There are some problems with relativism. For one thing, its claim of basic value differences implies there are fundamental, presumably irreconcilable divisions that cleave humanity. For another, it weakens the idea that our moral values have any objective sensibility or valid basis. Here relativism appears at least to flirt with, if not succumb to, nihilism.

In 1939, Karl Duncker published a critique of ethical relativism. He began with the unstartling fact that values tend to differ and change. Beliefs and practices deemed ethical by one group may be scorned by another. Upon this basis some conclude in favor of ethical relativism, "there is nothing invariable within the psychological content of morality" (p. 39). But value conflict does not in itself prove relativism. Duncker identified a critical but previously unacknowledged assumption of relativism, one now embraced by philosophy (see Brandt, 1961, 1967; Frankena, 1973; Ragsdale, 1985; also Ellis, 1992). To fulfill the demands of relativism's basic thesis, *descriptive relativism*, an object or situation that receives different valuations from different groups must have the same meaning to those groups. It is only when the meaning of a practice is constant despite differences in valuation that value differences are said to be absolute and relativism may be said to apply. Relativism requires that persons or groups who offer opposing valuations have in mind the same object of judgment (Asch, 1952, p. 420, see also Wertheimer, 1935/1961).

To determine whether descriptive relativism applies, one must consider the specific situational context of a practice. Where different contexts yield different valuations, one must ask whether the practice retains the same meaning in each case, or whether its meaning varies as a function of its context. If meaning constancy prevails, then value differences would appear to be absolute and descriptive relativism is indicated. If meaning covaries with valuation, then the contrasting Gestalt thesis would be supported. In that case, the meaning of a thing would not be an independent property, but a function of the thing's relation to a context of other things. And value differences would reflect, not basic ethical differences, but instead secondary differences in comprehension of the situation.

Duncker's key question was thus an empirical one: Does a practice that receives different valuations by different groups have different meanings to those groups? Duncker concluded that this was indeed the case. Reviewing instances of value conflict in the anthropological literature, he found consistent evidence of an "invariant relation between meaning and value." Where values differed, so too did underlying meanings. He concluded that neither value nor meaning are independent properties. The value (or valuation) of a thing depends upon its meaning. Its meaning in turn depends upon the context in which it is understood.

Duncker describes numerous instances where differences in valuation reflect corresponding differences in situational meaning. Examples include the sanctioned killing of infants or the aged, differences in standards of modesty in dress. Consider the practice of charging interest on money lent. In biblical days this constituted the sin of usury, while nowadays it is routinely accepted, even touted, as a bulwark of capitalism. Coinciding with this change in valuation of money-lending is a change in its meaning and role. In bygone days loans often arose out of vital need, whereas in capitalism loans are employed "as capital for profitable production" (p. 40). It is thus fitting to provide the lender a share of the profits:

> Interest no longer means an exploitation of necessities or passions. It has changed its typical meaning.... In our example we have not two different ethical valuations of usury, but two different meanings of money-lending each of which receives its specific valuation. (p. 41)

Let us examine a more current example. Consider the issue of abortion, and the polarization of attitudes into so-called pro-choice versus right-to-life camps. For this conflict to serve as evidence of a relativism of values, it must be shown that abortion has the same meaning for those with opposing views of its morality.

Yet this does not appear the case. The meaning of abortion tends to differ along with its valuation. The critical variable often concerns the context of beliefs about the status of the fetus: whether or not it is viewed as already a human being. One group may equate abortion with murder of a human being; another may see it as termination of a life form that is not yet a human being. Rather than support relativism, such co-variation of meaning and value lends support to Gestalt psychology's contrasting view of a "relational determination" of meaning and value (Asch, 1952).

To sum up, the traditional ethics of absolutism, which identifies concrete and unconditional rights and wrongs, is now opposed by a contrary assumption of ethical relativism, which denies the validity or universality of any moral code. These polar opposites share common assumptions of meaning constancy and elementarism. Objects and situations, or their component parts, are assumed to be independent facts. Gestalt psychology offers another way of looking at value differences. It posits a relational determination of meaning and value, which locates meaning, not in the thing itself, but in its relation to context. If so, then basic assumptions shared by absolutism and relativism are wrong. Meaning and value are not absolute, but relational facts. And the value differences that divide persons and groups are not absolute. A commensurability of sorts may exist across the full range of ethical valuation, finding room for all humanity within the same moral universe. This does not dispose of the metaethical questions of establishing validity, or normative questions concerning the clarification of actual moral demands. It does force a reformulation of the ethical problem so as to focus attention on underlying meanings.

Mahayana Buddhism

Let us now consider Mahayana Buddhism. The ultimate aim of Mahayana Buddhism is the enlightenment of ourselves and all other sentient beings. The motivation to follow this path is, or needs to be, a desire to relieve the suffering of all sentient beings. Personal enlightenment is a means to this compassionate end. Thus the basic intention of Buddhism may be seen as a moral one, manifested in the compassionate motivation to achieve enlightenment for the sake of others.

Enlightenment entails the perfection of both wisdom and compassion. By *wisdom*, Buddhists mean a fully integrated understanding of the authentic nature of reality. Our capacity for compassionate action ultimately depends upon the extent of this understanding, since it is the key that opens our heart most fully to others. Likewise our greatest expression of compassion is to awaken this wisdom in others as a basis for their own liberation. Thus we begin to see the interrelation and ultimate indivisibility of wisdom and compassion.

Before considering the nature of this wisdom, and the deviations from this understanding as represented in the error of the two extremes, we must realize that one does not set out on the bodhichitta path to enlightenment with a moral sense already informed by full awareness of the authentic nature of things. Buddhism requires an ethics for individuals short of such realization – which includes perhaps all of us. Lord Buddha possessed the "skill in means" to know just what a person needed to hear, based upon his or her level of realization, as a famous statement by Nagarjuna describes:

> Just as a grammarian [first] has students
> Read a model of the alphabet,
> So Buddha taught trainees
> The doctrines they could bear.
>
> To some he taught doctrines
> To turn them away from ill-deeds;
> To some, for the sake of achieving merit;
> To some, doctrines based on duality;
> To some, doctrines based on non-duality;
> To some, what is profound and frightening to the fearful –
> Having an essence of emptiness and compassion –
> The means of achieving [unsurpassed] enlightenment.
> (as cited in Hopkins, 1998, p. 90)

Progress on the path begins with a foundation of ethical conduct, and for this Buddhism offers an absolutist, deontological ethics (see Thurman, 1981). Thus the Ten-fold Path instructs practitioners not to take a life, not to take what is not given, nor commit sexual misconduct, nor lie, nor cause dissention, nor speak harshly, nor chatter foolishly, nor covet, nor harbor malice, nor hold wrong views. Later, at an intermediate level of development, Buddhist ethics focuses less on establishing restraint and more on cultivating virtue. It offers for example the Six Paramitas ("Perfections" or "Transcendences") of giving, ethics, patience, effort, concentration (or meditation), and wisdom. Yet the ultimate expression of Buddhist ethics is enlightenment itself, whose essence is emptiness and compassion. This ethical ideal cannot be achieved without realizing emptiness.

The central teaching of Buddhism is that of *sunyata* – translated as "emptiness" or "voidness" (see Hopkins, 1983, 1987, 1998; Napper, 1989; Thurman, 1981, 1984; Varela, Thompson, & Rosch, 1991). Authentic reality is said to have the nature of emptiness. Realization of this constitutes wisdom. Buddhism teaches that all things, self as well as others, physical entities as well as mental events, are empty of inherent, or independent existence. They do not exist "from their own side." Under analysis, the thing cannot be found. It is not the same as the parts that compose it, nor does it exist separate from those parts. Nor is it independent of the causes and conditions that give rise to it. Nor apart from name or use. On the other hand, the "unfindability" of any independent, self-existent thing does not imply utter non-existence. Things exist conventionally, but their existence is relational and interdependent.

While emptiness may be the fundamental nature of all things, this nature is not readily discernable in common experience. In fact, none of us – unless we happen to be a Buddha – can perceive this essential nature in our direct and ongoing experience of the world. We are trapped in habitual modes of experiencing that blind us to the ultimate nature of reality as empty of independent or inherent existence. This ignorance is the source of the suffering of *samsara*, from which Buddhism offers rescue through enlightenment.

Our pattern of misperception may take two forms. Thus Buddhists describe the error of the two extremes, which we may refer to as absolutism and nihilism. Each pole entails an absolutization of experience. With absolutism, one clings to a sense of things as really real, as possessing independent existence apart from other things. Here we are unable to digest the sheer contingency of existence, the dependence of all things upon causes and conditions beyond themselves, their interdependent origination with other things. We thus absolutistically confer upon things – including ourselves – an independent reality they do not have. Blind to the nature of self and other, we thus course in the samsaric existence of attachment and aversion as the price of our misunderstanding, and as the source of our hurtfulness to others.

Or we may fall into the other, nihilistic extreme. If we become disillusioned with absolutism, we may find ourselves clinging, not to being, but to non-being. We may mistake the absence of inherent or absolute existence for an absolute non-existence. We may end up rejecting the contingent truth that the thing may validly possess with respect to its own interdependent origination. That is, rather than allow for the conventional reality of a phenomenon relative to its own causes, conditions, constituent parts, etc., as may be established through valid cognition, we deny not just its absolutized, reified existence but its authentic, relationally grounded reality as well. What's worse, our negation of experience may lead us to reject its contents, to close our hearts to others and perhaps ourselves as well.

In between these two extremes is the middle ground of relationality, the authentic nature of reality, whose ultimate truth is emptiness, or absence, of *inherent* or *independent* existence. Let us consider some examples of emptiness, and explore some means by which Buddhism exposes our chronic blindness to it.

We need to begin where we live, in the world as it appears to us, which we take to be reality. Reality *appears* to be inhabited by real people and real things. The car I drive to work in is surely real. The "I" who drives it, who moves from one place to another with things to do and people to see, certainly seems real enough. It is this unexamined commonsense reality that Buddhism calls into question. While such facts of experience are by no means altogether unreal, the sense of reality we impute to them is exaggerated. We are challenged to look more closely into the nature of the things we construe to be real, including the self who does the construing. For this, Buddhism offers various formal reasonings that expose to us our habit of imputing absolute existence, as it reveals the very unfoundedness of this attribution (see Hopkins, 1987).

All such reasonings begin with an identification of a particular object or self (see Hopkins, 1987; Napper, 1989). We find that we automatically attribute to this object a sense of concrete, independent reality. It is so taken for granted in our experience that we remain largely oblivious to our reification. Since this imputation (of inherent existence) is determined to be in error, the object so construed is identified as the "object of negation." With this object of negation firmly in mind, we then set about to "ascertain the entailment," as follows:

If the object "really" exists (independently, in its own right), there are a limited number of forms its actual existence may take. Here we try to identify all possible forms, or logical possibilities that this absolute existence might take. One by one, we rule out each possibility. We "ascertain" that the inapplicability of each of these forms "entails" the conclusion that the object lacks inherent, or independent existence.

If our reasoning is effective, the logical analyses that follow from these questions awaken us to the startling realization that the object, as experienced, cannot be found within the experience. This is not to say that it is altogether absent, but that the kind of absolutized existence that we had taken for granted in the thing does not bear careful scrutiny. In the end our whole sense of reality may be turned inside out.

Consider the sevenfold reasoning provided by the Seventh Century Indian logician Chandrakirti

> A chariot is not asserted to be other than its parts,
> Nor non-other. It also does not possess them.
> It is not in the parts, nor are the parts in it.
> It is not the mere collection [of its parts],
> nor is it [their] shape.
> [The self and the aggregates are] similar.
> (as cited in Hopkins, 1987, p. 224)

While Chandrakirti uses the example of a chariot, we may prefer to think of a car. Our naive realism insists that the car standing before us is real, really real, a thing in its own right, existing "from its own side," independent of other things. The apparently inherently existing object – the chariot or car – is the "object of negation" (Hopkins, 1987, p. 223). The seven negations correspond to the seven hypothetical ways in which it might be said to possess absolute existence. We determine that if the object were to exist inherently, it would be in one of those forms. Next we deeply analyze each logical possibility to see if the object can be conceived within any of the modes of this presumably exhaustive list. If the object cannot pass muster within any of these modes, we may conclude that it lacks the kind of independent existence that we normally attribute to it. We discover that it does not *really* exist.

I will not try to flesh out the entire exercise. Consider instead the main part of the reasoning, concerning whether the chariot is the same or different from its parts. Note first that the chariot, or the car – like all productions – is a compounded entity. It is composed of parts: axle, wheels, body, etc. Yet is it the same as these parts? In pondering the question, we find that if the chariot were identical with its parts, then each part would be the chariot, and there would be as many chariots as there were parts. Or conversely, just as there is but one chariot, there would be but one part. Thinking through the various possibilities of relation between the thing and its parts, we find the chariot is not the same as its parts. It is not findable there.

If the chariot is not the same as its parts, then is it different from them? Notice that even in conceiving the question, we maintain a concept of chariot as distinguishable from its parts. Yet where is this chariot apart from its parts? The chariot, which is not findable in or as its parts, cannot be found apart from them either. While we might find ourselves clinging to a *concept* of chariot or car that would cover and contain its various parts, perhaps in the manner of a good paint job, we see that this notion is a reification that cannot pass the test of analytic findability.

While these glimpses of the unfindability of objects may prepare the way for insight into the emptiness of inherent existence, it is necessary, and apparently easier, to experience this unfindability with regard to the self. This same kind of reasoning applies here as well. Consider the fivefold reasoning of Nagarjuna. Here the object of negation is Buddha himself, the One Gone Thus, whose epistemological status is no different from that of any other self. The aggregates refer to the five parts (i.e., form, sensation, perception, mental formations, and consciousness) of which all experience is said to be composed, though the particular components are not critical to the analysis.

> The One Gone Thus is not the aggregates;
> The One Gone Thus is not other than the aggregates;
> The aggregates are not in the One Gone Thus;
> The One Gone Thus is not in the aggregates;
> The One Gone Thus does not possess the aggregates.
> What One Gone thus is there?
>
> (as cited in Hopkins, 1998, p. 58)

First consider the proposition that self and aggregates are one. The proposition in a sense contradicts itself, since it requires a distinction between self and part that it would deny. As Nagarjuna points out, it is senseless to assert a self as identical with its parts, since self would thus become a mere redundancy, utterly synonymous with its parts (e.g., mind and body), with no meaning aside from them (see Hopkins, 1987, p. 264). Also, as in the previous example, if self and aggregates were identical, there would be many selves. Here my nose is myself, my arm is myself, my leg is myself, my mind is myself, and I become an incredibly vast number of selves. Imagine that each part is "I," and as Hopkins suggests, try to figure out which "I" is to answer the door (1987, p. 266). Besides this is the problem that the proposition, in claiming an identity of whole and part, is bidirectional: Not only is my ear claimed to be myself, but myself is claimed to be my ear, in which case it becomes harder to assert that it is my eye.

The problem is redoubled when we consider the temporal continuity of "real" selfhood, to try to see how the self at one moment, subject to laws of cause and effect, and prone to change, is identical with the self of another moment. Is the self of yesterday, or the self at one's birth, or – if you will – the self of a former birth, truly the same as the self of today, or tomorrow? To say yes is to affirm a truly permanent self, incapable of change, and for that matter incapable of encounter or relationship, nor able to sow seeds or bear fruit of the law of karma.

Satisfying ourselves that the self is not utterly the same as its parts, we ask if it is utterly different. We find that it is as hard to assert utter difference as it is to assert utter identity. There is no self that we can find that is observable separate from its parts. Moreover, says Nagarjuna, if self and its aggregates were altogether different, self "would not have the character of the aggregates" (as cited in Hopkins, 1987, p. 272). Yet self does have the character of the parts that compose it. It has the characteristics of the mind and body. Selves do what minds and bodies do. We cannot find a self apart from its parts, any more than we can find a self as identical to its parts.

This deconstruction of the object of negation demands successful navigation past the Scylla and Charybdis of "extremist" views. If we define the object (of negation) too narrowly, we may negate too little, and remain trapped in the illusion of absolute existence. Defining it too broadly, we may succumb to the even greater danger of nihilism: We may negate too much and deny absolutely the conventional world, including the sentient beings we aim to help (see also Napper, 1989).

Here it is critically important to realize that this unfindability of things calls into question their *inherent*, or intrinsic, or independent existence. It exposes our mistaken reification of apparent reality, in which we superimpose a sense of absolute existence onto things that exist only relationally. It does *not* deny conventional reality, that is, the authentic existence of things as dependent upon causes and conditions beyond themselves – though our reifying minds can abide only so much veridicality. Thus the conventional truth of things is also a "concealer truth." It hides authentic reality behind false appearances (see Hopkins, 1983, pp. 400–421). Yet as the illusion of independent existence is overcome, it eventually becomes possible to have valid cognition and valid perception concerning the persons, places, and things of conventional reality, that is, an understanding of the conventional world that is informed by an awareness of its ultimate emptiness of inherent existence. Mind thus possesses the means, and nature possesses the order, for authentic insight into the nature of reality.

Especially since Buddhism is so often accused of the very nihilism it explicitly rejects, it bears repeating that its teaching of emptiness is not a nihilistic denial of existence or meaning. Let us take a closer look at nihilism and how it errs with its own implicit absolutism. This is described in recent work out of the West (Varela, Thompson, & Rosch, 1991): "The philosophical flight into nihilism... mirrors a psychological process: the reflex to grasp is so strong and deep seated that we reify the absence of a solid foundation into a solid absence or abyss" (p. 247). Mind, even as it rejects absolutism, is not necessarily disabused of the habit of further clinging to absolutes. Mind may cling to the absence of absolutes as itself an absolute.

Closer consideration of sunyata itself reveals the mistaken absolutism of nihilism from another angle. Sunyata means that all things – all ideas, concepts, feelings, percepts, physical objects, and selves – are "empty" of inherent existence. If all things are empty of inherent existence, then so too is the idea of emptiness itself. This has been described as *sunyatasunyata*, or the emptiness of emptiness (see Ramanan, 1966, p. 173). Emptiness itself is empty of inherent existence. Thus the idea of emptiness cannot itself serve as a refuge, to be clung to as though it itself had inherent existence, unless one misunderstands the meaning of the term. Nihilism represents such a misunderstanding. Nothing, not even emptiness, can be clung to as a reified absolute. The term serves as an invitation to let go of all traces of reification – however subtle – as may attend to any percept or concept, including the concept of emptiness itself.

There is yet another way in which the nihilistic extreme maintains the very absolutism it claims to reject. For our nihilistic rejection does not cause phenomena to disappear (see Ramanan, 1966). We continue to live in the world of demands and constraints, internal and external. Life presents a welter of phenomena that we must face. If we remain unable to fathom the relationality of these situations, we will by default remain trapped inside a naive realism that would conceptualize them as implicitly independent facts, even after we refute their absolutized existence. Imagine a person railing against God that He doesn't really exist. The denial not only fails to lay the matter to rest, it sustains it. Nihilism fails to dispose of the problem of how to respond to the very palpable events and situations it would explain away. Blind to relationality, mind remains attached to the very reifications it refutes. It is with respect to this tendency to persist in reifying that which one denies that the Prajnaparamitra Sutra says:

> If he knows the five skandhas as like an illusion,
> But makes not illusion one thing, and the skandhas another,
> ... Then that is his practice of wisdom, the highest perfection.
> (as cited in Conze, 1973, p. 10)

Skandha is the Sanskrit word for aggregates – in this case the parts that compose the person. We need not try to "disappear" the skandas as though such banishment were an appropriate response to the recognition of their illusory aspect. And if we do, we will have simply entered into another mode of clinging to them – or having their illusory appearance "adhere" to us – as though they were independently real. If we try to dispose of phenomena as *mere* illusion, rejecting not only their absolute existence but their conventional existence as well, we will maintain a reified sense of what we are discarding, without any means of relating to it outside this absolutized, non-relational viewpoint. We will continue to misperceive reality, committing a version of the very error we wish to refute. Nihilism's attempt to explain away the problem leaves us immersed in it.

Perhaps now we can catch a glimpse of what the Heart Sutra means when it says: "Form is emptiness; emptiness is form. Emptiness is not other than form; form is not other than emptiness" (in Lopez, 1988). Rather than preclude existence, emptiness – as the absence of absolute existence or inherent meaning – implies an unrestrained potentiality of things to become realized, and to gain meaning and functionality, on the basis of their infinite capacity to participate in relationship. Things exist in, and only in, this mutual interdependence.

Buddhism thus offers emptiness as the middle way between the two extremes of absolutism and nihilism. In it we find – not a nihilistic negation of experience and world – but a necessary condition for actual existence. For the only authentic existence of things is as relational events arising in dependence upon other things, and this is possible only because things are empty of independent existence.

Why is this so? First note that if things did possess independent existence, they would be independent of all other things, and thus incapable of entering into relations with other things, including the relations of cause and effect, even the relations of subject and object that allow us to perceive them. It is only because they lack independent existence that they can participate in the causal interrelations that allow them to come into being at all, or to have effects, or to be affected, or be perceived. Thus it is that the lack of inherent existence, rather than precluding existence, makes existence and meaning possible.

Consider next the nature of this actual existence. Buddhism teaches that the mode in which things may be said to exist is as *dependent arisings*. Things arise in dependence upon other things. Dependent arising and emptiness are mutually entailing facts: Because things are empty of inherent or independent existence, they are free to arise in dependence upon other things. And because they exist as dependent arisings, we can say that they are empty of independent existence. Emptiness and dependent imply each other.

Chandrakirti confirms the equivalence of emptiness and actual existence as dependent arising: Knowledgeable Ones, the meaning of emptiness, that is to say, the emptiness of inherent existence, is the meaning of dependent arising; it does not

> mean the non-existence of things, that is to say, an emptiness of capacity to perform functions. (as cited in Napper, 1989, pp. 182–83)

Likewise, dependent arising reveals the Buddhist middle way between the two extremes, as the Western scholar Jeffrey Hopkins (1987) notes: "Dependent-arising itself refutes both extremes at the same time. Things are dependent-arisings; that things are dependent refutes that they inherently exist; that they arise refutes that they are utterly non-existent" (p. 154).

As Napper (1989) points out, the mutuality of emptiness and dependent arising parallels and confirms the congruity of conventional and ultimate truth: "The compatibility of dependent-arising and emptiness is, in fact, a compatibility of the two truths, conventional truths and ultimate truths – the dependent-arisings of things such as sprouts, tables, persons and so forth being conventional truths and their emptiness of inherent existence being ultimate truths" (p. 40).

So what has any of this to do with ethics and social value? In fact, these twin compatibilities represent a sweeping conceptual condensation of an ultimately trans-conceptual understanding uniting mind and heart in unconditional compassion and ceaseless devotion to all beings. This transformation in consciousness that joins compassion with insight into emptiness entails profound change in moral understanding. Let us try to catch a glimmer of this moral view, and its difference from obstructed modes of consciousness. We may begin with the afflictive emotions and their source in our reifying ignorance.

We have seen that normal commonsense reality is trapped within the illusion of inherent existence. For such is the nature of our naive realism that all things appear to exist as independent, self-existent things. Buddhism teaches that this fundamental ignorance of authentic reality spawns the afflictions of hatred and selfish desire. Those three – hatred, desire, and ignorance – comprise the Three Poisons (Dalai Lama XIV, 1993). Each poison involves an absolutization of experience, based upon a similarly reified perception of the underlying situation.

It is worth noting that even before this desire takes shape, there is already an implicit attribution of inherent existence to the object, which is the basis for further absolutization around one's conscious desire for it (Dalai Lama XIV, 1993, p. 17). As desire takes hold, one's experience of the object may narrow to the terms of the desire. One understands it in the context of one's sense of need for it. Its meaning and valuation are frozen and absolutized within that fixed context. Persons as objects of desire may thus become objectified. Others who are seen to impede attainment may be reduced to mere obstacles. Moreover one may become possessive of the object. The "me" begets the "mine." This sense of entitlement is a breeding ground for conflict. The question also arises whether acquisition actually brings satisfaction. The incapacity of the object to fulfill one's felt demands leads to further cycles of craving, where too much is continually not enough.

Attraction, at least in its deluded form, is the flip side of aversion. Arising in relation to the other, each entails the other. In each case the prime culprit, the lynch pin of the delusional system, is the person's identification with a particular self-image, an imagined self that is implicitly taken to be one's actual self, which – by virtue of its being an image – requires steady maintenance. The image must be defended, and it must aggrandize itself, in compensation for the sense of inadequacy and insecurity that its very imposture entails.

These three poisons (hatred, deluded desire, and the ignorance underlying them), which we confront both in ourselves and in others, account for all human suffering. The next question is how to deal with these problems while still captive to the delusions that sustain them. Buddhism rejects the nihilistic response, even while debating its precise nature (see Hopkins, 1983, 1987; Napper, 1989). On the other hand, it offers an absolutist ethics, manifest in the Ten-Fold Path. Its ethics of restraint provides a foundation for developing an understanding that might eventually outgrow reliance upon any dualism, including that of its own absolutist teachings. Nagarjuna summarizes the moral standing and practical consequences of these three different orientations:

In brief the view of nihilism
Is that effects of actions do not exist.
Without merit and leading to a bad state,
It is regarded as a "wrong view."

In brief the view of existence
Is that effect of actions exist.
Meritorious and conducive to happy transmigrations
It is regarded as a "right view."

Because [inherent] existence and [conventional] non-existence are extinguished by wisdom,
There is a passage beyond meritorious and ill deeds.
This, say the excellent, is liberation from
Bad transmigrations and happy transmigrations.

A follower of non-existence goes to bad transmigrations,
And a follower of existence goes to happy transmigrations,
Through correct and true knowledge
One does not rely on dualism and becomes liberated.

(as cited in Hopkins, 1998, p. 50)

Nihilism, which would reject any valid basis for morality, denies the moral significance of actions. Absolutism asserts moral consequences, concretized around specific precepts and sanctions. Of the two extremes, nihilism is clearly the greater danger, in the moral license it would offer. Absolutism, though it wrongly imputes inherent existence, at least supports our connection to the conventional world. It thus preserves a basis for ethics and compassion, which are the foundation for further progress on the Buddhist path. And the karmic seeds sown by meritorious living may bring happiness within the cycles of birth and death. However, absolutist ethics is ultimately insufficient, compromised by its residue of absolutization. It cannot liberate us from conditioned existence. Liberation must await the perfection of wisdom that knows emptiness, which when joined with compassion, becomes Buddhahood.

Consider the reciprocal relationship between wisdom and compassion. When compassion is informed by insight into the emptiness of inherent existence, the result is Great Compassion no longer constrained by any conceptual blindness regarding self or other. As Nagarjuna says, "Without [an absolute] self, where will there be the property? Relieved from 'self' and 'property,' there will be no selfishness and no possessiveness" (as cited in Thurman, 1981, p. 16). With the reifying boundary between self and other erased, so too is any basis for cherishing self at the expense of another. Likewise, when one no longer harbors illusions of inherent existence concerning other persons or their actions or characteristics, there is no longer any basis for judgments that would withhold compassion from them. "Practice charity without regard to appearances," says the Diamond Sutra (1990, p. 20), and as one awakens to the authentic nature of reality as empty of inherent existence and thoroughly relational, this apparently becomes possible. When compassion is informed by this wisdom, it becomes unrestricted and unconditional.

On the other hand, where insight into emptiness is informed by compassion, we are less prone to reify emptiness, to impute inherent existence to the very notion that rejects all notions of the inherent existence. The reification of emptiness promotes nihilism. It activates a clinging to the distorted view, which may separate us emotionally from those we would seek to help. In contrast, a compassionate heart more readily fathoms the emptiness of emptiness. If our hearts are open to others, we are less disposed to garble our understanding of emptiness so as to employ it as a weapon or shield or excuse. This genuine insight sees through the false boundaries that otherwise condition our expression of love and care. Compassion thus appears as the implicit wisdom of the heart, naturally embodying an intuitive understanding of reality as relationship that anticipates the message of the fully illumined insight. Wisdom and compassion thus strive to fulfill themselves each in the other.

This Great Compassion stands in contrast to the dualistic morality of obstructed consciousness. We see that moral dualism is susceptible to some of the same benighted emotions as those it seeks to redress, where for example it would withhold care from those it might deem unworthy. Indeed there may be a naive moral dualism in our wrongdoing, whose narrowed perspective would attach moral justification to its excesses. As Solomon Asch notes, men "can hardly murder without invoking justice" (1952, p. 354). Ethical absolutism may also resist this mentality, and may be indispensable to our efforts at moral restraint, but it is not fully free of the blindness it opposes.

K. Venkata Ramanan (1966) contrasts this incomplete morality with Great Compassion.

> The highest kind of moral conduct, its perfection, consists in the non-clinging way, not clinging to sin or merit as absolute and unconditioned. The bodhisattva that enters deep into the truth of things, cultivating the contemplation of their *sunya*-nature, beholds with his eye of wisdom that sin and merit are not absolute and unconditioned. The excellence of moral conduct does not permit any attitude of despising the sinner nor any attitude of taking pride with regard to the merited. It is the non-clinging way imbued with the right understanding of things that gives perfection to morality. (p. 283)

Here we see that the moral categories (good and bad, right and wrong) that now sustain our sense of moral value, neither exist inherently, nor differ from each other absolutely. (If they did exist in absolute, mutually exclusive duality, they would be useless – even meaningless – to us, for we would be unable to relate to them.) Realization of the emptiness of inherent existence of these designations permits the moral sensibility that they can only imperfectly represent to shed the limits of its reifications, in a new and deepened tolerance for relationality. This awakening of consciousness, its transformation of ignorance into wisdom, is possible only because ignorance and wisdom do not inherently differ. Nor for that matter do samsara and nirvana. In this regard, enlightenment may be said to be, as Zen practitioners remind us, "nothing special." It is only when one sees through the illusion of *real* or *absolute* difference between ignorance and enlightenment, or between samsara and enlightenment, that liberation is possible. To think otherwise is eventually to chase in circles reified and thus deluded images.

In sum, we find that Buddha taught many things, in accord with people's varied capacities. This includes a foundation of absolutist, dualist ethics, which provides the needed concreteness to rescue minds that are unable to see beyond their own absolutizing distortions. Yet as persons grow in moral restraint, meditative stabilization, and insight, they need not rely so heavily upon concrete, restrictive rules to maintain and deepen their moral consciousness. And as insight into emptiness increases, there grows awareness that moral precepts themselves – like all other phenomena – lack absolute existence. One practical consequence of this is that there are times when an enlightened response would not accord with the precepts. Thus Thurman (1981) notes a discussion by the Eighth Century Saint Atisa that in exceptional situations, a bodhisattva may "kill, or steal or commit adultery, or lie, if his motivation is to benefit sentient beings, and if his causal awareness is such that he can prevent a greater amount of suffering on the part of his victim in future lives by thus depriving him of his present life..." (1981, p. 21). Of course we need to remember that such departures from the precepts assume great beings at high levels of realization. Those of us not utterly free of hatred and bad motivation would pay mightily in karmic consequences for such presumption. Despite this caveat, it is clear that Buddhist ethics and compassion cannot ultimately rest in specific rules or formal practices, any more than ultimate reality can be captured by finite concepts and discriminations. Buddhist ethics ultimately demands a fully integrated awareness of the emptiness of all phenomena, including precepts, of any absolute existence or independent truth.

And what has emptiness to do with ethics and social value? Buddhism locates hard-heartedness and malice ultimately in a false sense of reality. We imagine that things – including ourselves – exist in a way that they do not. We either absolutistically confer upon our experience a (inherent or ultimate) reality it does not have, or nihilistically reject the (conventional) reality it does have. These polar opposites of absolutism and relativism are united by a common absolutist assumption, revealed in the disposition to cling to things as though they were really real, to reify the contents of experience, even in our nihilistic repudiations of it. Thus we cling to false images as part of a defensive posture that exaggerates the nature of the boundaries between things, and between those things and the self. Those enforced boundaries between self and world dull our sensitivity to both. They ground a false sense of entitlement to withdraw care selectively from those we judge unworthy. Thus we harden our hearts to others and to ourselves.

The ultimate antidote for this blindness is a correct understanding of emptiness, which allows us to begin to see things as they are, erasing the enforced boundaries between self and other, ending the objectification of experience down to the subtlest forms of dualistic conceptualization, including ethical dualism, and opening us completely to self and other. It is here that wisdom and compassion are perfected and united in complete enlightenment – in unbounded, unconditional, spontaneous, and ongoing love.

Gestalt Psychology and Buddhism

Let us now compare Gestalt psychology and Mahayana Buddhism – specifically its Madhyamika school – first with regard to epistemology. Despite vast differences in cultural and historical context, the broad strokes of their message seem frequently to coincide. Each asserts the lack of independent reality of all phenomena, their dependence upon things beside themselves. In rejecting absolute existence, Gestalt theory asserts relational determination, while Buddhism offers dependent-arising or interdependent origination. They not only agree that existence and meaning are relational, but describe this relationality often in quite similar terms.

Both viewpoints thus reject naive realism, the spontaneous and unreflective attribution of independent existence to things across our perceptual world. Naive realism is the illusion of inherent existence run rampant. For what perception naively takes to be independent physical reality is instead phenomenal representation, dependent upon body (sense organs, nervous system) and mind. Phenomenal characteristics of percepts, which appear to be properties of things in themselves, maintained even in our absence, are instead relational facts, dependent upon an experiencing person. Consider the secondary characteristic of color. While appearing to be an independent physical property, color is instead a relational fact, arising in the interaction of light waves with our sensory-perceptual systems. Likewise the tertiary characteristics of meaning and value are relational facts, though our naive realism may blindly attribute them to objects or situations as independent, context-free properties. For while naive realism is clearly mistaken, its error is hard to fully appreciate and correct. As Köhler (1960/1971) notes, and as Mahayana Buddhism would heartily agree, "We are all naive realists most of the time" (p. 68).

Commonsense reality thus tends to ignore the dependence of our percepts on an experiencing person. Consider two particular aspects of relationality within the experiential field, concerning external interactions between things, and internal relations within them. First we see that objects of experience are not perceived independently of their context of other things. Phenomenal objects (percepts, concepts) do not exist in isolation. They represent parts of larger contexts, and their specific meaning is influenced by the role they play in completing this larger whole. Second, it appears that phenomena not only exist in contexts, but also *as* contexts. They depend upon internal relations of the parts that compose them. After all, if Gestalt psychology and Madhyamika Buddhism are correct, nothing exists as a whole and unitary thing. Such uncompounded elements have not been found to exist. Neither can we explain the existence of a thing as a summation or collection of elemental parts – as though its parts represented some ultimate reality – since parts are no more unitary than the entities they compose. Parts too are composite, and subject to further deconstruction. Thus both Gestalt psychology and Madhyamika Buddhism reject elementarism, the view that things are reducible to summations or collections of basic elements, which themselves are deemed to be independent and uncompounded, and in a sense more real.

For both Gestalt theory and Buddhism, relationality offers a middle way between the false extremes of absolutism and nihilism (cf. relativism). Absolutism (e.g., naive realism) reifies the existence of objects as though their meanings were a property of the things themselves, independent of other things. Nihilism, on the other hand, maintains its own implicit form of absolutism, by reifying the absence of any indwelling meaning, including meaning that is informed by awareness of relationality. It thus overextends its refutation of absolute existence to deny relational existence as well, succumbing to a version of the very absolutism it otherwise rejects. These extremist views share a common error: the human tendency to absolutize experience as though its contents represented independent facts. Elementarism seems to represent a blend of both absolutist and relativist errors. Its reduction of experience to discrete and self-existing units represents a nihilistic denial of the authentic relational existence of things, as well as an absolutist embrace of its notion of element as absolute and independent reality.

While this comparison is neither comprehensive nor conclusive, it certainly suggests areas of agreement in Buddhist and Gestalt epistemologies. However, we must not let general similarities blind us to important differences. To illustrate one difference, let us return the heart of the Madhyamika reasoning used to uproot the idea of inherent existence. Here we are invited to identify a seemingly inherently existing thing, such as a chariot, as the object (of negation), and to look for it – either in or as its parts, or apart from them. We discover – often jarringly – that we cannot find the object in either place. Compare this with Köhler's observation that the whole is different from the sum of its parts. Gestalt theory seems to echo the first half of Madhyamika reasoning. If in fact the thing is not the same as it parts, would Gestalt concur that the thing is not altogether different either?

The compounded nature of matter and experience has been a basic assumption of scientific thinking throughout the Twentieth Century. It was not composite nature that Gestalt theory rejected, but the atomistic reduction of phenomena to *mere* collections of aggregate parts, and to mechanistic views as to how those parts were associated in form and function. Gestalt theory pointed to "contexts in which what is happening in the whole cannot be deduced from the characteristics of the separate pieces, but conversely; what happens to a part of the whole is, in clear-cut cases, determined by the laws of the inner structure of its whole" (Wertheimer, 1924/1944, p. 84). The thing cannot be simply identified with the parts that compose it. And Madhyamika agrees: The thing is not the same as its parts.

Madhyamika next asks if the thing is altogether different from its parts. On the one hand, the inner structure to which Gestalt theory refers implies an internal differentiation of parts, and a corresponding dependence of the thing upon these parts. The structural characteristics of the whole are not separable from the coalescence of parts that give rise to it. The existence of the whole depends upon its parts, and thus seems to fulfill the second half of Madhyamika reasoning: that the thing (that is not altogether the same as its parts) is not altogether different from them either.

On the other hand, the Gestalt emphasis on structure or organization may imply a reality – albeit a relational one – that supersedes the parts that compose it. The Gestalt message focuses not so much upon the absence of inherent existence of all phenomena, even if such "emptiness" is implied, but in the presence of indwelling coherence and meaning based on internal relations of fittingness and external relations of differentiation across its "segregated wholes." There is a potential here to implicitly confer upon these segregated wholes a sense of independent existence. From the Madhyamika point of view, the Gestalt embrace of internal structure and organization may render Gestalt theory susceptible to a reification of its segregated entities of experience.

Here it is necessary to consider the historical and intellectual context of Gestalt psychology. Gestalt psychology was born as a protest against the elementaristic, mechanistic, and reductive explanations of early psychology. This traditional viewpoint – which largely persists today – may be rightly called nihilistic where it relativises away the human capacity for truth and value. Where psychology denies any genuine motivation for truth or value, and looks ultimately to forces of blind contingency (e.g., chance genetic mutation, conditioning by spatial or temporal contiguity) to explain order and apparent fittingness in experience, the result is nihilism. The course of Western intellectual history seems here to recapitulate the dialectic of extremes described in Madhyamika Buddhism, where early faith in absolute truth and categorical values, grounded in Judeo-Christian religion, came to be eclipsed by an equally absolute rejection of a valid or objective basis for truth and virtue, based upon a new set of myths given the imprimatur of science. Neither pole of the dialectic recognizes relationality as a middle way that avoids the absolutizing blindness of each. As Asch notes, both viewpoints agree that the "sole alternatives" are between themselves alone. Neither do they see that the grains of truth within each extreme become sensible only in the context of this middle way of relationality.

Enter Gestalt psychology. Recognizing both the logical inconsistency (e.g., Köhler, 1938/1966, 1944/1971) and the "relativistic defeatism" (Köhler, 1938/1966, p. 74) of scientific nihilism, it offers a vision and a program of empirical study to redress this scientific prejudice. Realizing that "science can have no more weight and sense than it itself attributes to human insight by which it is produced" (Köhler, 1938/1966, p. 38), it set about to reacquaint us with the human capacity for insight and value. It invites us to consider the essential order in nature and experience, based not on self-existing absolutes, but on the dynamics of relationality and self-organization. In uncovering a basis for objective truth and valid value, it offers an antidote to scientific nihilism, whose deconstruction of reality and experience left us adrift in a world without indwelling order, without beacons of truth and value even to strive for.

Given this historical context and moral priority, it is not surprising that Gestalt might tilt toward the side of realism or absolutism: not so much in advancing notions of absolute or uncompounded truth, but in overlooking reification of relational patterns themselves. While representing a greater level of truth than the views it sought to correct, it may not have fully confronted the implications of its own message of relationality. Instead it focused upon the need to clarify the case for valid establishment of truth and value, in an age in which these are systematically, if illogically, negated. Further deconstruction of implicit absolutism would seem impossible without first making room for the human capacity for truth that would endure it.

The situation for Gestalt psychology may not be entirely different from that of early Tibetan Buddhism, when the founder of its Gelupka School, Tsong Khapa, sought to organize disparate Buddhist teachings into a comprehensive view. He addressed the nihilism of his age (Napper, 1989, p. 37) with commentaries that stressed valid perception and valid cognition, in ways that exposed him to criticism of reification (see Dreyfus, 1997; Hopkins, 1983; also Dalai Lama XIV, 1993, p. 99). It would appear to be most difficult to do justice to the staggering dimensions of the Mahayana deconstruction of apparent reality, while likewise recognizing the human capacity for valid thought and perception, even though the task of overcoming ignorance inevitably demands, and thus implies, such intellectual and moral capacity, and its perfectibility. Gestalt theory may ultimately face the same tension of demands, whose seeming conflict nears the realm of paradox.

Thus, while the basic principles of Gestalt psychology echo Madhyamika teaching, some critical implications of its message of relationality may have been left unexplored. Perhaps as a result Gestalt theory has been hard-pressed to account for those frequent situations, mentioned earlier, in which the relational determination of meaning is not a matter of conscious insight – where it is substantially overlooked in favor of absolutist thinking. Thus while Asch acknowledges the human tendency to restrict relational thinking and to succumb to an absolutization of social knowledge, he largely passes on the question of why and how this occurs (1952, p. 442, but see p. 631). Recall also Duncker's observation of the tendency for value terms to succumb to reification as they become linked with static external behaviors. When circumstances change and those behaviors appear less fitting, the value itself – torn from its earlier context – may be disparaged. In the process, relativism gains a measure of face validity. Just why this kind of "cognitive freezing" (cf. Lewin, 1947) happens, or how it jibes with the relationality thesis, Duncker does not explain.

Buddhism may help shed light on these problems. From the Madhyamika point of view, Gestalt theory may have defined the object of negation too narrowly, and thus overlooked subtler levels of reification binding the relational structure, the gestalt itself, such it may appear to exist independently. After all, relational understanding is not an all-or-none proposition. The awareness of fitting relations that gives rise to a gestalt, which permits its perceptual or conceptual discrimination, and grants it truth-value up to a point, need not reflect the full extent of its relationality. Where further relational determination goes unrecognized – where it remains unconscious – the result may be a measure of absolutization. This absolutization of meaning and value may be needed for a time in the development of individual and social consciousness (see Neumann, 1969), but its benefits do not come without eventual costs, among them, alienation and enmity.

Thus while both Gestalt and Madhyamika accept a relational determination of value, Madhyamika further radicalizes the Gestalt message of relational understanding by extending it to subtler layers of reification that the Gestalt critique may not yet have penetrated. Consider naive realism. While Gestalt theorists have viewed it as an inevitable, albeit flawed, aspect of common thought, Madhyamika challenges us to let go of all manner of reification it entails. In raising the bar in this way, Madhyamika may help clarify the absolutizing tendencies that Gestalt theorists must acknowledge in their otherwise relational accounts.

Consider that the Gestalt rejection of absolutism and relativism in favor of relationality was based largely upon comparisons across absolutist viewpoints, that is, analysis by Duncker and Asch of contrasts in traditional cultural beliefs and values. These absolutist valuations evince relational determination in exposing the fitting relation between values and underlying meanings, and likewise between meanings and their context of beliefs and perceptions. Yet they still reflect significant absolutization, most clearly manifested in their clinging to their own specific meanings, which are reified and clung to as absolute truths. This absolutization of situated values – this attribution of absolute, context-free truth to culture-bound expressions, returns us to where we began, to the cross-cultural conflicts that emerge across those encrusted forms, where value differences may appear absolute.

This absolutization of meaning and value may involve, in Gestalt terms, insufficient insight into the contexts that govern their relational determination. Where meanings are shaped by contextual conditions that are effectively outside of awareness, the merely relational existence of those meanings is obscured, and they acquire a false sense of absoluteness. What is missing is insight into the basis of the meanings, that is, more penetrating awareness of their relational determinants, the contingencies both within and without the boundaries of the object, upon which its existence and meaning depend. If these bases were more accessible to consciousness, then the truth claims that proceed from them would be subject to critical examination, and meanings not fully attuned to their own relational basis might need to be modified, along with the valuations they support. This of course is what happens as layers of naive realism are seen through. One's understanding of the object is revised as properties previously attributed to it alone are discovered to be relational facts, dependent in part upon an experiencing person.

Thus conscious contexts may shape and support meanings, but within a constricted cultural universe that may have trouble seeing beyond itself to substantiate its own claims. This should come as no surprise. Cultural meanings are not necessarily assimilated purely on the basis of open-minded appraisal of their objective merits, or intelligent analysis of the truth-values of underlying beliefs. Nor does weak justification necessarily diminish one's emotional investment in them. There may be other demands at work besides those following from open appraisal of sensibility. We are all pressed to make sense of our world, regardless of our variable capacity to do so accurately. Born into human cultures with little initial understanding of how things work, we take much on faith. We embrace meanings partly because they are underwritten by the groups that we at least initially trust. In embracing their meanings, we avow our bond to those groups, which we seem desperate to maintain, as though failure to agree would sever a vital connection. Subsequent experience is organized in light of those received views, with the resulting interconsistency reinforcing our sense of the credibility of both. Even later reactions against these cultural meanings need not step free of their cultural determination, shaped and polarized as they are within the very cultural definitions they oppose.

It thus appears that cultural meanings may be powerfully shaped by contexts that are emotionally charged by investments in group membership and personal and social identity. Moreover, this functional aspect of contexts may be substantially unconscious, even resistant to conscious awareness. For to the extent that awareness of this further relational determination would threaten to reveal the contingency and artifice of our images of self and world and their connection, then those contents would appear to be ego-alien – offensive to the ego, which depends upon them for an identity.

The superimposition of absoluteness, at least at this gross level of reification, seems consistent with processes of depth psychology. Work by Erich Neumann (1949/1969) offers a valuable introduction to the role of unconscious processes in the attribution of meaning and value. He describes moral enculturation as a process of internalizing the values (and presumably underlying meanings) of one's group and suppressing or repressing what in oneself does not appear to fit. Repression begets projection of absolutized meanings onto others, and the incorporation of a fixed identity within the self, maintaining a rigid moral dualism.

This depth psychological viewpoint helps expose risks associated with the credulous application of absolute moral categories. In depth psychological terms, we are prone to project our own disowned darkness onto others, absolutize their moral difference from us, and elevate ourselves to a place of moral superiority to condemn those below. Thus an inflated and compensatory morality may demonize outer targets that correspond to our own hidden or disowned contents. Left to its own devices, this pattern generates endless repetition, as its dualistic moral censure perpetuates the conflicts it seeks to address. Within the world of moral absolutes, conflict is inevitable and never fully resolvable: Moral absolutization sets limits on both psychical integration and social reconciliation.

Are these hypotheses of depth psychology reconcilable with, and useful to, Gestalt theory? Elsewhere (Ragsdale, 1998) I have described how "projective contextualization" might lead to the false appearance of absoluteness and meaning constancy, while remaining in full accord with relational determination. The reification of meanings as seemingly context-free facts may involve a process of projection of fixed contexts onto their objects. Objects may become absolutized through an unconscious projection of contexts upon them. Likewise, introjection of contexts onto the self may solidify a particular self-image within the incorporated context. By this account, both fixity of meaning and our obliviousness to the process would fulfill an unconscious, ego-defensive function. As a result, the functional boundary between self and other may be transformed into a line of defense that reifies the entities it artificially divides. By this account, phenomenal self and other are, as it were, "coated" in unconsciousness. They are insulated within unconscious contexts that sustain the illusion of independent being, blinding us to the conditionality of their existence as a function of the parts that compose them, and their interdependent codetermination with that which their enforced boundaries would exclude.

Thus the self-construct may sustain an exaggerated sense of separateness and independence by means of an artificial insulation from the very causes and conditions (cf. context) that give rise to it. Were those causes and conditions to become conscious, the misapprehension of separateness would be exposed. Absent the intellectual understanding and emotional tolerance for utter relationality, the self courses in a dream-world of illusory absolutes, where enforced boundaries between self and other maintain an absolutization on both sides of the defensive border. Thus external objects that threaten this self-image are themselves imbued with equally false absoluteness by subjects that cannot yet bear this interdependent codetermination. These objects may indeed pose a threat, not perhaps to the authentic relational self, but to the precariously situated image of independent self to which we desperately cling – which may be all that we know.

Thus where relational understanding runs out, where it fails to penetrate all layers of relational determination with insight into fitting relations, perception may inevitably fall back into an absolutization within those deeper layers of meaning. Meanings would still be relationally determined, but determination would be partly unconscious, and that very unconsciousness – shared with, and connecting us to, the cultural communities with which we identify – would serve as a relational determinant for absolutization at that level of psychical processing. In this way it may be possible to extend Gestalt principles into the territory of depth psychology to suggest a means of reconciling the fact of absolutization with the likely truth of relationality. The approach may in turn offer a way of representing within Western psychological concepts some aspects of the Madhyamika view of emptiness and relationality amidst the illusion of inherent existence. As far as I can see, there is nothing in Gestalt theory to contradict such a formulation. Köhler, in his discussions of memory, argued for the role of unconscious processes in the determination of conscious experience, though he referred such causation directly to neural events rather positing an additional, inaccessible ("psychical but non-phenomenal") realm (1938/1966, pp. 183–184). Though clearly he did not have a psychodynamic unconscious in mind, I see nothing in Gestalt theory to rule out similar processes in the maintenance of personal and social identity.

If this analysis is correct, freedom from the illusion of absoluteness requires the work of psychological integration, through which one slowly outgrows reliance upon defenses to maintain a coherent self, and becomes increasingly able to bear – emotionally and intellectually – the truth of unbounded relationality. Relationality cannot be fully fathomed while the person maintains the enforced boundaries that generate the illusion of separateness in the first place.

So far our comparison has mainly addressed the epistemological problem, roughly corresponding to the first half of the Gestalt principle of relational determination – that context shapes meaning. The second half of that principle – that meaning shapes value – moves us from epistemological ground to its moral and social ramifications. Let us first recall what relational determination says, and what it does not say. Relational determination is not itself a moral claim. It neither asserts the validity of a particular ethic, nor prescribes norms of conduct. Applied to ethics, it simply offers an empirical claim that observed value differences reflect secondary differences in interpretation (based on corresponding differences in context) and not – as descriptive relativism would assert – primary differences in moral principle. Our first question is whether Buddhism concurs with this specific conclusion.

I believe that the invariant relation between meaning and value is implicit in Buddhist teaching. Its ultimate goal of enlightenment entails a transformation in the sphere of value, which is possible only through an awakening to the authentic meanings of self and world. (Consider here the Buddha's Four Noble Truths, which recognize ignorance as the cause of suffering.) These authentic meanings, freed of ignorance, consciously bear the insight of emptiness and dependent-arising. This entails – as though by definition – a full appreciation of the role of context in the relational determination of meaning, for context is the realm in which relationships arise. It moreover suggests a full conscious access to, and tolerance of, those contexts in unfolding experience. Liberation is relational determination made fully accessible to consciousness.

Assuming that Gestalt theory and Buddhism agree as to meaning-value invariance, attention may shift to the (metaethical) question of validity. Where conflicting meanings yield conflicting values, might certain meanings, with their corresponding valuations, lay claim to greater validity? And if so, upon what basis are those more valid meanings identified. While Gestalt psychologists clearly reject views of moral equivalence of meanings (cf. Wertheimer, 1935/1961), they postponed any attempt to define the precise moral axioms for assessing validity. This restraint seems well placed, since there is a risk that any such specification of decisive moral principle – any attempt to capture and concretize a universal moral sensibility in words – might commit the absolutist error of advancing itself as a context-free principle. What does Buddhism have to say here?

Here we see that Buddhism takes this need to avoid reification and – perhaps literally – turns it into a virtue. Non-reification becomes a property of "valid" meaning. Mahayana submits that the only meanings capable of doing justice to authentic reality are those that reflect *awareness* of, and tolerance for, its emptiness of inherent existence and the dependent arising of phenomena. Notice how the epistemological claim of relationality doubles back on itself to tender, in effect, a moral claim that its truth be realized. Relationality is true whether or not we realize it. Meanings not fully tolerant of it are compromised, along with ensuing valuations and behaviors. Our ultimate moral challenge is thus to awaken fully to emptiness and dependent-arising, such that resulting meanings may yield valuations and behaviors undistorted by assumptions of absoluteness that cloud awareness of the actual situation.

Buddhism thus picks up where Gestalt psychology leaves off. In awakening us to the ubiquity of relational determination in common experience, it exposes the pervasiveness of the absolutist error in everyday life, and proceeds to offer an ethical vision predicated upon conscious integration of relational understanding as the ultimate moral challenge.

Part of the difficulty in realizing emptiness and relationality concerns its intellectual demands. It takes (and perhaps makes) intelligence to see and understand relationships that are otherwise obscured by concretist thinking. However part of the problem may be more specifically emotional and interpersonal. The message of relationality challenges our entire structure of ego-defensive operations, which struggle to maintain a coherent identity by enforcing false divisions within and across selves. Psychological defenses are, after all, our admission that we can only bear so much reality. They expose the threat that relational determination poses to the fragile coherence of our still primitive consciousness and culture. It is ironic that this implicit sense of threat under which we all live, devolving from a substantial misunderstanding of the nature of self and world, is preserved by the very processes that serve to buffer that threat. As a further irony, it seems that the pain spun from this illusion must be emotionally borne for its baselessness to be fully realized.

Hopkins's (1987) description of the dawning of insight into the absence of inherent existence – which precedes the even more powerful realization of emptiness itself – speaks to the emotional difficulty of this path: "At ... times it seems as if you are carving out your own heart. You are rending the fabric of cyclic existence, and since this fabric is your own, it is difficult to bear" (p. 280).

It is reported, by the Fifth Dalai Lama and others, that this hurt – this sense of loss – is part of early realization, to eventually give way to deep consolation. For it may also be, in Hopkin's (1987) words, "just plain thrilling" to shed the burden of an identity as a would-be independent self.

This evolution of feeling and understanding seems compatible with depth psychological descriptions: If the illusion of independent existence is supported by psychological defenses, then the weakening of that illusion may involve a lowering of those absolutizing defenses, and a bearing of some of the accumulated pain those defenses had averted. Yet as one develops greater tolerance for previously unbearable contents, one's conception of the situation changes. Absolutized meanings give way to a deeper awareness of interdependent relations. This expanded perspective recognizes its higher level of truth, which has outgrown the need for previous levels of reification. In the process, some of the burden of standing guard over the illusion of an independent self is lifted. There is less and less of that shaky construction to protect from inner and outer threats. Thus the pain, perhaps grief, associated with early insight into the illusion of independent self may begin to give way to a new sense of peace and freedom, and a new openness to self and world.

One thus returns to the place one never *really* left, to our world and the sentient beings that inhabit it. In the shedding of progressive layers of reification, with their sequelae of hard-heartedness and deluded desire, compassion and lovingkindness are further released. The bodhichitta motivation to achieve enlightenment for the sake of all sentient beings crystallizes as a natural awareness of universal responsibility to others, not as a duty or chore, but as a pure and spontaneous response to the needs of beings we grow to love without exception or condition.

As we have seen, cultural context plays a critical role in this development. Societies may nurture or oppose the growth of individual minds, and perhaps all do at least a little of both. There seems to be a conservative tendency in all societies, and thus in each enculturated mind, to enforce their own cultural meanings as absolute. This requires the maintenance of a certain level of unconsciousness, with its own specific potential for stupidity and malice. Societies may also succumb to the nihilistic error, where members willfully deceive and exploit their fellows, often for money or power, and often behind a facade of social concern. These tendencies extend past criminality to the manipulation of public consciousness by the sanctioned agents of politics and/or commerce, to effect change by narrowing the mental field and discouraging open inquiry. It would be a worthy task for phenomenology to expose the cognitive and emotional meanings that support such cynical intentions, to which our culture largely acquiesces.

However, these harmful effects of cultures are balanced by other beneficial social forces. For the group identification that empowers a culture cannot last unless its members deem it well-meaning and credible on a more general scale. Cultural membership helps people sustain in their personal lives the qualities that they appreciate in their fellows. Individual effort and courage are often inspired by a sense of the greater good. Where pride in one's group is called into question, societies (and individuals?) tend to polarize to establish it in an opposing part. A measure of the quality of a culture is its ability to bear differences (cf. loyal opposition) within an overarching sense of shared identity, reflecting an equivalent capacity for relational as opposed to absolutized thinking among its members. This societal integration – whose good faith can face internal conflict without absolutism's *nihilistic* presumptions of irreconcilability – provides a basis to extend respect and cooperation outward to other groups. As our planet shrinks to more closely approximate a single social world and physical habitat, the need for this is heightened.

We are thus challenged to participate in the building of societies that best support the psychological growth of their members. Psychological growth is facilitated by relational understanding, which promotes respect for others and greater thoughtfulness in addressing value diversity. Where value differences are considered in relation to underlying meanings and contexts, a commensurability of values is suggested. Human beings may inhabit the same moral universe, within which value experience retains at least a measure of sensibility, in light of underlying meanings. This invariant relation of meaning and value provides a basis for ethical validity across its full range of expression (for our ignorance is never ever complete). Attention may then shift to the underlying meanings, whose truth-values may be examined more open-mindedly, without need to personalize differences or close one's heart to anyone.

This is a tall order for any society, whose moral absolutism, according to Erich Neumann, seeks scapegoats among its disenfranchised. Consider for example the very fashionable demonization of our prison population, or the ongoing social divisions – based on race, gender, and sexual orientation – that fuel hatred capable of murder. Of course some of our most reliable targets have been abroad, and they have at times been extraordinarily adept at justifying our worst doubts. Both Freud and Jung agreed that we do not project "into the blue," (Freud, 1922/1955, p. 226), that all projection requires a "hook" (Jung, 1960/1969, p. 53; see also Henle, 1982/1986, 1984/1986) and that hook has been well supplied by the institutionalized malevolence of some Twentieth Century regimes. Yet nowhere are we permitted the further attribution of absolute evil. For that would let us too much off the hook. As Pogo said, we have seen the enemy and he is us. And this is certainly true when we try to locate evil utterly elsewhere, or to deny it altogether, and thus preclude our own redemption. This recognition must be at the heart of any understanding of the relational determination of meaning and value. But, in closing, let us pause to appreciate what we have. Democratic cultures, which are home to most of us, offer a relatively safe haven to speak our truth, with reason to expect a relatively fair hearing. It is a mistake to take for granted this freedom, or the basis of mutual respect and trust from which it has grown. Others are not so blessed. It is a gift of previous generations, borne of a massive accumulation of individual struggle and sacrifice. This gift of democracy supports the further development of consciousness, as mind continues to discover its own indwelling freedom. Conversely, a continuing development of mind is necessary for the maintenance and further progress of free society. Societies and governments may never perfectly embody the values of freedom and equality, which must be re-earned, re-animated, and expanded by successive generations. Democracy sustains itself in its ongoing commitment to further realization, to extension of its principles to individuals and groups previously outside its social vision. To stand still is to regress. It requires an ongoing process of confronting inconsistencies and hypocrisies, and righting them (e.g., ending slavery, woman's suffrage, civil rights). These breeches represent blatant instances of absolutization, where false attribution of absolute difference (black vs. white, man vs. woman, gay vs. straight, Protestant vs. Catholic vs. Jew vs. Muslim, tall vs. short, smart vs. slow) ignites prejudice and denigration. Moral development of individuals and cultures requires that relational understanding supplant such misattributions of absoluteness. It often appears to be up to individuals and smaller groups to awaken the latent understanding and conscience of the larger culture, to confront the leaden force of cultural inertia and moral complacency with the deeper truth of undivided being.

Author's Note

This chapter is an expanded version of a paper originally presented at the 106th Annual Convention of the American Psychological Association, Aug. 15, 1998, in San Francisco, CA. I wish to thank Jeffrey Hopkins, Georges Dreyfus, and Robert Thurman for their immensely helpful comments on the sections on Buddhism. Timothy O'Brian, Ralph Ellis, Julie Barnes, Jeannie Russell, and Gabrielle Kelly have also earned my enduring appreciation for their wise counsel and unflagging support. Above all, I thank Mary Henle for awakening me to what psychology is and can be. Whatever merit this paper has is due largely to the contributions of these and other individuals. Where it falls short, responsibility is, of course, mine alone. Whatever merit that might not belong to others, I dedicate to all sentient beings.

References

Asch, S. (1952). *Social psychology*. New York: Prentice-Hall.

Brandt, R. B. (Ed.) (1961). *Value and obligation*. Harcourt, Brace, & World.

Brandt, R. B. (1967). Ethical relativism. In P. Edwards (Ed.-in-chief), *Encyclopedia of philosophy* (Vol. 3, pp. 75–78). New York: Macmillan and The Free Press.

Conze, E. (Trans.) (1973). *The perfection of wisdom in eight thousand lines & its verse summary*. Bolinas, CA: Four Seasons Foundation.

Dalai Lama XIV. (1993). *The meaning of life from a Buddhist perspective*. J. Hopkins (Ed. & Trans.), Boston: Wisdom Publications.

The Diamond Sutra & The Sutra of Hui-Neng. (1990). A. F. Price & W. Mou-lam (Trans.). Boston: Shambala.

Dreyfus, G. B. J. (1997). *Recognizing reality: Dharmakirti's philosophy and its Tibetan interpretations*. Albany, NY: State University of New York Press.

Duncker, K. (1939). Ethical relativity? (An enquiry into the psychology of ethics). *Mind, 48*, 39–57.

Ellis, R. D. (1992). Moral pluralism reconsidered: Is there an intrinsic-extrinsic value distinction? *Philosophical Papers, 21(1)*, 45–64.

Frankena, W. K. (1973). Ethics (Rev. ed.). Englewood Cliffs, NJ: Princeton-Hall.

Freud, S. (1955). Some neurotic mechanisms in jealousy, paranoia and homosexuality. In J. Strachey (Ed. and Trans.), *The standard edition of the complete psychological works of Sigmund Freud* (Vol. 18, pp. 223–232). London: Hogarth Press. (Original work published 1922.)

Henle, M. (1977). The influence of Gestalt psychology in America. *Annals of the New York Academy of Sciences, 291*, 3–12.

Henle, M. (1985). Rediscovering Gestalt psychology. In S. Koch & D. E. Leary (Eds.), *A century of psychology as a science* (pp. 100–120). Washington, DC: American Psychological Association.

Henle, M. (1986). On places, labels, and problems. In *1879 and all that* (pp. 36–45). New York: Columbia University Press. (Reprinted from *Social Research*, 1982)

Henle, M. (1986). Freud's secret cognitive theories. In *1879 and all that* (pp. 36–45). New York: Columbia University Press. (Reprinted from *Annals of Theoretical Psychology*, 1984)

Hopkins, J. (1983). *Meditation on emptiness*. London: Wisdom.

Hopkins, J. (1987). *Emptiness yoga: The Tibetan middle way*. Ithica, NY: Snow Lion Publications.

Hopkins, J. (1998). *Buddhist advice for living & liberation: Nagarjuna's precious garland*. Ithica, NY: Snow Lion Publications.

Jung, C. J. (1960/1969). On psychic energy. In R. Hull (Ed. and Trans.), *The collected works of C. G. Jung* (Vol. 8, pp. 3–66). (Original work published 1928)

Jung, C. J. (1964/1970). A psychological view of conscience. In R. Hull (Ed. and Trans.), *The collected works of C. G. Jung* (Vol. 10, pp. 437–455). (Original work published 1958)

Köhler, W. (1966). *The place of value in a world of facts*. New York: Liveright. (Original work published 1938)

Köhler, W. (1971). Value and fact. In M. Henle (Ed.), *Selected papers of Wolfgang Köhler*. New York: Liveright, 1971. (Reprinted from the *Journal of Philosophy*, 1944, *41*(8), 197–212)

Köhler, W. (1947). *Gestalt psychology*. (Rev. ed.). New York: Liveright.

Köhler, W. (1961). Psychology and evolution. In M. Henle (Ed.), *Documents of Gestalt psychology* (pp. 67–75). Berkeley and Los Angeles: University of CA press. (Reprinted from *Acta Psychologica*, 1950, 7, 288–297)

Köhler, W. (1959). Gestalt psychology today. *American Psychologist, 14*, 727–734.

Köhler, W. (1971). The mind-body problem. In M. Henle (Ed.), *Selected papers of Wolfgang Köhler*. New York: Liveright, 1971. (Reprinted from *Dimensions of Mind*, pp. 3–23, by S. Hook, Ed., 1960, New York: New York University Press)

Köhler, W. (1969). *The task of Gestalt psychology*. Princeton, NJ: Princeton University Press.

Lewin, K. (1951). *Field theory in social science*. New York: Harper.

Lopez, D. (1988). *The Heart Sutra explained: Indian and Tibetan commentaries*. Albany, NY: State University of New York Press.

Napper, E. (1989). *Dependent-arising and emptiness*. London: Wisdom.

Neumann, E. (1969). *Depth psychology and a new ethic*. New York: Putnam. (Original work published 1949)

Ragsdale, E. S. (1985). Ethical relativism in Milton Rokeach's theory of value. *Dissertation Abstracts International, 46*(06), 2123B. (University Microfilms No. AAC85–17173)

Ragsdale, E. S. (1999, August). *Wolfgang Köhler and the place of consciousness in nature*. Paper presented at the convention of the American Psychological Association, Boston, MA.

Ragsdale, E. S. (1998, August). *Beyond absolutism and relativism: Gestalt psychology, depth psychology, and values*. Paper presented at the American Psychological Association, San Francisco, CA.

Ramanan, K. V. (1966). *Nagarjuna's philosophy as presented in the Maha-Prajnamita-Sastra*. Delhi, India: Motilal Banarsidass.

Thurman, R. (1981). Emptiness that is compassion: An essay on Buddhist ethics. *Religious traditions: a journal in the study of religions*. (pp. 11–34). New South Wales, Australia: Department of Religious Studies, University of Sidney.

Thurman, R. (1984). *The central philosophy of Tibet: A study and translation of Jey Tsong Khapa's "Essence of true eloquence"*. Princeton, NJ: Princeton Univ. Press.

Varela, F. J., Thompson, E., & Rosch, E. (1991). *The embodied mind: Cognitive science and human experience*. Cambridge, MA: MIT Press.

Wertheimer, M. (1912). Experimentelle Studen über das Sehen von Bewegungen. *Zeitschrift Psychologie, 61*, 161–265. (Translation in T. Shipley (Ed.), *Classics in psychology*. New York: Philosophical Library)

Wertheimer, M. (1961). Some problems in the theory of ethics. In M. Henle (Ed.), *Documents of Gestalt psychology* (pp. 29–41). Berkeley: University of California Press. (Original work published 1935)

Wertheimer, M. (1944). Gestalt theory. N. Nairn-Allison (Trans.). *Social Research, 11*(2), pp. 81–99. (Original lecture 1924)

Part II

Healing and Psychotherapy

Alternatives in Psychotherapy

Chapter 4

Buddhism, Psychology, and Addiction Theory in Psychotherapy

G. Rita Dudley-Grant

There has been an explosion of interest in Buddhist philosophy, psychology and practices among psychologists within the past few years. Interest in Eastern religions is not new, however, Buddhist practices have been particularly well received within the more popular psychology or "self help" community. For example, movements such as EST and its' permutations, which are designed to help devotees improve psychological well being by becoming more self aware and here and now focused have deep roots in Buddhist thought. The interest has continued to expand and the commonalities are being studied from an ever-widening perspective.

It appears that a major source of the commonality stems from a shared focus and goal. The common vision is the study of the individual with the ultimate purpose of the alleviation of suffering. Both disciplines seek to delve into the depths of human functioning to explicate our realities. The psychological study of human behavior has developed a host of explanations for human suffering or "psychopathology", including theories of unconscious unmet needs or dysfunctional learning and/or environments. The practice of Buddhism also has sought to achieve absolute happiness or enlightenment to the individual and to society by a focusing on self and self-development. Buddhist tradition has contemplated and propounded various psychological theories as part of its' overall philosophical explanation of the ultimate nature of existence. Buddhist philosophies have attempted to address the issue of human suffering and it's relief. Shakyamuni, the person who first expounded Buddhism was moved to abdicate his princely life and engage in his Bodhisattva practices by his despair over the suffering of his people in India. It was his desire to relieve their suffering by coming to understand it at its most basic level which ultimately led to his enlightenment. His teachings aimed at sharing his insights and philosophies with the rest of humanity. His basic tenet was that suffering comes from attachment to transient aspects of life. It is posited that our vision is deluded and that it is this delusion, which results in our clinging to certain aspects of life, while rejecting others (Leifer, 1999).

The complexity of Buddhist doctrine is legendary. It is difficult to comprehend for many reasons. Of particular significance is that the doctrines are bounded by and a reflection of the Eastern culture where nonlinear, present reality thinking is highly valued. This is contrasted with the future focus, linear thinking of the Western culture. An excellent example of this dichotomy is provided by Fontana (1986) who pointed out that Western psychology studies human behavior, an external activity. Eastern "psychology" recognizes that the study has to start with the individual, the "self". Understanding of oneself ultimately promotes understanding of and the ability to help others.

All human sciences and theologies, secular and spiritual have promoted taking responsibility for one's own actions. However, the method by which one is taught to achieve that goal has varied significantly. Buddhism has tried to foster an awareness of the reality of life and life experience. Psychology too has studied the ways in which volition has developed and is manifested in the individual. These studies have converged or diverged based on the particular theoretical orientation. It is the intent of this chapter to foster a consideration of the commonalities between these two disciplines. It is hoped that this consideration will promote thought and continued dialogue, which ultimately will inform and enhance each of the disciplines. This chapter will further look at some of the commonalities inherent in these two great traditions, using the particular vantage points of self-control and addiction theory.

In this regard, psychological health and well-being has been a focus of study for mankind over the many centuries of our existence. Two traditions, the spiritual, and more recently the secular, have sought to analyze, guide and ultimately provide a path for optimal living. In earlier times, spiritual leaders played the central role in assisting man in his quest for the most meaningful existence. With the growth of science and technology, secular approaches, particularly those offered by practitioners in the field of psychology have gained prominence. The Judaeo-Christian ethic of reliance on an external "God" has conflicted with the more self, insight/behavioral oriented approaches of modern psychology. However, the Eastern philosophies, most prominently the Buddhist tradition has proven to be remarkable in its commonalities with the various psychological disciplines. Writers from both the psychodynamic as well as behavioral psychological approaches have written about commonalities between Buddhist psychology and their particular theoretical orientation.

To develop these concepts further, the study of psychoanalytic theory has continued to evolve since its inception. As a subset of the evolution, commonalities between Buddhism and psychoanalytic theory have been a popular area of study (Molino, 1998). The initial hypothesis of drive and instinct theory has, in more recent times given way to the focus on ego and self-psychology. The writings of Carl Jung are perhaps best known for their Buddhist influence, however, Karen Horney has also been reported to have incorporated Zen thinking, particularly considerations of the "real self", into her later writing (Morvay, 1999). More recently, Behavioral Psychology has turned to Buddhist practices and theories both for therapeutic strategies, such as meditation for anxiety disorders, as well as theories which speak to the development of optimal functioning in the individual (Csikszentmihalyi, 1990). So too, early Buddhist philosophy evolved as great teachers conveyed the principles and practices of the Buddha in new cultures.

Buddhism and Psychoanalysis

Classical Psychoanalytic thought comes from a tradition steeped in Western ideology. While Freud did consider Eastern philosophy, he did so with trepidation, as Epstein (1995) writes in his article on Buddhism and Psychoanalysis. Freud corresponded with the French poet and author, Romain Rolland, about the latter's experiences with Hindu teachers. Epstein feels that Freud's interpretation of Rolland's interactions led him to fundamental misunderstanding of the meditative practice and experience. Freud likened the experience achieved in a meditative state to the "oceanic feeling" found in early infantile experiences of helplessness and narcissism. Rather, Freud focused on the development of his instinct or drive theory which postulated that all behavior, cognitive, interpersonal, social, intellectual, and moral, to name a few, were the result of instinctual drives, primarily sexual and aggressive. As further explicated by Eagle (1984), Freud proposed that all behavior is on some level towards the service of drive gratification or the discharge of excitation. Psychological health was, in theory, to be found in the balanced gratification of these instinctual drives with all action and interaction ultimately serving that purpose. The focus was internal and individualistic, a reflection of the individualism of the Western ethos. Ray (1986) has explicated the commonality between drive theory and Buddhism as follows; "Buddhism stresses, as do dynamic psychologies, the importance of the 'fires' or passions as determining forces. Through these we remain attached to and immersed in the flood; only with their suppression can we escape" (p. 20). The flood she refers to is the "continuous and ever changing flux of events". Our lack of insight into this "stream of causality" keeps us locked into our karma and carried along in ongoing suffering due to delusions.

Further expansion of psychoanalytic theory came with the introduction by Hartmann (1958) of Ego Psychology. Hartmann's formulations suggested that there were large aspects of human behavior, thought, rationalization and other cognitive processes that were completely separate from instinct and drives. Comparatively, they developed out of the individual's biological maturation rather than any psychologically based function. In addition, Freud's drive theory did not address another instinctual behavior supported by the scientific observations of Bowlby (1969), and researched by Harlow (1958) and others for primary attachment to a mothering object. These theorists recognized attachment and interpersonal relationships as an essential aspect of human development. These scientific findings form, in part, the basis for Object Relations theory put forth by Fairburn (1952). Of course, Buddhism does not reject attachment in and of itself, but rather the craving after attachments, which ultimately result in unnecessary suffering.

Concepts of the "Self" in Buddhism and Psychoanalytic Thinking

Other challenges to Freud's strict id-ego model have also been explicated by Eagle (1984). "The core of these challenges is that certain critical issues and features of personality development and of psychopathology, having to do with object relations theory and self do not easily fit the basic id-ego model of traditional theory. [The most meaningful] descriptions of psychological development to many recent clinicians and theorists are ... accounts that focus on such dimensions as self-other differentiation, the move from symbiosis to separation-individuation, and degree of self-cohesiveness" (p. 18).

Similarly, the issue of the ego or "self" has been a central theme in Buddhism since its earliest inception. The initial conceptions, Hinayana teachings, reflected on the ego's attachment to illusion as a major source of all suffering. Nirvana was the goal to be attained, which represented the final nihilation of all "selfhood" and attachments, the causes of suffering. Later Mahayana Buddhism suggested that even Nirvana was not the ultimate goal. Rather the highest achievement was to transcend suffering in one's present condition as opposed to escaping it. The Nichiren sect of Mahayana Buddhism further explicates that rather than attempting to escape suffering, it is the challenging of one's earthly life, both positive and negative, that ultimately leads one to enlightened living (The Gosho Translation Committee, 1979).

Kohut (1971), a major leader in the development of the self-psychology model, proposed a theory based on the development of "healthy narcissism". In this psychoanalytic formulation, others are necessary as aids in development, but the ultimate goal is autonomous and independent functioning where one can be most productive and creative. This formulation is perhaps furthest away from

Nichiren Buddhist doctrine, which posits a healthy self who is both self sufficient and interdependent, completely integrated with others and the universe.

In Buddhism then, there has been a shift from the original conception of nonself. Ho (1995) while acknowledging that Buddhism has evolved into many sects described this original concept as follows, "at the heart of Buddhism is the metaphysical position that denies the ontological reality of the self. Therefore to speak of the self in Buddhism is a contradiction in itself" (p. 121). This conception reflects the previously mentioned Hinayana teachings, which posit mainly that one could escape suffering only by relinquishing all desires for attachments to transient phenomena. Transient phenomena were essentially characterized as all worldly phenomenon, even one's body and mind, fundamentally, one's "self" (Nichiren Shoshu International Center, 1984). However, Mahayana Buddhism based itself on the later teachings of Shakyamuni, in particular the Lotus Sutra, which he taught in the last eight years of his life. The Lotus Sutra reveals that the universe and the individual self are one and the same; that is, that our life is itself the macrocosm. Thus, the goal is an enlarged view of oneself, which exceeds the bounds of individualism and selfhood, a "universal self" that connects with all others. Nichiren Daishonin was a Japanese Buddhist Priest who founded the Nichiren Sect of Buddhism in 1272. Daisaku Ikeda, head of the lay organization of the Nichiren School, known as the Soka Gakkai International, explained, "Buddhism teaches that people's lives and society are inseparable. From this standpoint, the distortions in the age and in society reflect distortions in the people's lives" (Ikeda, Saito, Endo, & Suda, 1998, p. 20). Rather than the previously articulated goal of relinquishing all desires, the sixteenth chapter of the Lotus Sutra explains that "... to cast off all attachments ultimately results in the negation of life itself, for we survive through our various attachments and desires" (Nichiren Shoshu International Center, 1984, p. 49).

Object Relations theory seems to support this world view to a certain extent. Mahler (1968), Winnicott (1965), and others have expounded the introjection of the object as the necessary step for healthy development of separation and individuation. Disturbances in attachment and internalized "bad objects" are seen as leading to pathologies in psychological functioning as diverse as conduct disorder and borderline psychopathology. Thus while still focusing ultimately on the development of an integrated sense of self, Object Relations theory confirms the importance of relationships as an essential part of a functional self. It must be acknowledged however that the ultimate goal of Object Relations' theoretical formulation is the healthy and independent functioning of the self. The interconnectedness of all life has not been integrated into the theory. The self is seen as separate from the other, unlike the Buddhist teachings, which sees no separation between the two. Buddhist doctrine seeks to explain the interconnectedness of all things. One of the central tenants in Buddhism is "three thousand realms in a single life moment". The teaching, known as "*ichinen sanzen*", was developed by T'ien T'ai, who is revered as one of the greatest Buddhist scholars of all time. T'ien T'ai, who was also known as Chi-i, lived between 538 and 597 BC in Mainland China. He founded the T'ien-T'ai sect of Buddhism, which expounded the doctrine of *ichinen sanzen*. This theory explains in detail how each moment of life contains the entire universe in it. *Ichinen* indicates the life essence, and *sanzen* the phenomenon it manifests (The Gosho Translation Committee, 1979). Thus the healthy, independent "self" of object relations' theory is but a delusion or a partial reality from a Buddhist perspective.

Behaviorism and Buddhism

Behavioral Theory has also found itself in concert with Buddhist philosophy, and Buddhist practices. It is found that in both disciplines there is a fundamental belief that behavior change is possible (de Silva, 1986). Moreover, both Buddhism and behavioral psychology set out specific methods by which one's outward as well as inward behavior can be modified. One particularly interesting example was provided from the Dhammapada Commentary, which described the Buddha's recommended "treatment" for a King who had an eating problem, and who sought help from the Buddha due to his "slothful" and "drowsy" state after each meal. The Buddha set out a specific behavior modification plan, which included gradual reduction in food quantities, along with queuing, the systematic use of rewards, modeling and self-monitoring. Many other techniques now labeled as behavioral, but existing within Buddhist practice for centuries have also begun to gain acceptance in behavioral psychology. De Silva identifies at least eleven such techniques. In addition to the ones mentioned above, they include reciprocal inhibition, general behavior modification of dysfunctional behaviors, stimulus control, social skills training and cognitive skills such as thought stopping, thought switching, distraction and over-exposure.

Although Buddhism has developed and gone through many permutations in its spiritual theoretical understanding, the use of a "path" or particular techniques to achieve enlightenment or optimal living has been a mainstay of the teaching. Claxton (1986) has made a distinction between what he terms the "spiritual traditions" and religious practices, the former being in a sense prescriptions for living. Other techniques, such as the focusing taught in the Zen meditative tradition has found much success particularly in the cases of psychosomatic illnesses. Being able to tune into the body, recognize the feelings and set them apart from the sense of self has been found to be extremely helpful in addressing many psychosomatic illnesses (Ikemi & Ikemi, 1986). Thus, behavioral psychology and medicine continues to incorporate Buddhist technique and experience in the search for optimal functioning.

Self-Control

An essential element of the prescription for healthy functioning that is sought by both Buddhists and Psychologists is the ability to manage one's impulses and exert self-control over one's behavior, mental as well as physical. For classical Freudian thought, this control meant replacement of id instinctual impulses with mature ego modulated actions. From a developmental perspective, those id impulses were perceived as "ego dystonic", as opposed to the "ego syntonic" socially appropriate behavior exhibited in adulthood. Following this theoretical formulation, the goal of psychoanalysis is to have the ego gain control of these instinctual behaviors "... even to the point of renunciation, over certain instinctual impulses implicated in intra psychic conflict" (Eagle, 1984, p. 203). Using the later conceptualizations however, Eagle posits that a more functional goal is to enlarge the ego to incorporate these instinctual impulses, modifying them as motivators for positive growth.

For centuries Buddhist meditative and disciplinary practices proposed ever more vigorous eschewing of the everyday world, and turning towards reflection and considered action in all things as a means of improving one's life. In a sense, there has been a rejection of the base impulses and a turn towards solely higher paths. However, as Eagle has suggested for analytical thinking, so the Nichiren Shoshu School has suggested a more incorporative approach. In a concept called *hendaku iyaku*, or turning poison into medicine, one takes negative experiences and aspects of oneself, and uses them for personal growth and development. Thus Nichiren Daishonin points out that the Rokuharamitsu Sutra states that one should become the master of his mind rather than let his mind master him (the Gosho Translation Committee, 1979, p. 146). Moreover, in a related concept of *esho funi*, it is believed that we are one with the universe, thus as Dockett (1993) indicates, "Through controlling what is inside of us, we control what is outside as well." The issue of self-control is one that can be particularly well analyzed and theoretical constructs considered through the experience of addiction.

Addiction

Drug addiction has grown over the past several decades into one of the leading mental health problems around the world. The impact of illicit drug abuse and dependence can be seen to have changed society and contributed to increases in violence, the breakdown of the family structure, and a deepening change in the morals and values of individuals and societies. In cultures from Asia to America, and South America to Northern Europe, the impact has been both pervasive and devastating. Traditionally interventions have generated from within the substance abuse community, primarily with recovering addicts serving as addiction counselors.

More recently, psychologists and other mental health professionals have recognized the need to research, develop and implement paradigms of treatment which can draw upon the information from addiction research, as well as the newest approaches to intervention from psychodynamic and behavioral models. Genetics is also acknowledged as playing a role. The two major western psychological theories of addiction, psychodynamic and cognitive behavioral, currently provide the foundation for much of addiction research. A particular aspect of intervention with addiction is its relationship to spirituality, a long-standing aspect of recovery, which is more recently gaining attention from the research community (Carroll, 1993).

Buddhism also has addressed issues of addiction, from spiritual and theoretical perspectives. Buddhist doctrines, Eastern in origin, but having growing impact on Eastern culture and psychological thought, addresses craving and attachment, indicating that an appreciation of the impermanence of all things can inform our understanding of the causation and mechanics of addictions. Buddhist theories of the twelve-fold chain of interdependent origination have been used as a model for understanding addiction. More recently, the concept of the presence of the Ten Worlds has been considered in relationship to addictions. In this doctrine, the world of hunger or insatiable desire is one of the four lower worlds leading to the destruction of the human spirit.

Psychology, Buddhism and addiction are considered from two perspectives in this chapter. One is the theoretical understanding of the psychology of addiction from a Buddhist perspective. The other more subtle issue is the role of spirituality in recovery, and how the practice of Buddhism interacts with traditional understanding of that process. The theory of addiction within Buddhism is presented in the context of the discussion of the role of spirituality in recovery. Commonalties and contrasts between these two great Eastern and Western traditions can inform and enhance practitioners and researchers alike. It can move us beyond narrow, culture bound frameworks for understanding and intervention into a more inclusive theory which can address this world wide plague which has overshadowed the development of our global community and threatens to consume the forward development of all mankind.

Spirituality and addiction have been linked for many years, as exemplified through the growth and acknowledged success of Alcoholics Anonymous and other twelve step programs (McCrady & Miller, 1993; Spalding & Metz, 1997). Interest in the role of spirituality in recovery has continued to grow and has burgeoned to the point of national attention within the research community. For example, the National Institute on Alcohol Abuse and Alcoholism [NIAA] (Feb 18, 2000) in conjunction with the Fetzer Institute, a nonprofit foundation, released a Request for Funding to research the role of religiousness and spirituality in the prevention, treatment and recovery from alcoholism and alcohol-related diseases. While there has been a concerted attempt to distinguish religion from spirituality (Green, Fullilove, & Fullilove, 1998), spirituality has most frequently focused on belief in an external being or process, "power greater than ourselves to restore us to sanity" (Alcoholics Anonymous [AA], 1976, p. 59), following a Judaeo-Christian theology.

Conversely, as previously stated, the practice of Buddhism has sought to achieve absolute happiness or enlightenment to the individual and to society by a focusing on self and other. The meditative practices such as promoted within Zen and Tibetan Buddhism, can be seen as seeking to enable one both to concentrate and to use insight to achieve a deeper level of understanding and awareness (Epstein, 1986; Ross, 1991) as a means of achieving enlightenment. From a Tibetan Buddhist perspective, it is the obsession with attachments to all possessions or objects, both internal and external, which is the ultimate source of suffering. "The need to possess automatically creates anger and aversion resulting in defensiveness towards anyone or anything that threatens what one possesses" (Ross, 1991, p. 421). The path to enlightenment then can be seen as increasing freedom from possession. He proposes that enlightenment can and should be researched. The areas that could be studied for example are the Tibetan Buddhist definition of enlightenment. There are five basic hypotheses. 1. There exists a state of enlightenment. 2. Enlightenment is attainable by a person. 3. There is a method for attaining enlightenment. 4. There are discrete ordered stages leading to enlightenment. 5. Enlightenment is both a cognitive and an affective state.

Nichiren Buddhism charges each person with taking ultimate responsibility for one's life and following a path of faith, practice and study, which allows the individual to move ever forward on the path towards enlightenment or absolute happiness. Rather than ridding oneself of attachments, one uses these desires as motivation to continue the discipline of Nichiren practice. The act of chanting for a specific desire at first appears to be superficially seeking the gratification of a wish or need. However, with continued practice, one's wisdom, courage and confidence are heightened. Changes occur in the depths of one's karma bringing the individual ever closer to enlightenment. The concept of earthly desires equal enlightenment is explained by Nichiren Daishonin in his Gosho or teachings and is embodied in his writings to his followers (The Gosho Translation Committee, 1979).

These two examples from differing Buddhist sects, demonstrate how Buddhism focuses inward on the individual, rather than outward towards an external force or being to address suffering in one's life. From this perspective, it can be difficult to resolve Buddhist spirituality with the traditional understanding of the role of spirituality in addiction and recovery.

Psychological Theories of Addiction

One can look at the most generally accepted conceptual frameworks of addiction to resolve this dilemma. The major ones have included a biological orientation, or disease theory; a systems theory, which looks at the role of family and the environment in the development and maintenance of addiction; a psychodynamic approach; and a cognitive behavioral formulation. Each of these approaches has generated a specific set of interventions founded on that particular theoretical formulation.

The disease theory posits that alcoholism and drug addiction is a disease stemming from a biological substrate, which can be structural, chemical, neuropsychological, physiological, electrophysiological or genetic. While the actual physical marker has not yet been identified, studies have strongly suggested biological links, which may contribute to the development of alcoholism and other drug addiction in individuals such as found in family, twin and adoption research (Goodwin, 1979). For example, Dinwiddie and his associates (Dinwiddie & Cloninger, 1991; Dinwiddie & Reich, 1991) have reviewed the epidemiological literature and found that there is a significant interaction between genetics and the environment. This interaction often leads to the increased incidence of alcoholism in the children of alcoholics.

Systems theories have probably been the most heavily researched, particularly from the perspective of Adult Children of Alcoholics. Risk factor studies clearly show the higher prevalence of alcoholism and drug addiction in persons who have substance abuse in their family backgrounds. Moreover, addiction is highly associated with dysfunctional interactions in families including all types of abuses, physical, sexual, domestic violence and child abuse and neglect. The role of the environment in promoting and maintaining substance abusing behavior is also recognized. Hence, survey data indicates that while substance abuse appears to be abating among young adults, it remains entrenched among selected populations, particularly those in the inner city (Craig, 1993).

Behavioral approaches to the understanding of drug addiction tend to look at the strong reinforcers inherent in the substance itself, which serve to maintain the behavior despite its devastating impact. The cognitive behavioral model of addiction theory draws upon early learning and environmental experiences that negatively influences the individual. These early abuses and neglects result in excessively disparaging self-statements contributing to poor self-image, impulsive behavior including immediate gratification, and dependent helplessness. The consequence is the repetitive self-destructiveness of addictive behavior, despite knowledge of negative outcomes (McCrady, 1994).

From a psychodynamic perspective, addiction has been seen as resulting from a psychological process where the individual is trapped in infantile, narcissistic repetition compulsion. Immediate gratification is the sole method of functioning. Psychodynamic theories (Blatt, McDonald, Sugarman, & Wilber, 1984) look at unconscious processes, which result in and manifest the addiction. Theoretical constructs such as subconscious motivations and fixations can lead to psychic dysfunctions. The ensuring disorders such as repetition compulsions, affect dysregulation, ego pathology and low self-esteem are seen as psychological substrates to the development of addictive behavior. From a psychoanalytic standpoint, the addict can be considered to be one who is trapped in infantile, narcissistic repetition compulsion where immediate gratification of impulses is the sole method of functioning. These individuals are incapable of exerting delay of gratification, or any control over these impulses. Caught in the oral phase of development, the earliest and least mature, they live only for themselves and the fulfillment of their immediate narcissistic desires. Driving oral incorporative impulses leave them returning consistently to the dysfunctional behavior to satiate the craving which can never be met (Dudley-Grant, 1998). Psychoanalytic approaches have been taken to treat addiction (Yalisone, 1989). It has been suggested that the psychodynamic theories provide an area of commonality with Buddhist thought. Metzner (1997) compares psychoanalytical analysis of the levels of consciousness with Buddhist doctrines, which study the varying levels of consciousness. Both Buddhism and psychoanalysis seek to understand life and improve experience by a deepening awareness of subconscious and unconscious processes.

While there is merit in all of these theories, the argument has been raised that they are insufficient to understand or address the ever present and growing devastation of addiction in our society. In a study looking at medical students and patient attitudes toward religion and spirituality in the recovery process, Goldfarb, Galanter, McDowell, Lifshutz, and Dermatis (1996) report that there is an increasing appreciation for the role of spirituality in the recovery process. They exemplify this assertion by noting in their article that "the Joint Commission on Accreditation of Healthcare Organizations (JCAHO), which in its 1994 Accreditation Manual for Hospitals mandated that the assessment of patients receiving treatment of alcoholism or drug addiction specifically include 'the spiritual orientation of the patient' ... The patient's spiritual orientation may affect the success of this approach" (p. 549). Royce (1995) has suggested that it is a spiritual bankruptcy, which lies at the root of the unmitigated growth in drug abuse in our communities. Again, this premise is a major component of the most successful of the self help interventions, the twelve step anonymous programs, which have met with unprecedented success in treating alcoholism and other addictions (Khantzian & Mack, 1994; Warfield & Goldstein, 1996). It is suggested that a moral and spiritual devastation exists in the individual, which must be addressed through the twelve steps if recovery is to occur. In the twelve step philosophy, singular attention is paid to the insurance that no particular religious belief is promoted. However the message is clearly that a "power greater than ourselves", be it God in the traditional sense, a higher power of one's own choosing, even the power of the group is the only means by which recovery can begin to occur. Theoretically speaking, it is clear that whatever the chosen formulation of the illness, a spiritual intervention is usually perceived as coming from outside of the individual. In order to understand the role that Buddhism can play in addiction theory and recovery, it is necessary to understand the Buddhist formulation of substance abuse and addiction as part of the larger problem of craving (Metzner, 1996).

Buddhist Theories of Addiction

From a Buddhist perspective, inherent in human nature is desire, and it is fixation on this desire, which forms the psychical basis for addictions. Specifically, as previously noted, Ralph Metzner (1996) has shown the Buddhist concepts of the six worlds of consciousness and reality and the twelve fold chain of interdependent origination can serve as a model for understanding the addictive process. "… [I]n an addictive process, the individual does not cycle through the whole process moving through desire and craving to birth and becoming. Rather the addict gets fixated and continually repeats the behavior that satisfies the craving, looping back around the cycle again and again instead of going on to the next event, which might bring new and different sources of satisfaction" (p. 165). The concept of dependent origination is central to an understanding of Buddhist doctrine. It speaks to the interdependence of all things positing that nothing can exist outside of its relationship with another. All phenomena exist or occur solely through their relationship with other beings and phenomenon. In the twelve-fold chain, all phenomena, from birth and death to *upadana* or appetitive behavior and sensation seeking, arise because of their relationship to each other. This movement through the twelve steps of the chain represents the human experience. In healthy functioning one moves from the less developed events, such as *avidya*, or ignorance, blindness or unconsciousness, to the more creative conception and birth. The point of fixation for the addict then is the re-experiencing of the satiation of craving. Rather than the mind being able to regenerate new interpretations and representations, hence developing new experiences of birth and becoming, the addict cycles back through the same experience, stultifying growth, perception and meaning.

In order to understand self-control and the addictive process within Nichiren's Buddhism, one must understand the formulation of the Ten Worlds, (Soka Gakkai, 1998). The previously mentioned doctrine of *ichinen sanzen* or three thousand realms within a single life moment contains the concept of the Ten Worlds. These worlds are conditions or states of life which all persons cycle through on a continuous basis. The ten worlds are comprised of the six lower worlds including hell, hunger, animality, anger, tranquility and rapture. From the Nichiren Buddhist perspective, the addict is caught in the four lower worlds of Hell, Hunger, Animality, and Anger. Hell is a state of ultimate negativity and destructiveness often characterized by deep depression and feelings of helplessness, hopelessness and worthlessness. The individual is unempowered, but rather feels trapped in his life, with frequent desires to destroy him or her and everything around them. The state of Hunger is most closely allied with traditional perceptions of addiction in that it represents insatiable greed, whether it is for socially acceptable desires such as fame or fortune, or the more destructive ones of alcohol and other drugs. Any addiction can fall into this classification including work-a-holics, hunger for power and/or prestige, or even unhealthy, co-dependent relationships. While desire is a part of the human condition, in the state of Hunger one is at the mercy of one's cravings and cannot control them. This state does indeed correspond with the first of the twelve steps where the addict admits; "I am powerless over alcohol (narcotics, food, relationships etc.) and my life has become unmanageable" (AA, 1976, p. 59).

The world of Animality is the state where an individual is ruled by instinct. Morality nor reason have any impact on his or her actions, nor is there any ability to delay gratification. In this state, one takes advantage of the weak while abjecting oneself to the strong. Animality refers not to pure animal functioning but could correspond to pure id functioning; instinctual satisfaction with no modulation. Ikeda, in explicating Nichiren Buddhism describes the world of anger as not merely aggressive destructiveness but as characterized by a mind of perversity, one that is fawning and crooked, as well as one that arrogantly looks down on others seeking only its own aggrandizement (Soka Gakkai, 1998). In the world or state of anger, a person's ego is selfish, greedy and suspicious of others. They only value themselves while others are held in contempt. Their superiority is a dearly held belief requiring frequent reinforcement while the inferiority of all others must be constantly reasserted.

Along with the worlds of tranquility and rapture, the six lower worlds are considered to correspond to the six worlds of consciousness and reality. The world of tranquility is achieved when one is in a state of equanimity with oneself. Also referred to as the world of humanity, in this state the individual enjoys life and seeks harmony in all things. However, it is unstable as it is unable to manage the transience of all phenomena. Thus, the tranquility that is achieved is transitory, affected by suffering from without and within. Much has been written about the world of rapture or the Devil of the Sixth Heaven wherefrom we are manipulated by the attainment of any desire. This image has been defined as "the most powerful of the devils, which dwells in the highest of the six realms of the world of desire. He works to prevent believers from practicing Buddhism and delights in sapping the life force of others" (The Gosho Translation Committee, 1979, p. 309). This prevention of practice is brought about by the state of rapture, which this devil induces. The concept is designed to explicate the seductive but transient nature of heaven as conceptualized in the Ten Worlds doctrine. The rapture that one experiences in this world is the fleeting and illusive, but ever sought after satiation of a desire or consummation of a peak experience. In the six lower worlds, the individual is controlled and manipulated by the environment and events occurring at any given moment. A major aspect of self-control then is learning how to temper one's response to alleviate the suffering attached to these lower worlds.

The four higher worlds or four noble paths are Learning, Realization, Bodhisattva and Buddhahood. On these paths, the human condition is elevated beyond common experience, informing and refining consciousness and awareness of self and other. In the world of learning one studies and attempts to elevate one's life condition through the acquisition of knowledge. The discipline of study has been an important ingredient in the movement towards an enlightened life. The world of realization also speaks to the processes of insight found through chanting or meditation, which open's inner wisdom and clarifies perceptions helping to attain the paths of seeing and knowing. The Bodhisattva is one who has come to realize that our deep interconnectedness to all things requires a life that is devoted to caring for others. Attainment of Buddhahood is possible in this lifetime as the awareness of the ultimate reality and how to live happily within it, with unshakeable conviction and equanimity. Thus, Nichiren Buddhism does not propagate Nirvana, nor describe enlightenment as the absence of suffering. One does not seek to escape life's realities, but rather understands that Buddhahood, or unshakeable happiness is to be experienced and lived in daily life.

From a Buddhist perspective, the addict, however, is caught in the lower worlds of hunger, animality and anger, continuously cycling through them unable to move beyond. Nichiren taught that one could become enlightened in one's current state. The process of practice enables individual change through the development of insight and wisdom, or what Daisaku Ikeda calls a "human revolution". He goes on in the forward of his book of the same name to explicate "A great revolution of character in an individual will help achieve a change in the destiny of a nation and further, will cause a change in the destiny of humankind" (as cited in Soka Gakkai, 1998, p. 46).

Commonalities with Buddhist and Psychological Addiction Theories

These Buddhist conceptualizations of addiction are consistent with psychodynamic, cognitive and transpersonal theories. From a dynamic perspective, Buddhists conceive of the addict as being caught in a self-perpetuating negative process, which can feed upon itself to the point of extinction. As in psychological theories, these individuals are seen as functioning in lower, underdeveloped or infantile manners with inhibited growth and completely selfish or narcissistic orientation, the antithesis of Buddhist functioning. As one engages in Buddhist practice our delusions and attachments to the lower world are purified, our insight is enhanced, and we are able to function with more wisdom leading to less dysfunctional actions. In psychoanalytic theory, recovery is achieved through the catharsis that results from insight and the release from early life fixations. The addict in insight-oriented psychotherapy is able to identify the underlying causes of their addiction such as frustrated oral incorporative strivings. In each instance, Buddhist practice and dynamic therapy, insight leads to understanding and more functional behavior.

Similarly, from a cognitive behavioral perspective, a commonality with Buddhist theories is found in the attempt to explicate the cognitive dysfunctional reinforcers that the individual must address in order to overcome the addictive process. Cognitive Behaviorists suggest that the dysfunction of one's thoughts can lead to emotional dysfunction such as found in addiction. Nichiren Daishonin also speaks to the importance of one's mind. "While deluded, one is called a common mortal, but once enlightened, he is called a Buddha... A mind which presently is clouded by illusions originating from the innate darkness of life is like a tarnished mirror, but once it is polished it will become clear, reflecting the enlightenment of immutable truth" (the Gosho Translation Committee, 1979, pp. 4, 5). Thus, one's cognitions are key factors in healthy and enlightened functioning. In each instance, the practice of therapy and the practice of Buddhism purify one's thinking and modify behavior to enable evolution and growth thereby enhancing the quality of life.

Ross (1991) writes about a Tibetan Buddhist framework for psychology, enlightening the concept of possession from Buddhist and psychological perspectives. He indicates that in transpersonal psychology and Buddhism, identification with and attachment to both external and internal objects is considered a major source of suffering. He makes the analogy between possessing and addictive craving, indicating that in Tibetan Buddhism as in psychotherapy, the pathway to mental health is a process of cutting through materialism in all its variations to uncover a clear, egoless "awakened state of mind". He further distinguishes the state of being free from possessions as not an eschewing of material objects, love or relationships, but rather a neurotic preoccupation that motivates us to chase them, believing that in their possession we will find lasting happiness (p. 421). Thus, the path to mental health and an awakened state of mind can be seen as quite parallel if not synonymous.

Spirituality and Recovery

In order to recover one must achieve a higher life condition; break the cycling back through craving and satiation, and move oneself from control by the destructive impulsivity of the four lower worlds. Traditional spiritual aspects of recovery suggest that one must "surrender" to one's powerlessness over the addiction in order to break the cycle of the false sense of omnipotence, which is a cornerstone in maintaining it. On a superficial level then, it would appear that the Buddhist focus on the self would strengthen the narcissistic omnipotent core, thereby prohibiting rather than promoting recovery. Indeed, in a research project looking at the impact of religion and spiritual practices in preventing use and relapse, Green, M. T. Fullilove and R. E. Fullilove (1998) state "The most important element was that the something [or higher power that one believes in] be greater and more powerful than self" (p. 328). Those in recovery rejected a newcomer who did not believe that he was powerless over his addiction, "I believe in cause and effect, action, ... You are responsible for what you do. What is great is in me .... In their view, his intolerance toward spiritual principles was blocking his success in recovery" (p. 329). And yet his statements were accurate reflections of Buddhist philosophy and what one is ultimately trying to achieve, that is the taking of full responsibility for one's own actions.

Both the Zen and the Nichiren approaches to personal growth attempt to foster a belief in oneself and in the oneness of all things. A Buddhist who encounters the philosophy of surrendering to an external, higher power can be alienated from the process of the twelve step programs. The program can be seen as a direct contradiction to the paradigm of the acceptance of self in the present moment as being whole and complete, with the conceptualization of an internal higher power. Nevertheless, as in the example above, there are those who reject a theistic approach to recovery, yet can benefit from the twelve steps. There are Buddhists who do use their practice within the twelve step program, to recover from their addiction and/or emotional illness. As Buddhist doctrines deal with craving and attachment, the Buddhist emphasis on impermanence is pertinent to the causation and mechanics of addiction, (Groves & Farmer, 1994). In the context of the four noble truths, and the ten worlds, Buddhists can practice the twelve steps to assist in the recovery process.

In order to resolve the seeming paradox of a theistic external higher power, vs. the Buddhist empowerment through internal control inherent in the doctrine of the creation of karma based on cause and effect, one must re-assess what is meant by surrender, and taking responsibility. In fact, one can interpret the act of surrendering as the first step in taking responsibility for one's own actions.

Denial is the major defense system for the addict. All aspects of the disease and its impact on one's life are minimized as much and as long as possible. The addict believes that they can "control" their addiction, often holding on to this belief until they have lost virtually everything of value in their life. Surrendering to the fact that one is unable to manage their substance use is an extremely courageous and liberating step. The Buddhist who suffers from addiction must also acknowledge that the disease has overcome their clarity, self-discipline and wisdom. Buddhist practices can then be used to promote recovery in the same way that a Judaeo/Christian addict would seek "... through prayer and meditation to improve our conscious contact with God *as we understood him*" (AA, 1976, p. 59).

Meditation or chanting seeks to enlighten our current deluded state, opening our wisdom to a greater clarity and depth than we currently are capable of accessing. By harmonizing one's life with the rhythm of the universe one is embarking on a path of purifying one's life and seeking a more positive way of living (The Gosho Translation Committee, 1979). Whether an individual sees himself or herself as guided from without, or guided from within, it is acknowledged that one must seek more strength, hope and wisdom than is currently available in order to make the changes in one's life. As Epstein (1986) reports, Buddhist literature, specifically Abhidhamma in the Theravada school is replete with highly systematized texts of psychological thought that explain everyday mental states as well as how those mental states can be re-configured through the application of meditative techniques. Abhidhamma details the effects of sustained meditative practice, the lower concentration practices and the higher insight practices. These practices serve to improve one's sense of well-being, while gaining the ability to truly maintain one's understanding of the transient nature of all things. Thus, Buddhist practices can work as the addict follows other precepts of the program, in particular the twelve steps, to achieve long-term recovery.

In Nichiren Buddhism, the practice of gongyo and daimoku, recitation of parts of the fifteenth and sixteenth chapters of the lotus sutra and repetitive chanting of the title in a sonorous and rhythmical manner serves to heighten wisdom, develop courage and promote fortune in one's life (Soka Gakkai, 1998). Over time, these qualities can serve to lift the depression that is often associated with addiction, while at the same time motivating the person to make positive changes in their life.

Epstein (1986) reports that transpersonal theorists often suggest that the meditative practice of Buddhism may be too strenuous or psychologically debilitating for those with less than a fully developed sense of self. Conversely, he has argued that this position has not adequately considered how meditation can play a role in transforming narcissistic, infantile psychopathology. Bankart (Chapter 2 in this volume) reviews many of the studies on the effectiveness of meditation and concludes that while there may be "real and substantial psychophysiological and psychological benefits to be derived from a regular practice of meditation. These benefits, however, are not really of a different magnitude than those benefits that can be shown from a wide variety of similarly aimed interventions, including distraction" (p. 60). Similar concerns have been raised about the impact of chanting, invoking of the mandala in Nichiren Buddhism as a possible exacerbation of psychopathology in a fragile or immature ego structure. However, both practices have yielded positive results both in recovery from addiction and in psychological growth. Epstein (1995) reports that the strengthening of the ego ideal by the concentration practices leads to a sense of cohesion, and stability which can relieve narcissistic anxieties of emptiness and isolation, feelings also common in addiction. While chanting, the substance abuser can gain insight into the destructive nature of the addictive behavior and the courage to break free of those self-defeating actions.

A common but hidden aspect of all of these programs, the twelve step programs, the practice of Buddhism and the development of spirituality in the Judaeo-Christian traditions, is their emphasis on community. Each of these disciplines requires participation in a group, a community of fellow believers, practitioners or members with whom one shares the common bond and gains essential support. In fact, in each tradition, the focus is on helping others as well as oneself. In the Buddhist tradition, once the nature of reality and our interdependence in it is understood, we come to realize that we cannot benefit ourselves unless we focus on benefiting others. The twelfth step requires members to "carry this message to other alcoholics [addicts, etc.], and practice these principles in all our affairs" (AA, 1976, p. 59). Just so, the Judaeo-Christian tradition requires practitioners to "Love thy neighbor as thyself". It is clear that a focus on helping others is a very healing activity. It appears to relieve the narcissistic self-interest inherent in addiction. It fosters empathy and responsibility. A focus on others can be very empowering to the individual, healing their self-esteem and providing actions that are more altruistic. It appears to expand and improve one's life condition, harmonizing with the fundamental reality of oneness. This focus on caring for others as well as oneself, and group participation and membership are important aspects of research into understanding how spirituality can be so effective in helping addicts achieve long term recovery. It is essential that such research focus on the impact of commitment to others in the recovery process.

Summary

Buddhism and Psychology are great disciplines, which have concerned themselves with the highest development of human potential and the alleviation of suffering. This chapter has attempted to look at some of the contrasts and commonalities from the perspective of the issues of self-control and addiction. Drug and alcohol addiction continues to ravage our communities, particularly those that are most vulnerable. Research tries to identify effective interventions that can stem the tide of this scourge on our communities. Spirituality has been found to be highly correlated with achieving and maintaining long-term recovery. While spirituality has traditionally focused on the Judaeo-Christian orientation of a higher power which is external to the individual that can guide them in recovery, this chapter has examined ways in which a Buddhist view of paths to enlightenment can also support the process of recovery. Recognition of the value of the focus on others as well as oneself is consistent through all the traditions and may prove a fruitful area for further research. A spiritual understanding and pursuit of this line of research is exciting in that it offers a broadened approach to the development of all human nature, beyond addiction recovery to the ultimate attainment of enlightened living for all.

References

Alcoholics Anonymous, (AA) (3rd ed.) (1976). New York: Alcoholics Anonymous World Services.

Blatt, S. J., McDonald, C., Sugarman, A., & Wilber, C. (1984). Psychodynamic theories of opiate addiction: New directions for research. *Clinical Psychology Review, 4*, 159–189.

Bowlby, J. (1969). *Attachment and loss, Vol. I: Attachment.* London: Hogarth Press.

Carroll, S. (1993). Spirituality and purpose in life in alcoholism recovery. *Journal of Studies on Alcohol, 54*(3), 297–301.

Craig, R. J. (1993). Contemporary trends in substance abuse. *Professional Psychology: Research & Practice, 24*, 182–189.

Csikszentmihalyi, M. (1990). *Flow: The psychology of optimal experience.* New York: Harper & Row.

Claxton, G. (1986, reprinted 1996). The lights on but there's nobody home: The psychology of no-self. In G. Claxton (Ed.), *Beyond therapy: The impact of eastern religions on psychological theory and practice* (pp. 49–70). Dorset, England, UK: Prism Press.

de Silva, P. (1986, reprinted 1996). Buddhism and behavior change: Implications for therapy. In G. Claxton (Ed.), *Beyond therapy: The impact of eastern religions on psychological theory and practice* (pp. 217–231). Dorset, England, UK: Prism Press.

Dinwiddie, S. H. & Cloninger, C. R. (1991). Family and adoption studies in alcoholism and drug addiction. *Psychiatric Annuals, 21*, 206–214.

Dinwiddie, S. H. & Reich, T. (1991). Epidemiological perspectives on children of alcoholics. In M. Galanter & H. Begleiter, (Eds.) *Recent developments in alcoholism, Vol. 9: Children of alcoholics* (pp. 287–299). New York: Plenum Press.

Dockett, K. (1993). *Resources for stress resistance: Parallels in psychology and Buddhism.* Santa Monica, CA: Soka Gakkai International-USA.

Dudley-Grant, G. R. (1998). Individualism and collectivisim: Psychodynamic theories and commonalities with Budhist thought. In A. Marsella and G. R. Dudley-Grant (Co-chairs), *Buddhist and western psychological thought: Conceptual foundations and assumptions.* Symposium conducted at the annual convention of the American Psychological Association, San Francisco, CA.

Eagle, M. (1984). *Recent developments in psychoanalysis: A critical evaluation.* Cambridge, MA: Harvard University Press.

Epstein, M. (1986). Meditative transformations of narcissism. *Journal of Transpersonal Psychology, 18*, 143–158.

Epstein, M. (1995). Thoughts without a thinker: Buddhism and Psychoanalysis. *Psychoanalytic Review, 82*, 391–406.

Fairburn, W. R. D. (1952). *Psychoanalytic studies of the personality.* London: Tavistock.

Fontana, D. (1986, reprinted 1996). Mind, senses and self. In G. Claxton (Ed.), *Beyond therapy: The impact of eastern religions on psychological theory and practice* (pp. 31–48). Dorset, England, UK: Prism Press.

Goldfarb, L. M., Galanter, M., McDowell, D., Lifsutz, H., & Dermatis, H. (1996). Medical student and patient attitudes toward religion and spirituality in the recovery process. *American Journal of Drug and Alcohol Abuse, 22*, 549–562.

The Gosho Translation Committee, (1979). *The major writings of Nichiren Daishonin, Vol. 1.* Sendagaya, Sibura-ku, Tokyo: Nichiren Shoshu International Center.

Green, L. L., Fullilove, M. T., & Fullilove, R. E. (1998). Stories of spiritual awakening: The nature of spirituality in recovery. *Journal of Substance Abuse Treatment, 15*(4), 325–332.

Goodwin, D. W. (1979). Alcoholism and heredity: A review and hypothesis. *Archives of General Psychiatry, 36*, 57–61.

Groves, P. G. & Farmer, R. (1994). Buddhism and addictions. *Addiction Research, 2*, 183–194.

Hartmann, H. (1958). *Ego psychology and the problem of adaptation.* New York: International Universities Press.

Harlow, H. F. (1958). The nature of love. *American Psychologist, 13*, 673–685.

Ho, D. Y. F. (1995). Selfhood and identity in Confucianism, Taoism, Buddhism, and Hinduism: Contrasts with the West. *Journal of the Theory of Social Behavior, 25*, 115–139.

Ikeda, D., Saito, K., Endo, T., & Suda, H. (1998, July). Dialogue on the Lotus Sutra: The wisdom of the Lotus Sutra – A discussion on religion in the Twenty First Century. *Living Buddhism, 2*, 20–33.

Ikemi, Y. & Ikemi, A. (1986). An oriental point of view in psychosomatic medicine. *Psychotherapy & Psychosomatics, 45*, 118–126.

Khantzian, E. J. & Mack, J. E. (1994). How AA works and why it's important for clinicians to understand. *Journal of Substance Abuse Treatment, 11*, 77–92.

Kohut, H. (1971). *The analysis of the self.* New York: International Universities Press.

Leifer, R. (1999). Buddhist conceptualization and treatment of anger. *Journal of Clinical Psychology, 55*(3), 339–351.

Mahler, M. (1968). *On human symbiosis and the vicissitudes of individuation, Vol. 1: Infantile psychosis.* New York: International Universities Press.

McCrady, B. S. & Miller, W. R. (Eds.) (1993). *Research on Alcoholics Anonymous: Opportunities and alternatives.* Piscataway, NJ: Rutgers Center of Alcohol Studies.

McCrady, B. S. (1994). Alcoholics anonymous and behavior therapy: Can habits be treated as diseases? Can diseases be treated as habits? *Journal of Counseling and Clinical Psychology, 62*(6), 1159–1166.

Metzner, R. (1996). The Buddhist six-worlds model of consciousness and reality. *The Journal of Transpersonal Psychology, 28*, 155–166.

Molino, A. (1998). *The Couch and the tree: Dialogues in psychoanalysis and Buddhism.* New York: North Point Press.

Morvay, Z. (1999). Horney, Zen and the real self: Theoretical and historical connections. *American Journal of Psychoanalysis, 59*, 25–35.

National Institute on Alcohol Abuse and Alcoholism, (Friday, Feb 18, 2000). RFA: AA-00-002, Retrieved 2/24/00, from the http://www.ScienceWise.Com.

Nichiren Shoshu International Center, (1984). *Lectures on the Sutra, the Hoben and Juryo Chapters* (Rev. ed.). Sendagaya, Sibura-ku, Tokyo: Author.

Ray, C. (1986, reprinted 1996). Western psychology and Buddhist teachings: Convergence and divergences. In G. Claxton (Ed.), *Beyond therapy: The impact of eastern religions on psychological theory and practice* (pp. 17–29). Dorset, England, UK: Prism Press.

Ross, S. A. (1991). Freedom from possession: a Tibetan Buddhist view. *Journal of Social Behavior & Personality, 6*, 415–426.

Royce, J. E. (1995). The effects of alcoholism and recovery on spirituality. In R. J. Kus (Ed.), *Spirituality and chemical dependency* (pp. 19–37). New York: Haworth Press.

Soka Gakkai (SGI-USA). (1998). *The winning life: An introduction to Buddhist practice.* [Brochure] Santa Monica, CA: Author.

Spalding, D. & Metz, G. J. (1997). Spirituality and quality of life in Alcoholics Anonymous. *Alcoholism Treatment Quality, 15*, 1–14.

Warfield, R. D. & Goldstein, M. B. (1996). Spirituality: The key to recovery from alcoholism. *Counseling & Values*, 40, 85–89.

Winnicott, D. W. (1965). *The maturational processes and the facilitating environment.* New York: International Universities Press.

Yalisone, D. L. (1989). Psychoanalytic approaches to alcoholism and addiction: Treatment and research. *Psychology of Addictive Behaviors, 3*, 107–113.

Chapter 5

Suffering from Biobabble

Searching for a Science of Subjectivity

Polly Young-Eisendrath

In the last two decades of the twentieth century, our popular and scientific accounts of human suffering have been inching their way toward a new form of scientific reductionism: a knee-jerk biological determinism that I call "biobabble." This is the widespread tendency to use terms (e.g. adaptation) that come from various aspects of the biological sciences to attempt to explain human actions and moods without even a reasonable understanding of the term, the science, the associated theory (or lack of it), and/or the target of explanation. Biobabble names biological, evolutionary, and physical processes as the primary causes for many human traits and behaviors from the undesirable (like alcoholism and schizophrenia) to the sublime (like altruism and happiness). In my view, biobabble confuses and harms us in our attempts to understand and alleviate human suffering, on both an individual and a communal level.

By the term "suffering" here, I mean specifically the Buddhist notion of *dukkha*, which is typically translated as "suffering" in English. Dukkha literally refers to a state of being off-center or out-of-balance, like a bone slightly out of its socket or a wheel riding off its axle. I will use the word "suffering" in this paper to mean a state of being in which we are out of kilter because of a subjective disturbance that may be as mild as a momentary frustration or as severe as a depressive or psychotic state.

Buddhist discourses on dukkha are wide-ranging and deal with both physical and mental suffering. For my purposes, I am referring to the mental anguish that we create through our perseverations, distortions, evaluations, and internal commentary. Much of this anguish is rooted in our conscious or unconscious desires to have things go our own way, and the resultant feelings of humiliation and despair when they do not. This suffering is distinct from the pain and adversity that are inescapable and out of our control. Differentiating suffering from pain allows us to address the aspect of human adversity that is potentially under the control of an individual and can be ameliorated through a change in awareness or consciousness.

Such suffering arises from desires and intentions expressed through emotional habit-patterns that Western psychology calls "unconscious" conflicts, deficits, complexes, and defenses, as well as through impulsive actions, addictions, cravings and demands. The arguments laid down by psychodynamic theories, only about one hundred years old, are quite similar to ancient Buddhist accounts of suffering. But the importance given to unconscious conflicts, desires, and meanings in Western psychology has been rapidly shrinking, as biobabble has spread through media and popularized journalistic writing on science. The notion that people are responsible for their actions is disappearing from the popular imagination, along with the conviction that people can change their behavior by changing their minds.

Twentieth century scientific achievements have largely defeated the old metaphysics of Western Judeo-Christian religions. Widely regarded as a sign that humanity has grown up from a childhood in which human powers (agency, rationality, creativity etc.) were erroneously projected into an enchanted animistic world, enlightened secularism has had massive effects on our moral and ethical functioning. From a scientific perspective, we are now free to use the previously projected powers to understand ourselves and our accountability, responsibility, and limitations as agents in own lives and the world. And yet we can just as easily aggrandize ourselves and believe that *we* are now the gods and goddesses of the past, and should bring life and death under our own control. And/or we can avoid all accountability for our own actions and simply continue to project these vitalizing powers into things that are largely outside our responsibility and control (e.g. genetic predispositions).

Science offers its own metaphysics about the fundamental nature of reality, although it is a metaphysics that largely excludes human meaning. For example, matter and energy have replaced divinities as the ultimate principles of existence. Indeed, we educated Westerners put our faith in almost every "scientific" explanation whether or not we have any real knowledge of what is being explained or how it works. This in itself is not necessarily a problem; humans must employ a mythology, or bigger story, in order to know how to perceive "reality." And yet, if we are to make use of our powers of rationality and science, we must examine the social and cultural consequences of our current beliefs.

Merely replacing the metaphysics of religion with the metaphysics of science does not bring us closer to truth or knowledge. And most people suspect that there are ethical consequences of our scientific metaphysics, which have torn the social fabric supporting communities and families.

Biobabble, Buddhism, and Compassion

In the following, I look at some of the implications of biobabble in relation to explanations of human actions, especially as these have affected popular and scientific accounts of human suffering over the past two decades. As a clinical teacher in a department of psychiatry, I often feel overwhelmed by a *zeitgeist* that promotes the mystique of the mighty gene, genetic "predispositions," and biochemical explanations (that are not coherent theories) of mood and emotional disorders. As a psychoanalyst, psychologist, and psychotherapist (and ordinary citizen), I have been shocked at the recent popular shift away from personal accountability for our actions and motives to vague organic explanations (e.g. I am depressed because of my genes) that eradicate the complexity of personal meaning and responsibility.

Whether or not individuals understand what they are saying, when they speak biobabble, they eliminate the role of meaning and intentions in the development of societies and people. In this story the "master molecule" of the gene, falsely endowed with an autonomous power, overrides the effects of personal desires, intentions, and actions. The term "gene" or "adaptation" has in fact replaced intention, purpose, and morality in most popular psychological and psychiatric accounts of the ways in which people thrive or fail in their everyday lives.

All of our struggles, such as finding a mate or becoming a compassionate person, can be recast now in terms of their supposed advantages for our genes. Speaking biobabble, we sound like our genes are propagating themselves through us, and that *our* lives are meaningless without knowing what our genes are doing.

Many people who seek psychotherapy or analysis now come with such vague theories as "I am depressed because I inherited depression from my mother's family" or "I have an addiction because my genetic history is loaded for substance abuse" or "I have attention deficit disorder because of my genetic background" and so on. These people continue to feel hopeless *after* they have taken the appropriate medications and comforted themselves with the company of their ancestors because they still suffer. Of course, all of this can be addressed through effective psychotherapy, but for those who never consider psychotherapy – and most people do not – these vague organic explanations only block any desire to understand the personal motives and meanings that lead to their suffering.

A great deal of harm has already occurred as a result of our widespread biobabble. This is not to say that we should disregard the important advances that genetics and biochemistry have provided in helping us understand and medicate both physical illnesses and psychiatric conditions. It is to say that we need to be clear about the consequences of embracing an ideology that eliminates an account of our own intentions and actions in explaining our difficulties.

Unique among religions, Buddhism is rooted in empirical accounts and objective methods. Indeed, Buddhism is quite comfortable with scientific knowledge because many of its practices are grounded in dispassionate observation. Additionally, the Buddhist psychology of Abhidharma has developed systematic empirical investigations of the roots of human suffering and the nature of human subjectivity. Buddhism offers a unique opportunity for those in the human services to become acquainted with methods of studying subjectivity in ways that respect science, but are not inclined toward physical reductionism.

Moreover, Buddhism offers many skillful means for increasing our experience of subjective freedom in everyday life, based on a theory of the interdependent, impermanent, finite and changing nature of reality, which is remarkably consonant with Western post-modern philosophy of science. I believe that Buddhism and psychodynamic psychologies must, in the next decade or two, assist each other in diminishing the effects of biobabble by embracing a viable, scientific approach to the study of human suffering.

In a symposium, published under the title *Consciousness at the Crossroads* (Houshmand, Livingston, & Wallace, 1999), the Dalai Lama met with a group of prominent Western proponents of contemporary neuroscience. In the afterward (pp. 515–173), one of the editors reiterates a question posed to the neuroscientists by the Dalai Lama of whether strictly materialistic explanations of suffering will "critically undermine love and compassion?" (p. 173).

The neuroscientists claim, as anyone would, that a person is not a brain (malfunctioning or not), and should not be treated as such. And yet their biological determinism, used to explain mood and other emotional disorders, does not include any account of the "whole person" that could become a focus of compassion. Such a materialist account in Western scientific language takes the unit of the individual (for example, one brain and one body) to be the focus of study, but necessarily eliminates the experience of subjective life so that the person is described as an animal or organism.

Buddhism agrees with Western science that the "person" or "self" cannot be found in the heart or brain; in fact, no self can be discovered in a detailed ontological investigation of our physical functioning. Buddhism adds that, although we cannot find a self in our physical being, we really *do* exist "in profound interdependence." When this fact is fully investigated and developed, it yields "a far deeper sense of love and compassion than that" which is connected to a theory of humans as separate physical bodies or genetic programs (Houshmand, Livingston, & Wallace, p. 173). The interdependent nature of reality yields ontology of compassion in Buddhism, with ethical implications that are quite different from biological determinism, without any untenable "old" metaphysics.

Compassion – caring, kindness, affection – is considered to be a component of *reality* that is difficult for the individual to grasp because of the delusion of being separated from everything else through the experience of a separate self. Buddhism takes as its goal the direct experience and rational acceptance of this interdependence, which demonstrates that our kindness benefits everyone, ourselves as much as others. In advance of having such a direct experience, practitioners are encouraged to imagine or learn about compassion and interdependence through stories, teachings and other practices.

The Study of Intention and Subjectivity

Because Western culture has not stemmed the tides of biobabble in these past two decades, providers and teachers of human services now face a situation in which there is no viable dialogue between biological determinism and other scientific accounts of human subjectivity. Indeed, our clients and others appear to believe that proper medications or advice should alleviate suffering without any knowledge of how an individual or individuals create it. In the absence of such a dialogue, we may critically undermine love and compassion as the Dalai Lama suggests.

The epistemologies of the natural sciences (often called the "hard" sciences), which under gird biological determinism, necessarily eliminate all questions and accounts of human subjectivity and intention. To say this another way, the systems of knowledge used to study organic processes must exclude the experiences of the human subject. All epistemologies are limited and constrained; those used in the natural sciences cannot ask or answer questions about human intention and its meanings.

By the term "intention" I mean purpose, desire, or aim: what one consciously or unconsciously *wants or wants to do*. Psychoanalysis and psychodynamic methods and theories constitute a nascent science of human intention and meaning. This science depends on the practice of psychodynamic therapies, and on related scientific studies of personality, therapeutic change, and development. The psychodynamic science of intention comprises the following: a means to ameliorate human suffering through therapeutic treatment, a way of thinking about subjective life, and a set of testable hypotheses (contrary to Grunbaum, 1984) about such phenomena as defense mechanisms, attachment behaviors, motivations, core conflicts, therapeutic change, personality development, emotional memory, and more. By "science" I mean systematized knowledge – the product of agreed-upon objective methods of investigation – that becomes the basis for truth claims in a field of study.

Through our clinical work and scientific studies in the psychodynamic therapies, we discover the complex, conflicted and often-unknown intentions that are at the very core of personal suffering. I agree with psychoanalyst Strenger (1991) when he says the following about psychoanalysis:

> The assumption is that every aspect of human behavior is intelligible; i.e. behavior is seen as intentional action all the way down. Furthermore, it is assumed that by

> correctly understanding the meaning of actions, we help the patient to take full responsibility for who he is, and give him the freedom to change if he truly wants to. (pp. 62–63)

In order fully to develop and make use of this science, we need to expand and articulate further our models of the human psyche, especially through research that does not import whole cloth the epistemological categories of the natural sciences.

The sciences of numbers, objects, and processes – mathematics, physics, biochemistry, biology, and genetics – necessarily eliminate all traces of human intention in order to study their subject matter. Human subjective responses must be understood in terms that account for meaning and purpose and regard intentionality or free will as something other than adaptation to an environment. This goal is impossible to achieve through the natural sciences, even in such applications as systems theory and information theory, which are also constrained by the epistemology of process and reactivity. Only when we have achieved some solid foundation for understanding the complexity of human desires and intentions can we engage in a useful dialogue with biology, biochemistry and neuroscience to investigate such important topics as the nature and development of human consciousness.

As we have all been increasingly encouraged to explain more and more of our personal difficulties in terms of organic and biological processes, and less and less in terms of our own desires and actions, we providers of mental health services now risk obscuring the complexity of subjective life.

If we respond to questions about why we suffer, without any insight into human motivations, conflicts, and desires, we may short-circuit a question of meaning. And if we explain human moods, emotional difficulties, and other shortcomings mostly, or most adequately, in terms of biochemical or other organic processes, we will betray the thimbleful of social awareness of the role of unconscious intentions that has only recently become a part of Western culture.

When I was in graduate school in developmental psychology in the late 1970's, I studied the complexity of human desires in a seminar on motivation. In this and other seminars, I learned that human agency and language demand a non-reductive method of study. We were taught that the human freedom to think *abstractly* – to theorize even about one's thoughts and moods – sets humans sufficiently apart from other organisms and animals to create a "psychology of the person" that is rooted in meaning and intention, rather than process or reactivity. I was taught that it is dangerous to believe that humans are biologically *or* psychologically determined because an adequate theory of human action must account for intentions that go beyond determining forces. For example, when humans are condemned to horrific torture, some will continue to find a meaningful way to engage with their lives, as is illustrated in Frankel's (1984) *Man's*

Search for Meaning. Even when diagnosed with a terminal illness, a person is still free to see it as a personal adventure, rather than a doomed biological process, as writer Broyard (1992) shows us in *Intoxicated by My Illness*. These freedoms are not a by-product of organic or biochemical reactions.

In the late 70's, we psychodynamic types thought that cognitive-behaviorism was *the* reductionism to oppose. We did not see what was coming around the biochemical corner. A mere twenty years later, most popular and media accounts of science would concur with English journalist Appleyard (1998), who in a study of the ethical issues inherent in applying genetic methods to humans, states as a fact that "Almost every aspect of human life has a large and frequently decisive genetic component" (p. 15). Although Appleyard is a critic of genetic programs, he like most other popularizers of biological science is a true believer in the ideology.

All accounts of the biological basis of human action obscure the significance and complexity of desire and agency that cannot be reduced to reactivity. Even the human infant depends on intentional action rather than an adaptation to an environment. The infant cannot think for itself and yet it cannot live without thinking; so someone else must think for it. The infant cannot foresee its own needs and provide for them; so someone else must use foresight. Human beings develop in inherently personal relationships that include intention, meaning and reflection from the very beginning. Although our biology may affect how sensitive we are to certain interactions with others, our relationships and their meanings also affect how relevant these biological factors may be.

Thus, there is a massive distortion in using organic theories to explain human actions. Philosopher MacMurray (1961) says it like this:

> We are not organisms, but persons. The nexus of relations, which unites us in a human society, is not organic but personal. Human behavior cannot be understood, but only caricatured, if it is represented as an adaptation to environment; and there is no such process as social evolution but, instead, a history which reveals a precarious development and possibilities both of progress and retrogression. (p. 46)

When the facts and methods of studying organic life are applied by analogy to the human field, they deny us the possibility of understanding ourselves – in terms of intentions and actions. We transform our actions into organic processes, which automatically erase the freedom to change through self-reflection (whether changing for better or worse). Biobabble makes unintelligible any explanation of human behavior in terms of desire and intention, and transforms into gibberish the goal of subjective freedom through increased awareness, as found in psychodynamic and Buddhist practices.

For all of these reasons, I passionately believe that we must articulate a multileveled scientific study of the intentional and relational character of human subjectivity. Drawing on psychodynamic models and theories, and on the practices and methods of Buddhism, such a science would challenge the ideology of biological determinism.

As the Dalai Lama (1997) says, we need to use the complexity of human intelligence in a constructive way.

> of all the various species of animal on the planet, human beings are the biggest troublemakers.... It is therefore important that human intelligence be utilized in a constructive way. That is the key. If we utilize its capacity properly, then not only human beings would become less harmful to each other, and to the planet, but also individual human beings would be happier in themselves. (p. 132)

The study of human intentions, motivations, desires and inner conflicts is the path to understanding how human intelligence can be used for constructive purposes in understanding its own powers and limitations. The methods of Buddhist practice encourage us to pay attention to the effects of our desires on our contentment, our intentions on our actions, and our fears and anxieties on our states of mind. Similarly, psychodynamic therapies encourage sober self-reflection on our destructive emotional habits and our repetitive omnipotent longings to have things under our own control. Only the human sciences can provide the backbone for expanding and studying these approaches.

The Human Sciences

When I first encountered the philosophy of science, through the study of *The Structure of Scientific Revolutions* by Kuhn (1970), I was deeply impressed with the idea of scientific "paradigms" or exemplary models that are used as if they were reality.

Kuhn showed that the natural sciences, such as physics and chemistry, have grown through revolutionary shifts in these paradigms, rather than through linear accumulation of new knowledge or information. From time to time, some scientists discover and investigate anomalies in the exemplary model, and these anomalies eventually lead to a whole new worldview that topples the old paradigm and allows scientists to see data in a new way. Kuhn's theory appealed to psychological clinicians like myself because we believed that we were helping our clients shift their paradigms of reality by examining anomalies in their worldviews. But Kuhn strongly objected to applying his structural theory of the natural sciences to any understanding of the human sciences of psychology, anthropology, sociology, linguistics, economics or history. He believed that his theory belonged in the natural sciences, and was distorted in applications to the human sciences.

The original line drawn in the nineteenth century between the natural and the human sciences was as follows: the natural sciences explain events mathematically and organically in terms of the laws of nature, while the human sciences explain events in terms of human intentions. This distinction fundamentally came from one German philosopher: Dilthey who died in 1911. He claimed that the goal of the natural sciences is the discovery of causal principles and generalized physical laws, whereas the objective of the human sciences is to understand the purpose and meaning of human action. Because of this difference, Dilthey concluded that the natural sciences are inadequate for the study of human intentionality and experience at its most complex levels.

Throughout most of the twentieth century, philosophers of science have continued to debate the question of whether there are true differences between the natural and the human sciences and if there are, what they are. Is it the subject matter, the attitude of the scientist, or the method of study that makes two endeavors seem so different? There now appears to be some consensus among philosophers of science. There is a broad agreement that all sciences are hermeneutical or interpretive at base. This means that all of the assumptions and methods of science occur in particular contexts of meaning that are not necessarily generalizable from one to another. As philosopher Putnam (1989) states,

> We can and should insist that some facts are there to be discovered and not legislated by us, but this is something to be said when one has adopted a way of speaking, a language, a "conceptual scheme." To talk of "facts" without specifying the language to be used is to talk of nothing; the word "fact" no more has its use fixed by the world itself than does the word "exist" or the word "object." (p. 114)

We can no longer claim that the simple facts of *reality* are discovered, even by natural scientists, because no fact exists outside of some context of shared assumptions. Rather than discovering objective facts that are beyond interpretation, scientists are now understood to pursue their particular subject matter within a community of thinkers that share a worldview or a way of seeing something.

Is it still useful to maintain a distinction between the natural and human sciences? It is a necessity, in my view, from an epistemological perspective. The natural sciences are not capable of asking and answering questions of human meaning and desire. Nor are their methods designed to study the complexity of human intelligence, especially in its self-conscious and self-reflective aspects. This unique form of intelligence sets us apart from other animals and organisms, even those that have developed language. In adulthood, human self-reflective capacities give us, as a species, an unprecedented level of disengagement from our immediate experience and surroundings. This kind of decentering of our awareness allows us to perform complex abstract processes, to meditate on our own subjective experience, to develop theories about others, and ourselves and to explore and dominate our environment in a radical way. Self-conscious, self-reflective intelligence depends neither exclusively on chance nor necessity for its development and use. With these kinds of unique powers at our disposal, we have become the biggest troublemakers on the planet, and may eventually find that our tendency to dominate other life forms will become our greatest downfall as a species.

There are other philosophical reasons to maintain the boundary between the human and the natural sciences. In 1989, I heard Kuhn lecture on his own long-term conclusions about this issue. He claimed that the main difference between these two kinds of science is practical, in terms of what practitioners normally do, not how or what they study.

What natural scientists do, given their hermeneutic base, "is not ordinarily hermeneutic. Rather, they put to use the paradigm received from their teachers in an ... enterprise that attempts to solve puzzles like those of improving and extending the match between theory and experiment at the advancing forefront of the field." On the other hand, human scientists rarely work with such received knowledge. Their sciences "appear to be hermeneutic, interpretive, through and through. Very little of what goes on in them at all resembles the normal puzzle-solving research of the natural sciences. Their aim is ... to understand behavior, not to discover the laws, if any, that govern it" (Hiley, Bohman & Shusterman, 1991, pp. 22–23). Asking himself the question of whether the human sciences could eventually find paradigms that would support normal puzzle-solving research, Kuhn said he was "totally uncertain," stating that some aspects of economics and psychology already seem to use models that could be generalized in developing a puzzle-solving science. On the other hand, he himself wondered if it would be constructive to move further in this direction. When the unit of study is a social or psychological system, Kuhn wondered if there would be any real gain in abstracting principles that might lead to puzzle solving, rather than continuing to engage in a thoroughly hermeneutic enterprise.

Many psychological investigations that have emerged in dialogue with psychodynamic theories are already strong examples of a complex human science of subjectivity with strong records of reliability, validity and prediction. Those, which come easily to mind, are research programs in the following: (Loevinger's) ego development theory, affect theory and regulation, infant-mother observation, attachment theory, defense mechanisms research, psychodynamic psychotherapy outcome studies, some dream studies, and the core-conflict studies of psychotherapy.

All of these have contributed important new understandings and expanded old ones, while they have used hermeneutical or qualitative research methods to investigate human emotions and intentions.

Of course, it is also fruitful to draw on certain findings in the natural sciences. Many of these are useful as heuristics and analogies. But if we ground our theories of subjectivity in natural science paradigms (whether they come from biology or physics), as I described above, we will distort our views of intentional life and also do very bad science. Another contemporary philosopher of science, Taylor (1985) states that natural science explanations of our subjective experiences "end up in wordy elaborations of the obvious, or they fail altogether to address the interesting questions, or their practitioners end up squandering their talents and ingenuity in the attempt to show that they can after all recapture the insights of ordinary life in their manifestly reductive explanatory languages" (p. 1).

Biobabble in the Human Services

Biological determinism, as imported into the human services, is one such example of bad science. The typical way that this kind of thinking enters the fields of mental health services are through what geneticist Lewontin (1991) calls the "empty bucket metaphor." This metaphor depicts human beings as empty buckets of different sizes, waiting to be filled with the water of experience.

If the environment provides all of the necessary resources, then every bucket is filled to its capacity. Still, the metaphor implies, there will be differences in our abilities, capacities, and limitations because there are differences in how much water each bucket can hold. These differences are natural and inherent in the different sizes of the buckets from the start.

Lewontin (1991) claims that a major error is committed through the use of this metaphor because "A change in environment ... can change abilities by many orders of magnitude ... [and] the differences between individuals are abolished by cultural and mechanical inventions." For example, "Although there may be biologically based average differences in physique and strength between a random group of men and random group of women (and these are less than usually supposed), these differences rapidly become irrelevant and disappear from practical view in a world of electrically driven hoists, power steering, and electronic controls" (pp. 29–30). Environmental variation and genetic variation are not independent causal pathways; in fact, the interaction between the two is indissoluble.

Lewontin (1991) summarizes biological determinism as three main ideas: (1) that humans differ in fundamental abilities because of innate differences; (2) that those innate differences are biologically inherited; and (3) that human nature, therefore, guarantees the formation of a hierarchical society.

He then carefully reveals the profound flaws in the largest twin and population studies that make claims for major genetic tendencies in human behavior. These studies discover no causal laws (because their methods are correlational and statistical), but they claim to separate genetic and environmental influences for traits such as happiness and schizophrenia. In conclusion, Lewontin states that "[T] here is at present simply no convincing measure of the role of genes in influencing human behavioral variation." But we (scientists and public) have developed a problematic confusion "between inherited and unchangeable" (p. 33) in our beliefs about these studies.

Why do so many intelligent scientists then argue for the benefits of sequencing the human genome? Lewontin (1991) answers in two parts: these scientists are "so completely devoted to the ideology of unitary causes that they believe in the efficacy of the research and do not ask themselves more complicated questions" (p. 51). But he also adds, "No prominent molecular biologist of my acquaintance is without a financial stake in the biotechnology business" (p. 74).

The complexity of human desire, both conscious and unconscious, has played a determining role in our current version of biobabble and the story of the mighty gene. But this is not the first time that a theory of inherited traits has played a powerful role in persuading people that the roots of human misery are "in the blood" rather than in our intentions and actions. English journalist Appleyard (1998) traces the history of this notion from Plato who advocated an improved species as a necessary aspect of an ideal society, to the Christian Inquisition whose priests believed that faith and heresy were "in the blood," and finally to the modern Nazi Final Solution: the extermination of those people considered to be "genetically inferior." Without a science of human intention that fundamentally and convincingly presents a systematic understanding of the complexity of human desire, we are at risk to repeat the most destructive chapters of our history when the omnipotent longings of the few were supported by the many.

An Ethic of Human Suffering

Those people who practice psychodynamic therapies and those who practice Buddhism share in an ethic about human suffering: that one is the creator of oneself, and that whatever one does, one becomes heir to those intentions. In psychoanalysis, this is a belief that we create our suffering through the repetition of destructive emotional patterns that were, at some time, an apparently suitable response to our emotional and interpersonal environment. All practitioners of psychodynamic therapies are committed to understanding human beings as intentional persons, even when they do not understand themselves in this way.

Practitioners of all forms of Buddhism would agree with the famous words of the Buddha that open The *DhammaDada*:

> We are what we think.
> All that we are arises with our thoughts.
> With our thoughts we make the world.
> Speak or act with an impure mind and trouble will follow you as the wheel follows the ox that draws the cart.
>
> (Bryom, 1993, p. 1)

Buddhism teaches methods for observing the process through which our thoughts and intentions become our *karma*, the consequences that arise from our own actions and create certain patterns in our lives. In order to change this karma, we must change our thoughts and actions; according to Buddhism, our karma is fluid and emergent in our own thoughts and actions; it is neither wholly predetermined, as an adaptation to an environment, nor completely unpredictable and random.

The Buddhist theory of karma is consonant with psychodynamic theories and therapies about our tendencies to repeat the conflicts and emotional habits that are outside our awareness. To free ourselves from destructive emotional habits or change our irrational fears or reduce our discontent, we must come to know our own motives, especially those that we repeatedly project into others. I borrow some words from contemporary psychoanalyst Schafer (1978) who describes the course of psychoanalysis in the following way:

> The analysand progressively recognizes, accepts, revises, refines, and lives in terms of the idea of the self as agent. This is to say that, in one way or another and more and more, the analysand sees himself or herself as being the person who essentially has been doing the things from which he or she was apparently suffering upon entering analysis … (p. 180)

Buddhist and psychoanalytic practices have developed theories and methods for understanding suffering. This way of thinking leads to a set of moral principles or values that holds people accountable for their actions. It should be sufficiently clear that this ethic stands as a stark contrast to the ideology of biological determinism and the bad gene.

When the metaphysics of Western Judeo-Christian religions was overtaken by the metaphysics of Western sciences, the ethics of Western religions were lost in the process. The ethic of suffering that I expressed above could just as easily have been formulated from an account of the Ten Commandments or the Golden Rule. Western religions advocate close attentions to one's thoughts and actions in the practice of becoming an ethical human being. But the defeat of the metaphysics of religion by those of science in the West has also meant a loss of the ethical teachings of the religions in any form that might reach large numbers of people in order to have a major influence.

Americans seem baffled by the senseless acts of violence – homicides and suicides among them – carried out even by privileged young people living in our society and benefiting from all of our advancements of the natural sciences. We have seemed unable to grasp the consequences of our loss of an ethic of suffering. When human traits, from the sublime to the undesirable, are explained in terms of adaptations and genes, how can anyone who has developed during these times take seriously a belief in personal responsibility for oneself, let alone for one's community and society?

Within a human science of subjectivity, ethics and morality become part of the contemporary metaphysics of science; the study of personhood would certainly be on a metaphysical par with the study of organic processes. Surely we deceive ourselves if we believe that the humanities and religions can carry the burden of impressing young people with the ethic of suffering. Science *is* the spiritual adventure of our age and we have to engage its methods in order to bring validity to our pursuits. Maybe that will change in the twenty-first century, but if it does, the change will be the result of scientific investigations.

It is my hope that the early part of the twenty-first century will witness the convergence, of the objective methods of Buddhism with the clinical methods of psychodynamic theories and practices in a systematic study of subjective life. This pursuit should apply especially the methods that have developed through Western psychology, rather than the exclusively physiological and biological methods already used to study aspects of meditational practice. As I mentioned earlier, such psychological methods already exist and are used to investigate topics related to psychodynamic therapies. They include content analysis, narrative analysis, Q-sort, and other forms of self-report that produce predictable and reliable results.

Under the aegis of an adequate human science of subjectivity, we could begin to organize our selves, our relationships, and our communities toward an adequate account of the human development of responsibility, ethics, and compassion. Until we have this kind of scientific model of the development of the human subject in relationship, we cannot hope to use our contemporary metaphysics of science to understand ourselves. Unless we develop such a model, we are surely at risk for destroying the environment on which our species depends, as a consequence of our own disclaimed omnipotent longings.

References

Appleyard, B. (1998). *Brave new worlds: Staying human in the genetic future*. New York: Viking.

Broyard, A. (1992). *Intoxicated by my illness*. New York: Fawcett Columbine.

Bryom, T. (Trans.) (1993). *DhammaDada: The sayings of the Buddha*. Boston: Shambala.

Dalai Lama, H. H. (1997). *The four noble truths: Fundamentals of the Buddhist teachings*. London, UK: Thorsons.

Frankel, V. (1984). *Man's search for meaning*. New York: Washington Square Press.

Grunbaum, A. (1984). *The foundations of psychoanalysis*. Berkeley: University of California Press.

Hiley, D., Bohman, J., & Shusterman, R. (Eds.), (1992). *The interpretive turn: Philosophy, science, and culture*. Ithaca, NY: Cornell University Press.

Houshmand, Z., Livingston, R., & Wallace, A. (1999). *Consciousness at the crossroads: Conversations with the Dalai Lama on brain science and Buddhism*. Ithaca, NY: Snow Lion.

Kuhn, T. S. (1970). *The structure of scientific revolutions*. Chicago, IL: University of Chicago Press.

Lewontin, R. (1991). *Biology as ideology: The doctrine of DNA*. New York: Harper Perennial.

MacMurray, J. (1961). *Persons in relation*. Atlantic Highlands, NJ: Humanities Press.

Putnam, H. (1989). *Representation and reality*. Cambridge, MA: MIT Press.

Schafer, R. (1978). *Language and insight*. New Haven, CN: Yale University Press.

Strenger, C. (1991). *Between hermeneutics and science: An essay on the epistemology of psychoanalysis*. Madison, CN: International Universities Press.

Taylor, C. (1985). *Human agency and language: Philosophical papers, I*. Cambridge, UK: Cambridge University Press.

Chapter 6

Role of Responsibility in Daseinsanalysis and Buddhism

Belinda Siew Luan Khong

Introduction

Daseinsanalysis (commonly referred to as existential analysis in America) and Buddhism represent two systems of thought that are seemingly disparate. Daseinsanalysis as developed by the Swiss psychiatrist Medard Boss is a twentieth-century Western form of psychotherapy. Buddhism, more popularly understood as a religion and a spiritual pursuit, was promulgated by the Buddha around the sixth century BC. Despite these radically different geographical, historical, and cultural roots, the philosophy and the psychology of Buddhism (as opposed to the religion) and daseinsanalysis can enrich each other and psychology as a whole.

The term daseinsanalysis used by Boss for his psychotherapeutic work is grounded on the philosophy of the German philosopher Martin Heidegger. Boss's (1965) lifelong quest was to learn more about the nature of the human being. He was dissatisfied with the natural scientific model of the person, and he looked to Heidegger's ideas to help him gain a better understanding. Boss's (1979) intention was to take the human being out of the realm of the natural sciences into the existential one. In this respect, Boss was much taken with Heidegger's ideas and he collaborated closely with him for twenty-five years.

According to Boss (1963), daseinsanalysis is an approach or a way of thinking that encourages therapists to understand phenomena as they are immediately perceived and experienced by clients rather than through theoretical explanations and hypotheses. So, daseinsanalysts would not ask what the phenomenon represents, for example a phallic symbol or an unfulfilled wish. Instead they seek to understand what the phenomenon means in the context of the person's life. Daseinsanalysis also refers to a way of seeing and understanding the relationship between human beings and the world. This understanding is based on the Heideggerian notion of "Being-in-the-world," a notion which encapsulates the idea that the individual and world are not two separate entities, but form an indivisible whole.

Boss was also interested in Eastern philosophies, particularly Hinduism and Buddhism. He spent a considerable amount of time in India studying these philosophies and practised meditation (Boss, 1965). Privately, Boss was much influenced by his encounter with Eastern thoughts. Publicly, however he stayed with Heidegger's ideas. Although Boss had not explicitly incorporated Buddhist ideas and practices into daseinsanalysis, daseinsanalysis and Buddhism can contribute significantly to each other.

Today, comparing Buddhist ideas and practices with Western psychology no longer provokes curiosity or awe. It is generally acknowledged that Buddhism and psychology can provide new insights for each other and attempts to close the hiatus between Eastern and Western thinking are frequently undertaken in research, writings, psychology curricula and at conferences.

However, in relation to Buddhism, there is still a tendency in the West to focus on Buddhist practices and ideas as a means of attaining enlightenment. This tendency has given rise to the perception that Buddhism is more relevant to those seeking the spiritual path, but less relevant to everyday living. Such a perception has overlooked the psychological import of Buddhist thought, and the applicability of the Buddha's teachings to human concerns such as living and dying, and responsibility.

The Buddha teaches that to a large extent human suffering is attributable to psychological factors, and most of his teachings have therapeutic significance. According to de Silva (1996), Buddhist ideas and practices are particularly pertinent to psychotherapy as a prophylactic measure to prevent a dysfunction or problem from developing, and to improve a person's well-being and functioning, for example to overcome such existential concerns as alienation, anxiety and unsatisfactoriness associated with living itself.

It is in the second area that Buddhist psychology and daseinsanalysis have much in common. Both disciplines emphasize the individual's responsibility for his or her mental health and personal growth, and both perceive social responsibility as an essential component of our place in the world. Daseinsanalysis and Buddhism find common expression in alleviating human suffering by helping people to free themselves from delusion and to face the realities of life, and both take as their starting point the need for people to develop an understanding of the nature of human existence.

There are also important differences. Boss's main interest is in helping people to understand and deal with current impairments to responsibility in the therapeutic setting. The Buddha is more concerned with the question of why people get themselves into problematic situations, rather than helping them resolve specific dilemmas. As such, the Buddha does not promulgate an array of practices that deal with particular pathologies or neuroses. In this respect, daseinsanalysis can augment Buddhist psychology.

In this chapter I examine the stance that daseinsanalysis and Buddhism adopt towards personal and social responsibility. The parallels and differences between each approach are discussed when I look at their respective contributions. And finally, I illustrate with the case of Therese how these two approaches can be integrated. A comparison of these two disciplines will enable us to see the relevance of the Buddha's teachings to ordinary human concerns and how Buddhism can enrich psychology, and also how much further Boss could have taken daseinsanalysis if he had incorporated various important Buddhist ideas and practices.

Responsibility: An Overview

Daseinsanalysis and Buddhist psychology emphasise responsibility as a prerequisite for our mental health and well-being. It is true that the aim of most psychotherapies is to help people gain insight into the problems that have restricted their current functioning and to assist in them in taking the responsibility to overcome these blockages. Despite the emphasis on responsibility as a desired outcome of therapy, little is spoken as to what responsibility involves and what it means to be responsible.

Responsibility is usually understood as "accountability, answerability, care, charge, duty, obligation ... " (Mcleod, 1987, p. 852). Today we often hear calls for us to take responsibility – to be accountable for our lives, to fulfill our obligations and duties to our families and our countries, to care for the less fortunate, and for the environment. In this sense, responsibility is conceived primarily in terms of duties and obligations. Daseinsanalysis and Buddhism adopt a different approach. To them, responsibility involves the individual taking the responsibility to cultivate an attitude, that is a frame of mind, or a disposition which enables him or her to see things as they really are, and to permit the phenomena that are encountered to unfold naturally. According to daseinsanalysis, this sense of responsibility makes it possible for people to live authentically. And to the Buddha, taking responsibility is important in freeing the mind from remorse, that is to develop a sense of inner peace. In this chapter, I focus on how daseinsanalysis and Buddhism empower individuals to develop this sense of responsibility.

To understand the Buddhist and daseinsanalytic perspectives, we have to comprehend the difference between the ontological foundation for responsibility, and the ontic manifestation of responsibility. The difference between the ontological and the ontic is what Heidegger (1927/1962; 1988) refers to as the "ontological difference." The ontological refers to that which is primordial, fundamental to all beings, while the ontic is concerned with how the ontological is expressed in the ordinary everyday world. According to Heidegger, the ontological and the ontic are inseparable for the former provides the conditions for the possibility of the latter. For example, hearing is ontological, everyone has the capacity to hear. What each person hears is ontic, determined often by the emotions, culture and the environment. In terms of responsibility, the ontological difference means that human beings possess the ontological capacity for responsibility. How this capacity is manifested ontically varies with each individual.

In their philosophical and psychological explication of responsibility, what daseinsanalysis and Buddhism seek to do is to help people address such questions as – What are the ontological foundations for responsibility? To whom and for what are we responsible? How do we exercise responsibility? What gives rise to the ontic failure or the inability to take responsibility? How can people be assisted in taking responsibility?

Personal Responsibility

Daseinsanalysis

The ontological foundations for personal responsibility in daseinsanalysis are grounded on the Heideggerian notions of Da-sein, Being-in-the-world, Being-Guilty and the Existentials. Da-sein, meaning "Being-the-there" is used by Heidegger exclusively for human existence and denotes human existence as a clearing (*Lichtung*) (Craig, 1988; Heidegger, 1927/1962). According to Heidegger and Boss, the word "there" demonstrates that human beings are not just present bodily but that they exist as a realm of "world-openness," "apprehension" and "responsiveness" (Boss, 1988, pp. 63–64). What this means is that different phenomena can come forth and reveal themselves in the human clearing and that each person has the ontological capacity to perceive, respond and to care for what appears. The analogy given by Boss of a clearing is that of a space in the forest through which the light shines and illuminates everything on the ground. Therefore Da-sein, *Da* (there) and *sein* (being) refers to the open, worldly nature of human beings (Craig, 1988).

This idea of human existence as a clearing is also grounded on the Heideggerian (1927/1962) notion of "Being-in-the-world." Briefly, this notion emphasizes the indissoluble unity of human beings and world. Boss (1963), explains that "in" does not suggest "within" but "being with." Da-sein as Being-in-the-world signifies that it stands out in the world as an openness, and actively engages with the entities it encounters. The significance of this idea is that human existence is an ongoing process, continually evolving as it interacts with the world.

To whom are human beings responsible? The answer according to Heidegger and Boss is to Being. To understand this, we need to look briefly at what Heidegger means by Being. Being, Heidegger (1927/1962) explains, is not an entity, or a property. Heidegger perceived Being as Nothingness out of which all beings emanate, i.e., Being is the ontological foundation of everything. This is similar to the idea of Tao in Taoist philosophy. Understood in this way, Nothingness is not nihilistic, but rather a primordial source of creativity from which all things manifest themselves (Lee, 1995). Heidegger points out that while Being itself remains concealed, it is manifested through the clearing that is human existence. So when daseinsanalysts perceive responsibility as being responsible to Being, it means human beings have the responsibility to allow all beings that issue from Being to reveal themselves in their openness.

For what are human beings responsible? According to daseinsanalysis, they are responsible for any phenomenon that comes within the light of Da-sein. As a clearing, a person encounters different phenomena, and responsibility refers to the human capacity to respond to these phenomena and to enter into meaningful relationships with them (Boss, 1963). It involves responsibly taking over all the possibilities for world-disclosing relationships so that whatever shows up can come forth in its being in the best possible way.

According to Heidegger and Boss, individuals manifest their responses to what they encounter through the Existentials in different ways. When this response is impaired or blocked, the individual's Being-in-the world is narrowed, and the person's freedom to responsibly choose between different possibilities is restricted. The Existentials, Heidegger explains, are fundamental human characteristics that make up our humanness. The more obvious Existentials are temporality, spatiality, bodyhood, attunement or mood, historicity, Being-with and mortality (Being-unto-Death). Of therapeutic importance are freedom, responsibility, anxiety and Being-guilty (Boss, 1963; Heidegger, 1927/1962). According to Heidegger and Boss, the Existentials are ontological, but their ontic manifestation differs with each person.

The daseinsanalytic approach to personal responsibility is also informed by the Heideggerian notion of "Being-guilty," a human Existential. For Heidegger (1927/1962) Being-guilty does not involve moral or legal considerations, but simply the idea that one is owing or lacking something, and that one is responsible for what is lacking or owed. And what is owed is Da-sein's ability to fulfill all its existential possibilities. How is this indebtedness related to responsibility? Boss (1964) points out that the human openness is needed to serve as the clearing for every particular being (including possibilities) to come forth. Although human beings have this responsibility, Boss (1963) is cognisant that not all possibilities can be fulfilled or realised. Throughout a person's life, he or she has to select one possibility to the exclusion of others. So Being-guilty signifies to the individual the necessity of having to choose, and the realisation that the choices are finite. From a daseinsanalytic perspective, to be responsible means to take responsibility for the particular basis in which one finds oneself, and the particular choice that one makes on that basis (Muhall, 1996).

In Boss's view, although people are free to choose which life possibilities they wish to appropriate, some people are closed to specific possibilities. What gives rise to the ontic inability or the failure to take responsibility? According to Boss (1963), one reason for this is that Da-sein interprets its possibilities from the perspective of the "they," that is from what is conventional and comfortable. This brings us to the notion of "levelling down," which refers to the human tendency to gloss over the ontological with what is ontically familiar and public (Heidegger, 1927/1962). For example, Heidegger and Boss perceive human beings as "Being-unto-Death," meaning that mortality is an ontological characteristic of human beings. Yet ontically, people flee from this by rationalising death into something that will happen but not yet. Daseinsanalysts believe that if they can help their clients to comprehend how the ontological has been levelled down, clients can be assisted in taking responsibility for their present way of Being-in-the world.

This notion of responsibility is related to the idea of authenticity. For Boss and Heidegger, being authentic means being open to all possibilities but remaining content with the development of one. According to Heidegger (1927/1962), Da-sein exist authentically when its choice of existence does not hinge upon what is public and familiar, but upon its taking the responsibility to decide for itself how it wishes to live. Daseinsanalysis believe that by cultivating an attitude of seeing things as they are really are, people learn to differentiate between an "ontological self-understanding" which includes all knowledge about myself as a human being and an "ontical self-understanding," which is the understanding about myself as an individual in specific situations (Holzhey-Kunz, 1996, p. 97). This insight can assist people in comprehending what is changeable (the ontic situation) and what is not (the ontological situation) (Holzhey-Kunz, 1996).

Daseinsanalysis also recognises that the ability to take responsibility may be impaired in "neurotically troubled individuals" (Boss, 1988, p. 70). According to Boss, this lack of responsibility discloses an inability on the part of the individual to be addressed by a multiplicity of phenomena and to respond to them adequately. Take the example of schizophrenia. The daseinsanalytic understanding of this illness takes as its starting point that the human being is fundamentally a perceptive, responsive openness, and that in schizophrenic patients, this openness is impaired (Boss, 1979). In daseinsanalysis, illness is perceived as a privation or lack of health (Condrau, 1998). Boss (1979) explains that the privation in schizophrenics is their lack of possibility to act in an open manner towards the phenomena that they encounter, and to engage with them responsibly.

How do daseinsanalysts assist clients in taking responsibility? They do this by encouraging them to look directly at the phenomenon that is encountered rather than for things or meanings behind it. This manner of experiencing phenomena is founded on the Heideggerian (1969/1972) notion of "phenomenological seeing." The idea of phenomenological seeing is encapsulated in the maxim "to the things themselves" (Heidegger, 1927/1962, p. 58). This means allowing the phenomenon to show itself for what it really is, rather than relegating it to a secondary status in favour of theoretical explanations. Phenomenological seeing is associated with the Heideggerian (1930/1993a) notion of "letting be." For Heidegger, letting be does not imply indifference or neglect. Rather it involves engaging with the phenomena in a way that allows them to show up as what they really are.

In daseinsanalysis, employing the phenomenological approach means that the analyst permits the client's various modes of behavior to unfold on their own terms. In this way, the analyst is sensitized to the obstacles that are limiting the analysand's admission of behavior that had been previously avoided. Hence, clients are assisted in understanding how they have previously declined responsibility for their lives, and how this refusal continues to impede them presently (Condrau, 1995).

The application of this phenomenological approach to personal responsibility can be illustrated with one of Boss's cases (see Boss, 1979, p. 167ff). Boss's patient, Regula complained of the inability to form meaningful relationships with people, especially men. She frequently dreamt of being confined in a railway boxcar at the bottom of the ocean, naked and alone. According to Boss, he refrained from encouraging Regula to interpret the dream as an unconscious urge to return to an oceanic womb, or to view the ocean as representing the collective unconscious. Instead, he encouraged her "to do nothing ... except to attend to the elements of the dreams exactly as she perceived them ... [and] to ignore any meaning or context of reference that was not revealed to her perception by the things themselves in the dream" (p. 168).

Boss explained that in this straightforward manner of seeing the phenomenon, the patient was able to recognise that her whole being, dreaming and waking, was permeated by a mood of anxiety, isolation and abandonment. She also understood that her current way of Being-in-the-world has closed her off to relating to everything she encountered.

Buddhism

Let us now examine personal responsibility in the Buddhist context. The present discussion is based largely on the interpretation of the Buddha's teachings from the Theravadin tradition. The Theravadin school that has preserved the Buddha's earliest discourses is perceived as the most psychologically oriented (Rubin, 1996), and the psychology developed from these teachings is regarded as a prototype for the later schools of Buddhism (Goleman, 1988). However, references will be made to the perspectives developed by the other schools where such views enhance our understanding of the concepts under discussion.

Like Heidegger and Boss, the Buddha's teachings on responsibility take as his starting point, human existence, and the Heideggerian exposition of the "ontological difference" can assist us in understanding the Buddhist approach. Responsibility in Buddhism is based on the view that human beings are responsible for their sufferings, as these are consequent upon their own actions and it is within their own power to overcome them. The Buddha maintains that suffering is psychological, brought about by the human tendency to cling to experiences, beliefs and even to life, all of which are by their nature impermanent. According to the Buddha, if we take the responsibility to delve into the true nature of things, and apply this insight to the way we live our lives, we can learn to free ourselves. Comprehending the true nature of things involves understanding the three characteristics of existence (impermanence, non-self, and unsatisfactoriness), and dependent origination. These concepts provide the ontological foundations for personal responsibility in Buddhist psychology.

Although the Buddha emphasizes the three characteristics in relation to human beings, these hallmarks are not confined to human existence but apply equally to every phenomenon. The concept of impermanence (*anicca*) points to the idea that all phenomena including human existence is essentially changeable, in a constant of flux. The idea of non-self or insubstantiality (*anatta*) underlines the Buddhist view that the self is not a permanent entity and is made up of five aggregates (*khandas*), namely form, feelings, perceptions, consciousness and mental formations (Dhammananda, 1987). Each of these aggregates shares with all phenomena the quality of transitoriness. What this means is that the self is a process, constantly evolving and transforming as the person engages with the world. We can find echoes of this idea in the Heideggerian notion of Da-sein as a realm of openness, and as Being-in-the-world.

The third characteristic of existence, namely unsatisfactoriness (*dukkha*) forms the basis of the Buddha's teachings in the four noble truths. Although *dukkha* is usually translated in English as suffering, the term suffering fails to capture the philosophical and psychological underpinnings of *dukkha*, which while it includes ordinary suffering also incorporates the more profound ideas of impermanence, emptiness and insubstantiality (Rahula, 1978). Because of this, unsatisfactoriness is a more appropriate term for *dukkha*. In the four noble truths, the Buddha teaches that unsatisfactoriness exists; that it has an identifiable cause; that it can be terminated, and that there is a path by which unsatisfactoriness can be terminated. Underlying the idea of unsatisfactoriness is the notion of impermanence, and the message that the Buddha wants to convey is that everything is unsatisfactory because nothing remains the same forever.

In the first noble truth, the Buddha focuses on three types of unsatisfactoriness or suffering – the suffering associated daily existence such as death, aging, and disease; the suffering associated with the impermanence of sensation and experiences, and the suffering associated with the impermanence of conditioned states. The third type of suffering refers to change which takes place at the imperceptible level, for example in human bodies when each cell "rises" and "dies" naturally. No secondary condition is needed to bring about the third type of suffering, as it occurs spontaneously.

The final concept that provides the ontological foundation for responsibility is the doctrine of dependent origination. Applied to human existence, this doctrine highlights a series of psychological factors and shows how they are conditionally related to each other, that is how one thing leads to another. The importance of understanding this causal process, the Buddha says, is to give the individual the option of interrupting the cycle, so that things could be otherwise. For example when we encounter an unpleasant situation, we may react with anger. This reaction could snowball into more feelings of anger, fear and anxiety. However if we understand that anger is perpetuating all the other negative feelings, and take the responsibility to interrupt the process, either by letting go or working through the anger, the associative feelings could dissipate.

The principle of dependent origination originally applied to the aggregates that constitute the human being has been extended by the Mahayana school to everything in the phenomenal world through the concept of emptiness (*sunyata*). According to this concept "nothing exists in itself or by itself… but is dependent upon and related to everything else" (Jacobson, 1983, p. 64). Hence the Buddhist view of the world enunciated in the doctrine of dependent origination, and extended by the concept of *sunyata* is one of inter-relatedness. In recognising that everything is inter-connected and changeable, we learn not to cling to the past or be fearful of the future. In this way, we take responsibility for ourselves in the present. As Jacobson (1983) points out, in comprehending the transitoriness of life, people develop an awareness that "what is really real is each fleeting momentary now (p. 38) and learn to value each moment. We find similar sentiments expressed in Heidegger's and Boss's explanation of Da-sein as "Being-unto-death," and Boss's (1979) advice to people to take responsibility for the present as no two moments remain the same.

What gives rise to the ontic inability to take responsibility? Buddhism maintains that this is related to our failure to come to terms with the nature of reality, and is grounded on ignorance, delusion and craving. Because people are ignorant that everything is ontologically impermanent, devoid of self-existence, and unsatisfactory, they delude themselves into thinking that if they could somehow manipulate things, including life, they could find a measure of satisfaction.

This leads to the craving for and the attachment to symbols of permanency in the quest for certainty.

How does Buddhism assist the individual in taking personal responsibility? According to the Buddha by encouraging the person to see things as they are, and to respond appropriately. This takes us to the heart of the Buddhist conception of responsibility. From the Buddhist perspective, responsibility involves *respond-ability*, that is the ability to respond appropriately and skillfully. Our responsibility lies in being aware of what unique response is called for in each unique situation (Batchelor, 1990). The idea is to let go of "what should or ought to be" and to respond judiciously as opposed to acting from habitual tendencies.

Developing the ability to respond appropriately is emphasized in the ontic manifestation of responsibility and brings into play the Buddha's teachings of karma and the eightfold path. Karma means volition or action. The concept of karma involves the idea that every action produces a reaction. As Dhammananda (1987) explains, karma is not an entity but a process, "it is our doings reacting on ourselves." (p. 89). Karma also helps to address the question, "to whom and for what are we responsible?" In the Buddhist context, the "whom" and the "what" refers to the individual's responsibility for freeing his or her own mind from remorse. According to the Buddha, our actions have effects not only upon others, but more importantly on our own states of mind. In psychological terms, it means that the suffering or the happiness that we experience is a result of our own deeds, and that we are responsible for our actions. The idea of karma underscores the importance of personal responsibility and self-reliance in Buddhism.

To understand the effects of our actions, the Buddha points out that we need to learn to see things as they are. To develop this attitude of openness, he advocates a way of life lived according to the eightfold path (the fourth noble truth). According to Batchelor (1997), in this path, the Buddha recommends for the individual "not something to believe in, but something to do" (p. 17). In this sense, it is an ontic application of the Buddha's teachings concerning the cessation of human suffering, and encapsulates his teachings concerning personal responsibility.

The eightfold path consists of three aspects, namely morality, mental culture and wisdom. The morality aspect which comprises the behavioural categories of right speech, right action and right livelihood represents the ethical foundation of the path (Epstein, 1995). The word "right" used to qualify each of the eight factors of the path does not refer to moral judgments or constraints imposed from outside. It concerns taking responsibility for one's speech, actions and mental attitudes so that one gains a sense of inner peace and harmony. In this sense, right is synonymous with harmonious. In the context of morality, the Buddha advocates self-reflection and self-discipline. He counsels people to continually reflect on the consequences of their actions before proceeding and to refrain from actions that is not conducive to harmony in each situation. This is in line with his teaching that responsibility involves the ability to respond appropriately.

In the wisdom category, the Buddha advises developing right understanding and right thought. This means understanding the three characteristics of existence, the workings of karma and dependent origination. Right understanding frees us from ignorance and enables us to gain insight into ourselves and the nature of reality.

Mental culture, more commonly understood as meditation, the third aspect of the path, deals with the training of the mind to develop the wisdom and insight to overcome psychological suffering. It involves the development of right effort, right mindfulness and right concentration. In all his teachings, the Buddha emphasizes personal responsibility. But nowhere is this sense of responsibility and self-reliance more prominent than in mental culture, where the individual's opportunity for growth and happiness lies in his or her taking the responsibility to develop the mental discipline for clear thinking. We can see a parallel between the Buddha's advice to people to cultivate this frame of mind and phenomenological seeing advocated by Heidegger and Boss.

Social Responsibility

Daseinsanalysis

Social responsibility in daseinsanalysis is grounded on the following Heideggerian notions:

- Da-sein as the "shepherd of Being"
- Fourfold
- Letting be

It may be recalled that Heidegger and Boss emphasize Da-sein's ever-present concern for its own Being, and the Being of everything that it encounters (Craig 1988). In other words, Heidegger considers human beings indispensable to Being and perceives "man [Da-sein] as the shepherd of Being" (Heidegger, 1947/1993b, p. 234). According to Heidegger and Boss, seeing themselves in this guardianship role helps to motivate people to take responsibility for other beings.

Additionally, both men seek to promote social responsibility by entreating people to perceive everything as inter-related. This notion of inter-relatedness is captured in Heidegger's (1952/1971a) concept of the "fourfold" which comprises earth, sky, divinities (gods) and mortals. To understand the fourfold in relation to social responsibility, we need to look briefly at Heidegger's distinction between technological (calculative) and meditative thinking; and his idea of "letting be."

For Heidegger (1941/1993c), technological thinking refers to the utilitarian attitude that human beings adopt towards things, perceiving them as "standing reserve" (p. 17) to be used in the service of something else. This attitude,

Heidegger (1959/1966) points out, has given rise to calculative thinking, that is thinking that continually computes things in terms of means-ends. To move away from this materialistic attitude, Heidegger recommends meditative thinking, that is the adoption of an attitude that reflects on the meaningfulness of everything, and permits this meaningfulness to show itself to us. Meditative thinking, Heidegger (1959/1966) explains, allows us to dwell in the world in a totally different way, by "letting be" (p. 61). For Heidegger, "letting be" in relation to social responsibility does not infer indifference or passivity. Instead it entails fostering a contemplative attitude towards the phenomena that we encounter and allowing them to unfold naturally. In this sense, "letting be" is a corollary of phenomenological seeing.

According to Heidegger, people let things be by permitting them to manifest themselves as a unique confluence of the fourfold (Cooper, 1996). In his oft-quoted example of the water-jug, Heidegger (1950/1971b) explains that the outpouring from the jug, whether of wine or water, reflects the gathering of the four elements – "the earth nourishment," "the sky's sun" (p. 172), the beneficiaries (human beings) who consume the wine, and the divinities (gods) to whom it offered as libation. Hence, the fourfold represents a way of appreciating interrelatedness. When we see things as assemblages of the fourfold, we learn to care for things as part of a whole and comprehend their relationship with everything else. Heidegger and Boss believe that this caretaker's role lessens people's tendency to impose their will on things and to conceive of the world in utilitarian terms. It promotes a meditative attitude of letting things be and encourages people to become socially more responsible.

Buddhism

In Buddhist psychology, social responsibility is grounded on the notions of:

- *Karma*
- Interrelatedness (dependent origination, *sunyata*)
- Compassion

In the discussion on personal responsibility, we have seen how the concept of karma, the "law of cause and effect" encourages people to be mindful of the effects of their actions so as to avoid triggering off a chain of negative reactions o the detriment of their own peace of mind. In the social context, people are also encouraged to be mindful of the effects of their actions on others. This is not because human beings are responsible for others, but because by living "right" their actions are less likely to engender negative consequences for others.

The application of karma in the social arena is an extension of the concepts of dependent origination and *sunyata*. It may be recalled that the ideas of dependent origination and *sunyata* emphasize the indissoluble unity of human beings with all other beings, and the inter-connectedness of all phenomena. Collectively, these three ideas reinforce the need for the individual to take social responsibility. When we understand that we are not an enclosed entity, but are intimately connected with all beings in the universe, we learn to be responsible to ourselves and to others.

Comprehending the inter-relatedness of everything leads to compassion, another important theme in the Buddhist approach to social responsibility. In Buddhism, every form and phenomenon is considered to have equal merit (Zimmerman, 1993). The practice of compassion is based on this equality of self and others (Batchelor, 1983). The Dalai Lama (1997) explains that genuine compassion is not founded on pity or love, but from "a respect for all beings, and a realisation that others have a right to be happy and to overcome suffering just as you" (p. 134). Out of this sense of empathy and an awareness of the organic unity of the world we develop a sense of caring and responsibility that is extended spontaneously to all beings.

The parallels and differences between the daseinsanalytic and Buddhist perspectives on responsibility point to various major contributions that Buddhism and daseinsanalysis can make to each other.

Enlargement of Responsibility

With personal responsibility, daseinsanalysis is more concerned with responsibility in terms of choices. Although Boss recognises that not all human possibilities can be carried out, he maintains that nevertheless, it is the individual's responsibility to make choices on the basis of his or her particular existence. Buddhism on the other hand is more concerned with appropriate responses. In the Buddhist context, there is less emphasis on individual resolve and will. Here, the relevant question is not "What are my possibilities and how do I choose," but rather "What is an appropriate response to the situation or the phenomenon that I am encountering." Sometimes this calls for action, and sometimes for non-action. In my view, our *ability to respond* grounds our *ability to take responsibility*.

The differences between the daseinsanalytic "responsibility" and the Buddhist "respond-ability" suggest how our understanding of responsibility can be refined and enlarged. In Western psychology, responsibility is generally conceived in pro-active terms, as doing something, rather than refraining from actions. Non-action and passivity are often disparaged as indifference. The Buddhist notion of respond-ability shows that restraint is a positive way of being responsible when it is warranted by the situation (Khong, 1999).

In terms of social responsibility, there are many parallels between the Heideggerian, daseinsanalytic and Buddhist perspectives concerning inter-relatedness. Heidegger, Boss and the Buddha promote social responsibility through a profound appreciation of the oneness of everything. In this sense, all three have much in common. There are two important albeit subtle differences. These differences point to the ways that Buddhism can expand the scope of social responsibility in daseinsanalysis.

The first difference relates to the role that Heidegger and Boss envisage for human beings in the grand scheme of things. Both men place humankind at the apex, as having the responsibility for other beings, and in the unique role of acting as a clearing for Being. Although, this approach is evidently a step in the right direction in reducing humankind's tendency to impose their will upon nature and the environment, it is still relatively anthropocentric and hierarchical. In this respect, the Buddhist stance on social responsibility can make a significant contribution.

Pivotal to the Buddha's teaching is the parity between all sentient beings (Gyatso, 1995). From this perspective, the human being is important, but only as a link in the chain, and not as the most essential one. We can well imagine Heidegger or Boss saying to a person, "You are important and you have responsibility *for* other beings." On the other hand, the Buddha would probably say to the same person, "You and other beings are equally important, and your responsibility is to ensure that your own actions do not engender negative consequences for other beings." The Heideggerian and daseinsanalytic approaches to social responsibility have an element of a hierarchy of sentience which is absent from the Buddhist perspective.

The other important difference lies in the emphasis that Buddhism places on social responsibility as a continuum of personal responsibility. The Buddha teaches that "protecting oneself, one protects others, protecting others, one protect oneself" (Samyutta Nikaya V:148). So from a Buddhist perspective, responsibility starts with the individual. Understanding the law of cause and effect, interrelatedness, non-self and compassion, this sense of responsibility for oneself is extended *reflexively* to all beings to whom we are inextricably connected socially and ecologically. This intimate relationship between personal and social responsibility appears to be absent from Heidegger's and Boss's approaches to social responsibility. As I pointed out earlier, their promotion of social responsibility is intended to reduce people's technological attitude. In this sense, social responsibility is regarded as an invaluable addendum to, rather than a spontaneous extension of personal responsibility.

Foundation for the Psychology of Change

Both the daseinsanalytic and Buddhist expositions on the human concern with impermanence and change complement each other in so far as they show that this concern is a universal phenomenon. However there is a significant difference. Daseinsanalysis focuses on the transitoriness of human existence, Buddhism on the transitoriness of all phenomena.

As I pointed out earlier, Boss and Heidegger counsel people not to avoid or level down the contemplation of their own mortality, but to accept death, the ultimate change, as a real possibility and to take responsibility for their lives. The Buddha encourages people to take responsibility because nothing remains the same, period. As Zimmerman (1993) puts it, in Buddhism, "no particular moment is privileged" (p. 255). Death per se does not feature as prominently in Buddhist thinking as it does in daseinsanalysis. People are counselled to live responsibly in spite of death, rather than in anticipation of it. This difference in focus leads to the difference in the advice proffered by daseinsanalysis and Buddhism on how to cope with change.

According to Boss, if we *accept death as natural and inevitable*, we can learn to deal with our ontic attempts to avoid it. Resolutely anticipating death, Boss notes, helps people live authentically, since it inculcates in them the ability to look at their lives holistically, and to evaluate future possibilities in the face of this eventuality. Hence daseinsanalysis encourages people to be aware of changes, and the necessity of making choices in light of these changes. By emphasizing choice however, the idea of having to change could be construed as one of many possibilities. Perceiving change as a possibility can delude people into thinking that changing is optional. In this way, it conceals the inescapable nature of change and gives the illusion of choice when there is really none. In reality, whether people elect to change or not, change impinges. Take the example of aging. There is tendency in contemporary society for people to delude themselves that they have a choice about aging, triggering off such associative thinking as "Why me?" or "How can I prevent it?" Consequently, we see frantic attempts by people to stay young, and to stave off the process of aging.

The Buddha posits another way of helping people to deal with change – by showing that our inability to cope with it is part of our failure to come to terms with impermanence. In Buddhist psychology, people are assisted in dealing with change, not by seeing it as a possibility, but by understanding change as ontological and inevitable, i.e., that it is in the nature of things. The Buddha teaches not just living with the awareness of change, but living with change per se. If *we accept change as natural and inevitable*, it can help us to overcome the fear of change. Then we move on and respond to changes of all kinds. In the case of aging if we accept that aging impinges on everyone and that it is a natural and inevitable process, we learn to respond to it, rather than resist it.

The Buddha's intention is to help us accept change gracefully and to let go of things when they come to pass. Its meditative practice of mindfulness increases our awareness of the nature of the mind and of reality, and enables us to experience change as ontological and spontaneous. It also helps us to realise that change *per se* does not cause suffering. It is our attitude toward change that can. By contemplating life in a more open and accepting manner, rather than focusing on specific issues, we learn to appreciate the relativity of the situation, and to refine our responses to each passing moment. The Buddhist approach can provide a radical and profound foundation for the psychology of change, not only for daseinsanalysis, but for psychotherapy in general.

Daseinsanalytic and Buddhist Practices

In daseinsanalysis, Heidegger's phenomenological approach has been adopted in therapy. Boss (1963) explains that the phenomenological approach of returning "to the things themselves" allows both analyst and analysand "to remain with the [person's] undistorted perceptions, and to let the phenomena speak for themselves and show us their ... meanings." (p. 59). The attitude of "even hovering attention" that Freud recommends for therapists to adopt towards their clients has also been incorporated into daseinsanalysis (Condrau, 1995). Boss explains that for the therapist it encompasses amongst other things, the ability to be clear-minded and "to hear" beyond what is being verbalized. (Boss, 1984–1985, p. 122).

These daseinsanalytic approaches require both analyst and analysand to maintain an open attitude and accords with the Buddha's call for us to see and accept things as they are. Both disciplines promote a spontaneous awareness of experience without linguistic filters and conceptualizations. Boss points to the need for such an attitude but did not articulate a method for fostering it. We know that our responses to what we perceive and experience are often colored by our psychological makeup. Rubin (1996) argues that it is a fallacy to think that we can listen and observe in this open manner "without quieting the mind" (p. 124). Given the emphasis that Buddhism and daseinsanalysis place on returning to the things themselves, Buddhist meditative techniques are highly appropriate for both therapists and clients, and Buddhist meditation can complement the daseinsanalytic therapeutic approach.

In meditation and in particular with the practice of mindfulness, a person learns to focus the mind on one object to the exclusion of others. In this way, the mind is trained to settle down by letting go of internal running commentary. This can aid the kind of quiet listening so crucial to phenomenological seeing and constant attentiveness. According to Epstein (1995), if a therapist can sit silently with a client without an agenda, without anticipating what is going to happen next, clients are encouraged to enter and to explore new territories, or revisit old ones at their own pace. The silence fostered in meditation can contribute to an environment that can facilitate the openness that Boss recommends for therapists to adopt.

Additionally, during meditation, people are encouraged to remain detached towards what is being observed, neither rejecting, repressing nor identifying with them. They are given the barest of attention. In this way, people develop the ability to "stand back" and separate their experiences from their thoughts, feelings and emotions. For both therapist and client, mindfulness enables them to focus on what is experienced in a non-judgmental way and enhances the capacity for quiet listening.

When meditation is practiced alongside phenomenological seeing, the result is that you have a powerful and incisive therapetic "tool" for clients to use, to isolate the core phenomena from their emotions and feelings, and for the therapists to understand clients' experiences free from theoretical explanations and assumptions. In this way, Buddhist meditation can provide a practical hands-on-approach for the phenomenological stance recommended by Boss.

While Buddhist meditation can strengthen daseinsanalytic therapeutic practices, daseinsanalysis can also contribute to Buddhism. As I noted earlier, Buddhism lacks the techniques for dealing with specific impairments that prevent people from taking responsibility. Kornfield (1993) notes that certain developmental issues and unhealthy psychological defenses may require the help of a skilled therapist to uncover and resolved. The advantage of daseinsanalysis is that it addresses specific impairments that often meditation alone cannot overcome. For example, the daseinsanalytic practice of assisting clients to see the ontic ways by which they have avoided taking responsibility, and how this refusal continues to impede them is particularly useful in helping people to deal with blockages that have arisen.

The other advantage of daseinsanalytic practices lies in their helping the client to understand the meaningfulness and therapeutic significance of his or her experiences in relation to the person's whole existence. In the case of Regula discussed earlier, Boss helped her to see that her dream experience of being stuck in a railway boxcar, alone and naked, shows that she perceived the world as dark and desolate, and herself as a forgotten piece of merchandise. He also helped her to become aware that as a consequence of her attunement of anxiety and insecurity, and her feelings of abandonment, she was unable to form healthy relationships with people. Gaining insight in her restricted way of Being-in-the-world, Regula was able to take responsibility for a different way of behaving. This approach towards understanding and dealing with specific impairments is absent from Buddhism.

Empowerment of Clients

According to Condrau (1995), the daseinsanalytic method of "analytical self-recognition" (p. 347) is designed to take the patient to the point where he or she is able to assume personal responsibility. However, without equipping clients with the means to sustain phenomenological seeing, it could be difficult for them to assume this responsibility beyond therapy. Clients clearly need to develop the skills to "decipher" their own experiences. Unfortunately, current daseinsanalytic practices do not equip them with the techniques do so. Buddhist meditation on the other hand, promotes a "do-it-yourself" approach, and insight is perceived as coming from self-observation, rather than from the therapist. Additionally, as meditation can be practised in any setting, clients will be able to sustain this phenomenological seeing. Meditation can therefore serve as a lifelong adjunct for helping people to take responsibility beyond therapy.

In empowering clients to take responsibility, we need to distinguish between the ability to see the problem, and the ability to bear the problem that this insight brings. In addition to learning to see things realistically, the Buddha also encourages people to accept them as they are. Acceptance does not imply becoming passive or fatalistic. It means learning to see the situation realistically and to come to terms with what the situation calls for. Take again the example of death. Daseinsanalysis believe that people cannot transcend existential anxiety concerning death. At best, they can become aware of their fear of death (Boss, 1962). Adopting a different approach, Buddhism maintains that people can learn to accept death without anxiety while they are still alive (Rhee, 1992). Acceptance involves the insight that transitoriness or impermanence affects not only human beings, but every phenomenon in the world. As Dhammananda (1995) expresses it poignantly, "Inevitably I am going to die – so does every plant, every form, every living being.... Soon it will be autumn, the leaves will fall off the trees. We do not cry, it is natural, that is what leaves are supposed to do at the end of the season. Human beings experience the same thing" (p. 27). In other words, if I understand and accept *now* that I am not exempt from what the Buddha refers to as possessing the nature "to rise and pass away" (Samyutta Nikaya. I: 158), then the anxiety concerning this happening to me can dissipate.

The Case of Therese

Therese was diagnosed with cancer about five years ago. After receiving medical attention, she sought counselling to come to terms with her illness psychologically. Therese spoke of her varying emotions regarding her illness, such as anger, fear, and resentment, and wanted to find a way to prevent these negative thoughts from spiralling into depression.

Using the concentration techniques of Buddhist meditation, Therese trained her mind to calm down. She also learned to simply observe and accept what she was experiencing from moment to moment without falling into the habitual tendency of judging these experiences as good or bad. In this phenomenological and mindful way of seeing things, she able to experience each emotion for what it is, for example "anger as anger," and "fear as fear." By making space for these responses, but not reacting to them, Therese was able to isolate the core phenomenon, i.e., her illness, from her responses to her illness. She was experiencing a different way of being in the world, one that entailed action, but more importantly, restraint when appropriate.

Therese was encouraged to observe and experience change in nature. She reported that once when she was feeling depressed about her increasing loss of hair, she focused her attention on a deciduous tree that was shedding its leaves, and observed the changing forms of the passing clouds. Her experiences with impermanence in nature were deeply moving and profound and she gained the insight that change, including death, is natural and inevitable. In Buddhist terms, Therese had realised for herself the Buddha's advice that if a person can see and accept change universally, it will be easier to accept change at the personal level. Experiencing change in this way, she spoke of a feeling of oneness and interrelatedness with the universe, and a lessening sense of isolation and alienation. Therese appeared to have cultivated a way of understanding and relating to the world that Heidegger would describe as meditative thinking.

Therese is now in remission. She attributed her "cure" to the fact that while the medical profession helped her with her physical symptoms, her priest with her spirituality, meditation and her meditative attitude towards life helped her gained an inner peace of mind. Therese has succinctly summed up an approach to mental health that Marsella (1982) would term as "harmony among parts." (p. 366).

Therese's case evinces the efficacy of integrating comparable daseinsanalytic and Buddhist practices and ideas into an approach that helps to empower the individual to take responsibility. The daseinsanalytic practice of phenomenological seeing and the Buddhist meditative practice of concentration and mindfulness enabled her to separate her illness from her fear of dying. However being able to see the issues does not ensure that she accepts her situation. The Buddhist practice of experiencing change as ontological assisted her in coming to terms with the knowledge that she is not exempt from this natural and inevitable process. This insight helped her to relate the ontological situation (that everything is impermanent) to her ontic situation (that she is impermanent) and enabled her to let go of her attachment to life. Hence, for Therese, the possibility of dying no longer poses an issue and she was able get on with living.

Conclusion

This comparative analysis demonstrates that daseinsanalysis and Buddhism are fundamentally compatible and that there is a genuine basis for an authentic, healthy engagement through an enlarged notion of responsibility, since each perspective is made more meaningful by an understanding of the other. The Buddha's teachings relating to impermanence, non-self, unsatisfactoriness, karma, compassion, and inter-relatedness can expand the scope of responsibility in daseinsanalysis. The Heideggerian notion of the ontological difference (i.e., the difference between the ontological and the ontic) facilities our understanding of responsibility in the Buddhist context, while daseinsanalytic therapy augments the Buddhist lack of techniques in dealing with specific impairments of responsibility and lends itself as a vehicle for the application of Buddhist ideas in psychotherapy. An integration of these two disciplines will make their ideas and practices more accessible to communities outside their traditional domains. The daseinsanalytic and Buddhist perspectives relating to personal and social responsibility provide us with valuable philosophical and psychological insights into this very important human phenomenon and show us practically how individuals can be assisted in taking responsibility for every moment of their existence, and to develop a sense of respond-ability to different situations. As Therese's case demonstrates, responsibility is not an option but a prerequisite to self-understanding and personal growth.

References

Batchelor, S. (1983). *Alone with others.* New York: Grove Press.

Batchelor, S. (1997). *Buddhism without beliefs.* New York: Riverhead Books.

Boss, M. (1962). Anxiety, guilt and psychotherapeutic liberation. *Review of Existential Psychology and Psychiatry, 2*(3), 173–207.

Boss, M. (1963). *Psychoanalysis and daseinsanalysis.* (L. B. Lefebre, Trans.). New York: Basic Books.

Boss, M. (1965). *A psychiatrist discovers India.* (H. A. Frey, Trans.). London: Oswald Wolff.

Boss, M. (1979). *Existential foundations of medicine and psychology.* S. Conway & A. Cleaves (Trans.). New York: Jason Aronson.

Boss, M. (1984–1985). Is psychotherapy rational or rationalistic? *Review of Existential Psychology and Psychiatry, 19*(2–3), 115–127.

Boss, M. (1988). Recent considerations in daseinsanalysis. In E. Craig (Ed.), Psychotherapy for freedom: The daseinsanalytic way in psychology and psychoanalysis. [Special Issue]. *The Humanistic Psychologist, 16*(1), 58–74.

Condrau, G. (1995). Daseinsanalysis as psychotherapy. *Proceedings of the 16th International Congress of Psychotherapy* (pp.341–347). Seoul, Republic of Korea: Korean Academy of Psychotherapists.

Cooper, D. E. (1996). *Thinkers of Our Time: Heidegger.* London: Claridge Press.

Craig, E. (1988). Daseinsanalysis: A quest for essentials. In E. Craig (Ed.), Psychotherapy for freedom: The daseinsanalytic way in psychology and psychoanalysis [Special Issue]. *The Humanistic Psychologist, 16*(1), 1–21.

Dalai Lama. (1997). *The four noble truths.* (G. T. Jinpa, Trans.). Hammersmith: Thorsons.

De Silva, P. (1996). Buddhism and behavior change: Implications for therapy. In G. Claxton (Ed.), *Beyond Therapy* (pp. 217–231). Dorset: Prism Press.

Dhammananda, K. S. (1987). *What Buddhists believe* (4th ed.). Kuala Lumpur: Buddhist Missionary Society.

Dhammananda, K. S. (1995). *Life is uncertain-death is certain.* Malaysia: Buddhist Missionary Society.

Epstein, M. (1995). *Thoughts without a thinker*. New York: Basic Books.

Goleman, D. (1988). *The meditative mind*. Los Angeles: Jeremy. P. Tarcher.

Gyatso, T. (1995). *Universal responsibility and the good heart*. (4th ed.) Dharamsala: Library of Tibetan Works & Archives.

Heidegger, M. (1962). *Being and time*. (J. Macquarrie & E. Robinson, Trans.). Oxford: Basil Blackwell. (Original work published 1927)

Heidegger, M. (1966). *Discourse on thinking: A translation of Gelassenheit*. (J. M. Anderson & E. H. Freund, Trans.). New York: Harper & Row. (Original work published in 1959)

Heidegger, M. (1971a). Building, dwelling, thinking. In *Poetry, language, thought*, (A. Hofstadter, Trans.) (pp. 145–161). New York: Harper & Row. (Original lecture given in 1952)

Heidegger, M. (1971b). The thing. In *Poetry, language, thought* (A. Hofstadter Trans.) (pp. 165–186). New York: Harper & Row. (Original lecture given in 1950)

Heidegger, M. (1972). *Time and being* (J. Stambaugh, Trans.). New York: Harper & Row. (Original work published in 1969)

Heidegger, M. (1988). On adequate understanding of daseinsanalysis (M. Eldred, Trans.). In E. Craig (Ed.), Psychotherapy for freedom: The daseinsanalytic way in psychology and psychoanalysis [Special Issue] *The Humanistic Psychologist, 16*(1), 75–98.

Heidegger, M. (1993a). On the essence of truth. (J. Sallis, Trans.). In D. F. Krell (Ed.), *Martin Heidegger: Basic writings* (pp. 115–138). (Rev. ed.). London: Routledge. (Original lecture given in 1930)

Heidegger, M. (1993b). Letter on humanism (F. A. Capuzzi & J. G. Gray, Trans.). In D. F. Krell (Ed.), *Martin Heidegger: Basic writings* (pp. 213–265) (Rev. ed.). London: Routledge. (Original work published in 1947)

Heidegger, M. (1993c). *Basic concepts* (G. E. Aylesworth, Trans.). Bloomington: Indiana University Press. (Original lectures given in 1941)

Holzhey-Kunz, A. (1996). What defines the daseinsanalytic process? *Journal of the Society for Existential Analysis, 8*(1), 93–104.

Jacobson, N. P. (1983). *Buddhism and the contemporary world: Change and self-correction*. Carbondale: Southern Illinois University Press.

Khong, B. S. L. (1999). *A comparative analysis of the concept of responsibility in daseinsanalysis and Buddhist psychology*. Unpublished doctoral dissertation. Macquarie University. Sydney, Australia.

Kornfield, J. (1993). *A path with heart*. New York: Bantam Books.

Lee, Z. N. (1995). Tao in view of daseinsanalysis. In *Proceedings of the 16th International Congress of Psychotherapy* (pp. 365–369). (Rev. ed.) Seoul, South Korea: Korean Academy of Psychotherapists.

Marsella, A. J. (1982). Culture and mental health: An Overview. In A. J. Marsella and G. M. White (Eds.), *Cultural conceptions of mental health and therapy*. (pp. 359–388). Dordrecht: D. Reidel Publishing Company.

McLeod, W.T. (Ed.). (1987). *The new Collins dictionary and thesaurus*. London: Collins.

Muhall, S. (1996). *Heidegger and being and time*. London: Routledge.

Rahula, W. (1978). *What the Buddha taught* (Rev. ed.). London: The Gordon Fraser Gallery.

Rhee, D. (1992, May). *The Tao and empathy: East Asian interpretation*. Paper presented at the 136th annual meeting of the American Academy of Psychologists.

Rubin, J. B. (1996). *Psychotherapy and Buddhism. Toward an integration*. New York: Plenum Press.

Samyutta Nikaya, (Ed.) K.S. Dhammananda (1994) *Treasure of the Dhamma*. Kuala Lumpur: Buddhist Missionary Society.

Zimmerman, M. E. (1993). Heidegger, Buddhism, and deep ecology. In. C. E. Guignon (Ed.), *Cambridge companion to Heidegger* (pp. 240–269). Cambridge: Cambridge University Press.

Chapter 7

Classical Buddhist Model of a Healthy Mind

Richard P. Hayes

Introductory Remarks

Since the Buddha taught in India more than 2500 years ago, his followers have divided into countless divisions over dozens of issues, both practical and theoretical. To speak of Buddhism as a whole is therefore to run the risk of making the error that each of the blind men made in the famous Buddhist parable, namely, making the mistake of thinking that what is true of a part of an elephant is true of the entire animal. Let me say at the outset, then, that what follows is an attempt to be true to the contemplative and scholastic traditions of Buddhism with which I am most familiar. Other Buddhists would almost surely describe Buddhist practices, and perhaps even some Buddhist goals, differently.

The principal concern of the Buddha as he is portrayed in the canonical texts of India and Southeast Asia is the elimination of frustration. Frustration, observed the Buddha, arises when people (and other living beings) fail to get what they strive for, and when they are confronted with what they do not welcome. The task of reducing frustration could be approached in either of two ways. One way would be to devote most of one's energy to getting everything that one wishes to have and avoiding everything one finds unpleasant. This strategy involves, in effect, making the universe conform to one's will. Given that the universe is a large place, and notorious for being difficult to bend to one's will, this strategy is more likely to increase one's frustrations than to reduce them. The Buddha, therefore, suggested that a more successful strategy would be to adjust one's expectations to conform to reality. Rather than striving to acquire everything that one wishes to have, said the Buddha, one should strive to reduce one's wishes. Similarly, rather than working to rid the world of everything that one finds obnoxious, one should work to rid oneself of the tendency to find things obnoxious. If one succeeds in making the necessary changes, the result is a mentality that is flexible enough to adapt to changing realities. Such a mentality is open to a wide range of possibilities and competent to heal itself and benefit others. In short, such a mentality is said to be *kusala*, a Pali word that means healthy, fit and capable. This type of mentality is also the goal of psychotherapy. Modern psychology recognizes the frustrations identified by the Buddha and offers therapies to reduce them. This chapter will present the Buddha's path to the healthy mind sought by both Buddhist practitioners and those who practice psychotherapy.

Changing one's mentality, as everyone knows who has tried to do it, is not an easy task. It requires more than simply deciding to improve. Because the task is complex, Buddhists devised a number of programs to help people improve their outlooks and cultivate more realistic expectations. What will be described below is an outline of a representative classical Buddhist program for transforming the human mentality from one that is rigid, closed and prone to injuring itself and others to one that is healthy and resilient. As I hope will become clear, the traditional Buddhist methods of self-cultivation are at every stage closely connected with taking care of others. Ideally there is in the Buddhist view no distinction, and certainly no conflict, between serving one's own best interests and serving the best interests of others.

The Classical Program

Traditionally the Buddhist path has been divided into three phases: ethics, contemplation and wisdom. Ethical guidelines, which have to do with the individual's interactions with other human and non-human beings, help the practitioner avoid actions that naturally lead to guilt, shame, remorse and other unpleasant mental states. A mentality that is relatively free of such negativity is said to be more capable of enduring the demands of contemplation. This is a process of quiet reflection leading to a heightened awareness of one's own physical and psychological conditions. This quiet reflection then culminates in the cultivation of wisdom. Wisdom itself also has three phases: study, reflection and cultivation. Study involves learning what various sages have had to say about the successful conduct of life. Reflection involves making an honest inquiry into fundamental questions of value by comparing one's own life to the standards set by sages and becoming aware of what specifically one has to do to make one's life more harmonious and contented. Cultivation consists in making the determination to change one's thinking by acquiring those attitudes that lead consistently to fulfillment. This leads in turn to changing one's habits of acting and speaking. When the path is pursued to the end, it comes full circle to where it began: living ethically in the world. The difference between ethics at the beginning and at the end of this process is that the initial stages tend to be consciously governed by following prescribed rules and guidelines, whereas ethics at the end pours spontaneously out of habitual and deeply ingrained feelings of love, joy and compassion. This process reflects the commonly expressed Buddhist conviction that one cannot benefit oneself without benefiting others, and one cannot benefit others without benefiting oneself. With that as a quick overview, let me now look more closely at some of the features of this traditional program.

Ethics

The beginning of the Buddhist path involves developing good habits *(sãla)* or good character. Good behavior begins with good intentions, a good intention being the wish to do what benefits oneself and others. The most fundamental kind of karma consists in just this motivation. According to Buddhist theory, all pleasant feelings and all comfortable experiences ultimately arise from one's moments of wishing well for self and others. Conversely, the fact that experiences are perceived as unpleasant and uncomfortable originates in an attitude of some kind of negativity. The negativity may take the form of greed, of resistance or of confusion – these three mental factors are said to be the principal source of all other forms of negativity. Other forms of negativity that are commonly listed are competitiveness, dogmatism, irresolution, laziness, excitement, shamelessness and immodesty.

The positive or negative valence of one's intentions usually manifests as speech or bodily actions. For example, negativity, such as competitiveness (the compulsion to compare oneself to others and one's achievements to those of others), may give rise to belittling others by drawing attention to their shortcomings or even by fabricating unflattering stories about them. Negativity such as resistance may take the form of anger or even hatred, which may manifest itself as sarcastic or scathing speech, or as inflicting physical harm or even death on another living being. From positive intentions, on the other hand, spring acts of generosity and other actions that promote feelings of harmony in oneself and others. These observations are summarized in the often-quoted opening verses of the Dhammapada (1987, p. 13):

> Preceded by perception are mental states,
> For them is perception supreme,
> From perception have they sprung.
> If, with perception polluted, one speaks or acts,
> Thence suffering follows
> As a wheel the draught ox's foot.

Preceded by perception are mental states,
For them is perception supreme,
From perception have they sprung.
If, with tranquil perception, one speaks or acts,
Thence ease follows
As a shadow that never departs.

The first steps to be taken towards speaking or acting "with tranquil perception" are to follow the behavioral guidelines offered in the ten precepts. These precepts are usually given in the form of kinds of conduct to avoid. Three kinds of physical misconduct to be avoided are killing, stealing and harmful sensuality. Four kinds of verbal misconduct to avoid are lying, harsh speech, slander and idle chatter. Three kinds of mental incompetence to avoid are covetousness, malevolence and wrong views. All ten of these forms of incompetent use of the body, speech or mind result in negative feelings, such as remorse, that make it difficult to concentrate the mind. More to the point, they produce a generally unpleasant mindscape that is liable to be uncomfortable to inhabit when one's defenses have been lowered through the elimination of external distractions. On the other hand, when one's external behavior is less harmful, then feelings of guilt and remorse decline, and spending quiet time with oneself becomes less daunting.

Meditation

Despite the constantly growing body of literature available on Buddhist meditation, some misconceptions about it continue to circulate. Perhaps one of the most persistent of the inaccurate notions of Buddhist meditation is that it is a passive process of keeping the mind blank. In fact, there are many types of contemplative exercise used by Buddhists. All of these types fall into two broad categories on the basis of the immediate goal of the person doing the practice.

The first of these broad categories includes exercises that one does for the sake of achieving a state of dispassionate calm. Specifically, the first goal is to arrive at a flow of mental states that are relatively free of five kinds of hindrance: sensual desire, restlessness, irresolution, laziness and hatred. Before one can begin to work on eliminating these states, of course, one has to recognize when they are present and what effects they are having. So the most fundamental principle of Buddhist meditation is that one must be fully honest with oneself about what one is observing in one's own mind. When one is irritated, then one must know and admit that one is irritated. When this irritation is allowed to evolve into anger or hatred, then one must fully acknowledge that fact.

Once a hindrance to tranquility is recognized, then one can employ various methods to work on getting past it. One may, for example, reflect on ways in which the mental state feels uncomfortable. Just feeling how unpleasant a mood feels may be sufficient to make one drop it. Alternatively, one may think of real or imagined characters that are admirably free of these negative tendencies. Many Buddhists find it helpful just to look at a statue of a meditating Buddha with a slightly smiling serene countenance. Others may reflect on descriptions of the Buddha, or a living teacher or even a character from a novel or play or cinema, as a person with a remarkably calm and friendly disposition. The method by which one achieves the elimination of the hindrances is less important than the result of being free of them. The hindrances are so called because they hinder the ability of the mind to concentrate on a single object. Once the mind is capable of maintaining a focus on a single topic, it may begin to feel deeply contented and restful, open to watching whatever arises without fear or judgment.

Although achieving a state of calm and focused alertness is very pleasant, the Buddha repeatedly made it clear that being in this state is not the end of contemplative practice. It is a valuable state to be in, for it gives one a direct experience of how pleasant it can be to be even momentarily free of worry, longing and disapproval, and this pleasantness may inspire one to strive to be in such a state of mind much more often. It may even help one form the habit of getting into that state quickly. Despite these benefits, being in a state of concentration does not in itself do much to eliminate the more deeply rooted habits of thinking that get one into troublesome moods when events do not conform to one's wishes and expectations. Uprooting deeply entrenched habits requires a change in the way one sees experience, and this change is best achieved by the application of insight. Gaining insight is the task of the second broad category of Buddhist meditative exercise.

As we saw above, a principal observation of the Buddha was that frustration arises when people fail to get what they strive for. It is also be said that frustration arises when people do get what they strive for but then grow tired of it or find that getting it leaves them feeling still unsatisfied. Insight consists in seeing clearly, by reflecting on one's previous experiences, what kinds of accomplishment are, and which are not, capable of providing satisfaction. Much of the Buddhist program of meditation is based on the observation that very little, when examined carefully and honestly, provides the degree of satisfaction that it first shows promise of delivering. To recognize that this is so, and then to have the courage to stop striving for what finally yields only frustration, is to enter the domain of wisdom.

Wisdom

As was mentioned above, wisdom is traditionally said to evolve in the three phases of study, reflection, then cultivation. Study consists in hearing or reading discussions of virtue. Reflection entails thinking about those teachings and applying them in some detail to one's own living situations. Cultivation involves developing in oneself the virtues that one has heard discussed and making them a habitual part of one's own character. Wisdom means realizing virtue, in the sense of making it real or actual. Wisdom is said to be the antidote of fruitless outlook.[1] The stock formulation for fruitless outlook is to entertain the following thoughts: "There is nothing given, nothing offered, nothing sacrificed; no fruit and result of good and bad actions; no this world, no other world; no mother, no father; no beings who are reborn spontaneously; no good and virtuous recluses and Brahmins who have themselves realised by direct knowledge and declare this world and the other world" (*The Middle Length Discourses of the Buddha*, 1995, p. 381). According to traditional commentaries, all these propositions have some connection to denying that one's actions have eventual consequences either in this life or in some future life. The propositions concerning parents and recluses and Brahmins amount to denials that one has mentors from whom to learn what is important about the cultivation of good character.

It is said in many Buddhist texts that the ultimate source of frustration is ignorance about virtue. This ignorance is said in some texts to arise from associating with the wrong kinds of people. The elimination of ignorance, therefore, requires that one begin to seek out associations with good people (*sap-puriso*), with people who are true friends *kalyàõa-mitta*). It could be said that the principal purpose of the Buddhist community is to be a collection of good friends who together show the rest of the world the joyous benefits that arise from living together in harmony. This is true of the community of monks and nuns, but it is no less true of the community of lay Buddhists.

A Good Society of Good Friends

The early Buddhist literature naturally set the tone for most of the forms of Buddhism that later evolved. This early literature is filled with advice for those who renounce the world to lead a homeless life, but it also contains much of value for those who choose to remain in the world to raise families and pursue careers. Much of this advice is given by means of narrative accounts of early times. Such stories bear many of the marks of satire and irony and were probably meant to amuse as well as to edify. Some of the stories are obviously parodies of stories found in earlier Indian literature, such as the Veda and the Upanishads. Like all myths, these stories were meant to instill values in their hearers. Several of the early Buddhist myths deal with the ideal society. One of the most important of these is a text called "The Lion's Roar on the Turning of the Wheel" (Cakkavatti-Sãhanàda Sutta).

[1] The Pali term *micchà-diññhi* is usually translated "wrong view." Some have rendered it "distorted vision." The word *micchà* has several meanings, among them "false, wrong, counterproductive, fruitless, barren." Given that many people tend to think of views as opinions or doctrines, I prefer to translate the second word as "outlook," since, as we shall see, the propositions here have more to do with a basic outlook on life than with articles in a creed.

(*Thus I Have Heard: The Long Discourses of the Buddha*, 1987a).[2] This is one of several texts in the Pali canon that gives advice to kings and other heads of government.

Advice for a Government

Without retelling the entire story in the "The Lion's Roar on the Turning of the Wheel," let me summarize the essential points. This text tells the story of a king who lived long ago. Concerned about keeping his kingdom intact, he sought the advice of wise men, who told him that everything would be fine so long as he sought the counsel of sober people of high integrity and so long as he made sure to provide for the needs of the poor. The king followed this advice, and for seven generations his descendants followed his example. Eventually, however, one of his descendants began to neglect the poor. As a consequence of this neglect, poverty became increasingly widespread. As poverty spread, the poor had no means of making a living, so some of them began to steal from those who had what they needed. In order to forestall the increase in theft, the king introduced capital punishment for theft. Thieves then began to arm themselves to protect themselves from the police. This led to a general increase in weapons among the populace, for people with property took up arms to protect themselves against the thieves. As more and more people took up weapons, murder increased among the population. As crime increased, law enforcement became more stringent. People fearing arrest began to lie. Meanwhile, some people saw an opportunity to get their rivals into trouble with the law and began making accusations against their neighbors. This eventually led to a breakdown in people's trust for one another. As trust eroded, animosity increased. As animosity increased, people's thinking became more careless. This carelessness led to people no longer respecting their parents and teachers. As respect for wise and experienced people decreased, so did the human lifespan. Soon the kingdom was beset by shortages in pleasant-tasting food and then of nourishing food. Eventually the very idea of "good" disappeared, and people began to regard one another as animals, with the result that there was incessant strife among the population.

The text offers a dismal portrayal of the human condition that eventually results from neglect of the poor, and the narrative emphasizes several times that all this social chaos came about gradually as an inevitable consequence of

[2] This text is found in *Thus Have I Heard: The Long Discourses of the Buddha*. Translated by Maurice Walsh. London: Wisdom Publications, 1987. Pp. 395–405. A translation also appears in an appendix in Steven Collins, *Nirvana and Other Buddhist Felicities: Utopias of the Pali Imaginaire*. Cambridge: Cambridge University Press, 1998. Collins provides an excellent discussion of Buddhist visions of the ideal society in his chapter entitled "The perfect moral commonwealth? Kingship and its discontents."

neglecting the needs of the poor. Having made that point, the text then provides a narrative of how the situation was eventually reversed. People grew tired of chaos. Some people simply decided to live differently. They went away to a relatively secluded place and began to live in harmony together. Eventually, other people saw that those who lived in harmony were much happier and more prosperous than those who fought with one another. And so gradually all the conditions were reversed, with the result that finally a government was established that saw the advantages of looking after the poor. Those first people who grew tired of strife are described as living lives remarkably like the life that the Buddha recommended for monks and householders. The obvious but unstated message of the sutta is that the Buddhist community should strive to set a positive example of harmonious living for the rest of the world. The task of the Buddhist, then, is not to add to the chorus of conflicting opinions about how to live, but rather to show people how to live by actually living in a way that obviously leads to peace and contentment for all who choose to live that way.

Advice for Family People

Keeping a harmonious society is not the sole responsibility of the head of state. According to several Buddhist texts, one of which we have looked at above, the government does have the responsibility of levying enough taxes to cover the expenses of protecting citizens and caring for the poor and weak, and it also has the responsibility of setting a good example of integrity for the people. The smooth running of a society, however, requires more than good government; it also requires the good conduct of citizens. Although some members of society may take the option of remaining celibate so that they can dedicate all their time and energy to learning and teaching, only a minority can or should do this. The majority of people should dedicate themselves to family life. Realizing this, the Buddha provided guidelines for the laity as well as for world-renouncing monks.

One of the best-known texts for householders is called the Sigàlaka Sutta (*Thus I Have Heard: The Long Discourses of the Buddha*, 1987b). In this sutta, it is said that a Brahmin youth named Sigàlaka had promised his father that every day he would perform certain ablutions in the sacred waters near his home. His ritual required him to face each of the four directions and offer a prayer and sprinkle some water in that direction, then offer water upwards and downwards. One day he was doing his purification rituals, when the Buddha happened to see him and inquired what he was doing. When Sigàlaka explained the promise he had made to his father, the Buddha commended him for his loyalty and advised him to continue doing the rituals. He then explained that Sigàlaka could honor the six directions in an additional way. He could think of each of the directions are representing a kind of social relationship.

The Buddha advises Sigàlaka to let the east stand for his parents. In addition to offering prayers and water towards the east, he should honor the east by honoring his parents and being a good son. Similarly, the south can be honored by honoring teachers, the west by honoring spouse and children, the north by honoring friends, the space above by honoring employers and the space below by honoring subordinates. This leads to a long discussion of the particular ways in which one might honor all these people with whom one has a social relationship.

In this text and in many others like it, the Buddha talks about the benefits of true friendship, that is, friendship with beneficial companions. Good friends, says the Buddha, are those who offer help when one is in need, remain loyal in bad times as well as in good times, offer advice about what is best for one, and provide sympathy. Each of these four ways of being a good friend is then expanded. Helping a friend, for example, may take the form of looking after the friend's property when the friend has become careless or indisposed, or it can take the form of providing comfort in times of fear and distress. Remaining loyal consists in such things as being a trusted confidant and listening to confessions, and so on.

Contrasted to the true friend is the companion who entices one to waste time, spend money foolishly, pursue frivolous goals, and indulge in gossip and small talk. The false friend is the companion who offers flattery rather than criticism, and temptation rather than sound advice.

It is said in the canonical writings that the Buddha's cousin and faithful attendant, ânanda, once said "I think that good friendship is half the religious life." The Buddha responded "Don't say that, Ânanda. Good friendship is not half the religious life; it is the entirety of the religious life." Nothing is more important than being a good friend to everyone to whom one is related, whether as a kin, as a business associate, as a neighbor, as an elder or as a junior. Just attending to the quality of all these relationships, it is said, is a means by which one can go the full distance to liberation from the petty-mindedness that leads inevitably to frustration and discontent.

Conclusions

What we now call Buddhism was called the middle path by the Buddha. As he explained the name, his method of achieving an end to frustration was one that avoided extreme self-denial and extreme self-indulgence. If we look at his path from the perspective of social activism, we could also call Buddhism a middle way between one extreme of complete withdrawal from worldly affairs and the other extreme of an overly intense involvement in political struggles. As anyone who has engaged in social and political reform or in environmental work knows, it is easy to become so overwhelmed by the enormity of the task that one becomes discouraged into a state of paralysis. This phenomenon of becoming "burned out" may result from paying too much attention to external events and too little attention to the internal architecture of one's own mentality. As the Buddha put it, one cannot get others out of quicksand when one is mired in the quicksand oneself. It is essential to build a solid foundation for oneself before embarking on the task of rescuing others in distress.

The essence of the middle path is to keep these two aspects of life in a careful balance. Paying attention only to external factors can lead, as noted above, to burning out. Paying attention only to internal factors, on the other hand, may lead to becoming so self-absorbed as to be of little value to others. The key to finding this balance is to situate oneself in a network of relationships with other people, and with other sentient beings. One begins by finding a small circle of true friends whom one can trust and who offer one support and encouragement and guidance. And gradually one expands that circle to include others. By learning to expand one's circle of friends by befriending more and more people whom one once regarded with fear, suspicion and uneasiness, one gets oneself into a proper perspective, neither bloated with pride nor shriveled up with diffidence. If one patiently works at expanding the circle of friendship to include all of humanity, and then all of life, before one knows it, fear gives way to trust, despair to hope, arrogance to confidence, competitiveness to cooperation, anxiety to serenity and folly to wisdom. And then, without giving the matter any further thought, one shines as a beacon by which others can also find their way.

References

Collins, S. (1998). *Nirvana and other Buddhist felicities: Utopias of the Pali imaginaire.* (Appendix). Cambridge: Cambridge University Press.

Dhammapada: A new English translation with the Pali text and the first English translation of the commentary's explanation of the verses with notes translated from Sinhala sources and critical textual comments. (1987). (J. R. Carter & M. Palihawadana, Trans.). New York: Oxford University Press.

The middle length discourses of the Buddha: A new translation of the Majjhima Nikàya. (1995). (Bhikkhu Ñàõamoli & Bhikkhu Bodhi, Trans.). Boston: Wisdom Publications.

Thus Have I Heard: The Long Discourses of the Buddha. (1987a). (Maurice Walsh, Trans.) (pp. 395–405). London: Wisdom Publications.

Thus Have I Heard: The Long Discourses of the Buddha. (1987b). (Maurice Walsh, Trans.) (pp. 461–470). London: Wisdom Publications.

Part III

Empowerment, Responsibility, and the Challenges of Change

Chapter 8

Buddhist Empowerment

Individual, Organizational, and Societal Transformation

Kathleen H. Dockett

There is no greater good than empowering humanity and revitalizing society. Like politics, economics, and education, religion is devoid of meaning unless it contributes to this process.

DAISAKU IKEDA (1999, p. 25)

Empowerment has emerged as a vital construct for understanding the development of individuals, organizations, and communities (Zimmerman, 2000). In the nearly three-decade period from 1974 to 2001, citations on empowerment in the psychology literature (PsycINFO) increased from 96 to 1,201. Although empowerment has been defined in many ways, most definitions imply a process by which people, organizations, and communities gain mastery over the issues of concern to them (Rappaport, 1987).

Religion is a source of empowerment for most people (Hood, Spilka, Hunsberger, & Gorsuch, 1996, p. 381). Religion plays a central role in meeting our basic motivational needs for meaning, control, and self-esteem (Hood et al., 1996). It provides an enhanced sense of power and control over what is taking place, and is therefore an important resource for coping and adjustment (Hood et al., 1996).

Despite the plethora of empowerment studies and religion's central role, the study of religious empowerment has been neglected. The term "empowerment" typically does not appear in the index of psychology of religion books. A search of the psychology literature (PsycINFO) from 1982 to 2001 produced only 45 citations that combine empowerment with religion or spirituality or faith (out of 1,201 empowerment citations and 20,034 religion/spirituality/faith citations). Moreover, when the terms Buddhism (397) and empowerment (1,201) were combined, no citations emerged.

This paucity suggests several things. First, there are probable limitations in the way both religion and empowerment are being conceptualized, with "religion" being associated more with individual development and "empowerment" with political-economic community development. To the contrary, however, religion's potential as a resource for the empowerment of individuals and communities is beginning to receive attention. Notably, a sizable proportion of that attention is coming from community psychologists who are studying religion and spirituality from the perspective of empowerment (cf., Maton & Salem, 1995; Moore, 1991; Pargament & Maton, 2000; Rappaport & Simpkins, 1991; Speer, Hughey, Gensheimer, & Adams-Leavitt, 1995), prevention and health promotion (cf., Dockett, 1993; Maton & Wells, 1995), community building (cf., Jason, 1997, 1999), and social change (cf., Cohen, Mobray, Gillete, & Thompson, 1992; Dockeki, 1982; Dockett, 1999a). Kloos and Moore (2000) provide a review of empirical findings within the framework of key constructs of community psychology.

Second, Buddhist empowerment is clearly a neglected variable in the literature of Western psychology. This is a serious omission given Buddhism's long and rich history of empowering individuals and transforming communities. Several factors are responsible for this neglect, not the least of which is how Buddhism is perceived and used in the West. In the United States, Buddhism has been perceived more as a solitary quest for self-enlightenment than as a vehicle for social reform. It has been used more as a personal psychotherapy (Imamura, 1998) than as a strategy for social and community change (Dockett, 1999a).

Yet there are schools of socially engaged Buddhism and Buddhist scholar-activists deeply committed to macro level change through the application of Buddhist principles to ethical, social, political, and economic problems (cf., Kotler, 1996; Thurman, 1999). These themes resonate with community psychology and it's goals of promoting well-being, increasing empowerment, and preventing the development of problems of communities, groups, and individuals (Solarz, 2000).

Also noteworthy is the consistency in definitions of empowerment and engaged Buddhism. Empowerment is described as a "construct that links individual strengths and competencies, natural helping systems, and proactive behaviors to social policy and social change" (Perkins & Zimmerman, 1995). Engaged Buddhism is described as "the connection between personal and social-political transformation, and its expansion of traditional teachings and practices to apply to contemporary social settings" (Rothberg, 1992). These definitional commonalities point to the possibilities of an exciting intersection between community psychology and socially engaged Buddhism, suggesting the potential for a collaborative partnership to inform the processes involved in empowerment and social change (Dockett, 1999a). However to realize this potential will require, as Marsella (1999) has noted, that Western psychologists become more open to exploring paradigms that differ from their own.

The main thesis of this chapter is that Buddhism represents a potential resource for empowerment at the individual, community-organizational setting, and societal levels. To advance our understanding of the processes and structures through which empowerment may work at these levels, I will draw from my case study of a particular Buddhist faith community to describe: (1) how Buddhist philosophy and practice may promote stress resistance and empower persons to feel in control of their lives; (2) how Buddhist-inspired organizational structures and processes may promote collective empowerment at the community setting level; and (3) how socially engaged Buddhism *of various types* seeks to promote empowerment at the societal level. Where possible, Buddhist approaches will be examined from a psychological perspective, noting their consistency with Western psychological theory and research. The goal is to inform our conceptual models, enrich our understanding, and guide future research.

Over the past 12 years I have studied the United States branch of a lay Buddhist society, the Soka Gakkai International (SGI)-USA. Based on the Nichiren school of Mahayana Buddhism, the Soka Gakkai is a form of engaged Buddhism that has been described as a social movement for world peace (Hurst, 1998; Prebish & Tanaka, 1998). It has grown rapidly in the 32 years it has been outside of Japan to include 177 countries and territories around the world, and claims a membership of approximately 12 million, including over 300,000 in the United States (Eppsteiner, as cited in Hammond & Machacek, 1999; McCloskey, 2001). The Soka Gakkai holds the distinction of being "the largest and most racially diverse Buddhist organization in America" (Chappell, 2000, p. 299). This organization was selected for case study because of its exemplary efforts in developing empowerment at the individual through the societal level, and because of my in-depth knowledge of its teachings and organizational practices. Using participant-observation methodology, interviews, and doctrinal analyses, I have examined the stress buffering and empowerment potential of this faith community (Dockett, 1993, 1999a, 1999b). To begin, it is important to clarify what empowerment is and briefly examine its historical origins.

The Concept of Empowerment

In its essence, empowerment is a process that enables people, organizations, and communities to gain control over issues of concern to them (Rappaport, 1987). However, empowerment has many meanings because it is a multilevel and multifaceted concept. It can be applied at the level of the individual, the organization, the community, and the society. Depending upon the level involved, the empowerment values, goals, processes, and outcomes may differ. This can be seen in the following definitions.

- *Individual empowerment* or "psychological empowerment" focuses on increasing one's feelings of value, self-efficacy, and personal control (Zimmerman, 1995). This includes gaining access to resources and

competencies needed to have control over one's life and to achieve one's personal goals (Alinsky, 1946; Kroeker, 1995; Maton & Salem, 1995).
- *Organizational empowerment* focuses on changing the power structures of society as they are manifested in a group or in a specific community. This might include creating alternative settings or empowering organizations within a neighborhood (Kroeker, 1995). An "empowering organization" involves "processes and structures that enhance members' skills and provide them with the mutual support necessary to affect community level change" (Zimmerman, 1995). In contrast, an "empowered organization" involves "improved organizational effectiveness by effectively competing for resources, networking with other organizations, or expanding its influence" (Zimmerman, 1995).
- *Community empowerment* involves "individuals working together in an organized fashion to improve their collective lives and linkages among community organizations and agencies that help maintain that quality of life" (Zimmerman, 2000).
- *Societal empowerment* or political empowerment focuses on changing the larger social structures and institutions that maintain positions of powerlessness and poverty (Albee et al., 1988; Alinsky, 1946; Freire, 1970; Rappaport, 1986, as cited in Kroeker, 1995). This would include national and international structures that influence resources and policies.

From a historical perspective, the concept of empowerment grew out of its opposite – conditions of powerlessness. Early social activists such as Paolo Freire (*Pedagogy of the Oppressed*) and Saul Alinsky (*Reveille for Radicals*; *Rules for Radicals*) are known worldwide for defining the principles of empowerment based on their work in disadvantaged communities. Empowerment became the way to help people who were poor, disadvantaged, oppressed, and otherwise not in control of their lives or their environments, to gain power. In many third-world countries and in the industrialized nations as well, there are groups of people and entire countries that do not have control over their natural resources, living conditions, and opportunities for development. Especially people living in extreme poverty, they do not have control over their lives. They do not have self-determination or participation in the decision making of the community.

To reverse the conditions of powerlessness (in the minds of the people and in their actual ability to control their personal lives and environment), the concept of empowerment emerged. The goals of empowerment are to give the "power to the people." This calls for change on three levels: personal change, organizational change, and societal transformation. Strategies for empowerment (or social change) include grassroots activism, citizen participation, community development, community organizing, education and information dissemination, and public policy activities to change the laws (Duffy & Wong, 1996).

Some have asked why psychologists would be interested in empowerment. Whether a psychologist is a clinical therapist or a community activist, both are interested in helping people gain a sense of personal control over their lives. Whether working with an individual person or an entire community, the issue of control remains. When people feel they can control their personal lives and what happens in their neighborhood/community/society, they have better psychological and physical adjustment. When organizations, communities, and societies expand their influence and control over access to resources, they can improve the quality of life of their citizens. Community psychologists are interested in empowerment as a means of fostering healthy individuals and healthy communities, and a growing number are interested in the role of religion in this regard.

Empowerment at the Individual Level

Psychological Perspective

Individual empowerment, or psychological empowerment, refers to a process through which individuals gain control over their lives (Rappaport, 1981). It focuses on increasing self-perceptions of competence and control, understanding one's environment, and taking actions to produce change (Zimmerman, 1995). It also "includes a concern for the common good and a sense of connectedness to others" (Zimmerman & Rappaport, 1988, p. 747).

Personal control is also a central trait in Suzanne Kobasa's (1982) "hardy" stress resistant personality and, for purposes of this paper, psychological empowerment will be discussed within that context. Based on her research in highly stressful situations comparing persons who did not develop psychological or physical illness with those who did, Kobasa identified a hardy personality style that is unusually resistant to stress. According to Kobasa, hardy persons have a general orientation toward life that is characterized by three traits: commitment, control, and challenge. Essentially, hardy persons are those who have:

- a deep sense of personal commitment to self, family, relationships, work, and other stabilizing values.
- a belief in personal control over the events in their lives.
- an orientation toward life change as a challenging opportunity for growth, rather than a threat.

Commitment. Deeply held commitments, especially to self, provide a sense of purpose and meaning to the activities of one's life. Commitments denote what is important to the individual. They underlie the choices one is willing to make to achieve one's goals, and motivate the individual to persist in pursuing a goal in the face of repeated obstacles. It is a strong sense of purpose that prevents highly committed individuals from giving upon their goals and on themselves in times of stress. In this way, commitments serve as a generalized buffer against the harmful effects of stress.

Control. Control refers to the belief that one has personal control over the outcomes of events in one's life. Our expectations regarding control are a powerful determinant of our behavior according to an extensive body of research based on the social learning theory of Julian Rotter (1966). For example, the likelihood that a person will seek public office, or apply for a highly desirable job, or attempt to repair an important relationship depends upon their *expectation* that they will be successful in those instances. Based upon our experiences of success and failure within the different domains of our lives, we form generalized beliefs about being able to control events. These generalized expectations are called locus of control (LOC) and are defined as a basic personality trait consisting of our beliefs about the nature of the world and the causes of events, and specifically about how reinforcement or rewards are controlled (Rotter, 1966).

There are two types of LOC, internal and external. When persons believe they control the outcomes of their behavior, and that their abilities and personality characteristics determine their success in achieving a goal, this belief is labeled internal LOC. "Internals" believe that outcomes in a particular endeavor are contingent upon their own behavior. On the other hand, when persons believe that outcomes are not contingent upon their own behavior but are the result of luck, chance, fate, or powerful external forces over which they have no control, this is called external LOC. "Externals" believe that no matter what they do, they cannot control what happens.

In general, the perception that one has control of his or her life is associated with successful adjustment, while the perception that external forces are in control is associated with negative outlooks and outcomes (Lefcourt & Davidson-Katz, 1991). Behavioral differences are apparent between internals and externals. Internals tend to be more active in mastering their environment, more effective in influencing other people, and higher achievers, while externals tend to be more passive and apathetic, feeling powerless to control or change their circumstances. Extreme externality can have dangerous consequences for one's mental health. Externals often blame their environment for events that occur (e.g., "I got a poor grade because the teacher is unfair." "There's no use applying for this job because they won't hire me anyway."). While this defensive maneuver protects the ego from experiencing failure, the danger is that when we externalize control over the outcomes of our behavior, we place ourselves in the posture of a victim, inviting feelings of helplessness.

The connection between external LOC and feelings of helplessness, hopelessness, and depression has been demonstrated in the extensive animal research of experimental-clinical psychologist Martin Seligman and his colleagues (1967,

1968). In a typical experiment, dogs were exposed to an electric shock from which escape was either possible or not. The dogs that experienced two inescapable shocks within a 24-hour period developed a chronic failure to escape. When placed in the condition in which escape was possible, these dogs sat passively, enduring up to 50 seconds of severe shock without making any effort to escape. Seligman termed this behavior learned helplessness – a disempowering psychological state that frequently results when events are uncontrollable. The dogs had developed an expectation that termination of the shock was not contingent upon any response they could make. That is, they developed a generalized expectation of external LOC that was so powerful that they perceived themselves to have no control even when they actually did. Helplessness studies done with human beings and with entire communities report the same finding (Rappaport, 1977). When people are repeatedly exposed to uncontrollable situations, they too develop learned helplessness. Understandably, therefore, a major approach to behavior change is to help people change their expectancies by teaching internal LOC.

Challenge. Persons with a challenge orientation welcome change as a natural part of life. They view change as a challenging opportunity to grow and to shape the outcome of events. Consequently, they focus on the potential for gain inherent in demanding situations, experience pleasurable emotions of excitement and exhilaration, and vigorously interact with changing circumstances to produce the outcomes they want. Like highly committed persons, their strong motivation to endure in the face of crisis is thought to buffer the effects of stress. In sharp contrast are persons who are threatened by change; they tend to focus on the potential for harm and experience the associated negative emotions of anxiety, fear, and anger, which lead to negative behavioral responding.

Kobasa (1982) found that individuals with this stress resistant style are far less likely to become ill, either physically or psychologically, when faced with a stressful situation. Her work suggests that one's general orientation toward life and characteristic interests and motivations influence the way any stressful event is handled and, therefore, the impact that event has. Having briefly reviewed psychological perspectives on stress resistance and personal control, we now examine Buddhist teachings that foster the development of these traits.

Parallels to the Philosophy and Practice of Nichiren Buddhism

The philosophy and practice of Nichiren Buddhism embodies a system of beliefs through which individuals develop stress resistance and gain control over their lives. This is particularly well illustrated in the Buddhist teachings of the bodhisattva imperative, dependent origination (Jap. *engi*), the oneness of self and environment (Jap. *esho funi*), karma, and changing poison into medicine (Jap. *hendoku iyaku*). These concepts will be examined within the context of Kobasa's model of stress resistance.

Parallels to Commitment. Corresponding to Kobasa's findings that deep commitments buffer stress, the practice of Nichiren Buddhism is based on a set of overarching goals that provide profound purpose and meaning to the activities of one's life. These goals are articulated in Buddhist doctrine as the "bodhisattva imperative." A bodhisattva is a person of great compassion who is motivated by a commitment to "complete self-transformation and complete world transformation" (Thurman, 1996). Growing out of the bodhisattva's great compassion for the sufferings of others is the imperative to delay his or her own entrance into Nirvana in order to help others achieve enlightenment. For practicing Buddhists, this imperative translates into a serious commitment to actualize the Buddha nature inherent within one's own life, while simultaneously helping others to do the same. Practicing to develop one self and others (Jap. *jigyo keta*) is so essential that it has been institutionalized as one of the three pillars of Nichiren Buddhist practice.

Given that we live in a society and era largely characterized by egoism, it is important to understand the Buddhist rationale for altruism. At a most profound level, the imperative of the bodhisattva to alleviate the suffering of others is rooted in the deeply ecological Buddhist principle of *dependent origination*, (Jpn. *engi*). Dependent origination is a fundamental doctrine of the interdependence of all things, which teaches that all beings and phenomena exist or occur only because of their relationship with other beings and phenomena. From this ecological perspective, practice for one self and for others are inextricably interconnected because one's own happiness cannot exist separate from the happiness of others within one's environment. Describing dependent origination as "the web of life that binds all people," Soka Gakkai International President Daisaku Ikeda (1993, p. 54) states:

> Nothing in this world exists alone;
> everything comes into being and continues in response to causes and conditions.
> Parent and child.
> Husband and wife.
> Friends. Races.
> Humanity and nature.
> This profound understanding
> of coexistence, of symbiosis –
> here is the source of resolution for
> the most pressing and fundamental issues
> that confront humankind
> in the chaotic last years of this century.

Citing the parable of "Two Bundles of Reeds," Ikeda states,

> Only by supporting each other
> can the two bundles stand straight –
> if one is removed, the other must fall ....

The most important implication of this teaching is that we do not exist alone. The meaning of our lives and our happiness arises through our interconnectedness with those around us, our community, and the world. This realization, of the interdependent nature of our existence, is expected to naturally foster a sense of responsibility and appreciation for others, which is manifested in altruistic behavior.

Thus, the bodhisattva imperative, based on the rationale of *dependent origination* and expressed through a committed practice for the development of oneself and others, is the overarching goal of Nichiren Buddhists. With this imperative as a guiding mission, SGI members develop a deep sense of commitment to themselves and to their relationships with others in all spheres of life. It is this kind of strong commitment to self and others that, according to Kobasa, provides the motivational drive that buffers the harmful effects of stress.

Parallels to Control. A belief in internal locus of control lies at the very core of the Buddhist philosophy of life. This parallel is well illustrated by the doctrines of the oneness of life and its environment (Jpn. *esho funi*) and karma.

Esho funi explains the relationship between human life and its environment. Westerners typically see the world as divided into two parts: everything from the skin inward we call *self*, and everything outside the skin we call *not self*. Thus, we divide the world into self and objective environment. In Buddhist terms, *eho* or the objective environment, and *shoho* or the living subject, are contracted into *esho*, which means life and its environment. Buddhism teaches that these two exist in a relationship of *funi*, which means they are two but not two.

Most of us readily understand that individuals and their environment are two separate entities, which means we see the distinction between them. We also understand how closely interrelated they are. An example is psychology's findings of the bi-directional influences that operate in parent-infant bonding, where the responsively of each influences the receptivity of the other and the quality of the attachment that develops between them. Yet, no matter how closely interwoven these mutual influences are, traditional Western thought holds that living beings and their environments still belong to the realm of two separate entities. However, Buddhism teaches that there is a realm in which the private world of self and external reality are "not two" but are one and the same; a dimension of human life that is one with the entire cosmos itself. This dimension Buddhism calls the true aspect of all phenomena – the ultimate truth of life that is the Buddha nature or the Mystic Law (*Seikyo Times*, 1988, p. 18).

The implications of the oneness of self and environment are profound. Because the individual and the environment are fundamentally one, whatever internal life condition the individual manifests will be simultaneously manifested in his or her environment. For example, persons whose basic life tendency is characterized by hellish suffering will bring forth anguish and misery in their surroundings, whereas persons with a basic altruistic state will enjoy protection and support from the world around them. To illustrate further: a person whose basic life tendency is characterized by animality will perceive other living beings as animals, and the world as a jungle in which only the strong survive. Based on this worldview, the person will act in animalistic ways and elicit animalistic responses in return. Thus, the way we perceive, think, and behave are all a reflection of our internal life condition.

Accordingly, Buddhism teaches that life condition is *reflected* in the environment; *environment does not determine life condition*, although it does influence it. This is what Nichiren meant when he wrote "environment is like a shadow and life, the body. Without the body, no shadow can exist, and without life, no environment" (*The Writings of Nichiren Daishonin*, 1999a, p. 644). And when he wrote in On Attaining Buddhahood (*The Writings of Nichiren Daishonin*, 1999b, p. 3), "Life at each moment permeates the entire realm of phenomena. To be awakened to this principle is itself the mutually inclusive relationship of life at each moment and all phenomena." In the same writing, Nichiren stated, "unless one perceives the nature of one's life, one's practice will become an endless, painful austerity" (p. 4). In other words, individuals cannot change their karma unless they realize that all causes are internal and are created by and under the control of the individual.

These examples illustrate that the core philosophy of Nichiren Buddhism as revealed in the concept of *esho funi* embraces the notion that we are coextensive with the universe. Through controlling what is inside us, we control what is outside as well. Realizing that we and our environment are one and that we can change our objective environment by changing our internal life state is, I believe, synonymous with an internal locus of control.

A belief in internal locus of control is also inherent in the Buddhist doctrine of karma. Teachings on karma assert that the effects of our prior actions find expression both in ourselves and in our environment. Thus, Nichiren states, "if you want to understand the causes that existed in the past, look at the results as they are manifested in the present. And if you want to understand what results will be manifested in the future, look at the causes that exist in the present" (The *Writings of Nichiren Daishonin*, 1999c, p. 279). This doctrine promotes self-responsibility for both the causes and the effects in our life. Here we also see another important aspect of karma. Karma or destiny is not viewed as a fatalistic finality that cannot be changed. The creation of karma is a continuous process under the individual's control. An empirical relationship between this "process" view of karma and internal LOC was reported in Fazel and colleagues' (cited in Pargament & Park, 1995) study of Hindus and Tibetan Buddhists. Tibetans who viewed the creation of karma as an ongoing process reported a more internal LOC and greater life satisfaction than the Hindus who viewed karma as a fixed life debt to be paid.

In summary, through teaching the concepts of the oneness of life and environment (*esho funi*) and karma, Buddhism promotes a belief in complete personal control and self-responsibility for the causes and effects in one's life (Dockett, 1993). This personal control is synonymous with the definition of psychological empowerment, which involves increasing perceptions of competence and control, understanding one's environment, and taking action to produce change.

Parallels to Challenge. A challenge orientation, the third trait in Kobasa's stress-resistant personality, consists of viewing change as a natural part of life and as an opportunity for growth rather than a threat. Numerous Buddhist writings teach the "challenge orientation." For example in the writing, "Happiness in This World," Nichiren states:

> Though worldly troubles may arise, never let them disturb you. No one can avoid problems, not even saints or worthies .... Suffer what there is to suffer, enjoy what there is to enjoy. Regard both suffering and joy as facts of life and continue chanting Nam-myoho-renge-kyo, no matter what happens. (The *Writings of Nichiren Daishonin*, 1999d, p. 681)

In the Gosho "A Ship to Cross the Sea of Suffering," Nichiren states:

> In the Latter Day of the Law, the votary of the Lotus Sutra will appear without fail. The greater the hardships befalling him the greater the delight he feels, because of his strong faith. Doesn't a fire burn more briskly when logs are added? All rivers run to the sea, but does the sea turn back its waters? The currents of hardship pour into the sea of the Lotus Sutra and rush against its votary. The river is not rejected by the ocean; neither does the votary reject suffering. Were it not for the flowing rivers, there would be no sea. Likewise, without tribulation there would be no votary of the Lotus Sutra. As T'ien-t'ai stated, "The various rivers flow to the sea, and logs make a fire roar more briskly." (The *Writings of Nichiren Daishonin*, 1999e, p. 33)

Socialization as a Buddhist involves learning how to take any hardship and use it as a source to nourish growth. Buddhism teaches that negative events especially provide the opportunity to develop, to purify one's life, and to change negative karma. This viewpoint is embodied in the Buddhist principle of "*changing poison into medicine*" (Jap. *hendoku iyaku*). This phrase was originally used in describing the Lotus Sutra, the highest teaching of the historical Buddha of India, Shakyamuni Buddha, as "the great physician that changes poison into medicine." In a broader sense, it refers to the capacity of people who embrace the Lotus Sutra to transform sufferings that derive from negative karma and illusions of desire into the virtues of the Buddha's life.

Changing poison into medicine involves cognitive reframing and is consistent with psychology's cognitive approaches to converting negative events into positive outcomes (Beck, 1976; Ellis, 1977; Finkel & Jacobsen, 1977). From the trauma-strengthening conversions of Norman Finkel, to the rational emotive therapy of Albert Ellis and the cognitive restructuring therapy of Aaron Beck, cognitive therapies assist clients in restructuring the irrational beliefs that cause them to emote and behave in maladaptive ways. According to Pargament's (1997) review of 40 studies, positive religious reframing has been found to be a helpful type of coping activity.

Buddhist doctrine requires the individual to cognitively reconstruct traumatic experiences in ways that accord with the true reality of life and therefore foster psychologically healthy adaptations. A key to performing these reconstructions seems to lie, in part, in internalizing the teachings of (a) the oneness of life and its environment (*esho funi*), (b) karma, (c) changing poison into medicine (*hendoku iyaku*), and (d) viewing crisis as an opportunity for growth. This process is the equivalent of training in Finkel's trauma strengthening conversion process – a reframing of the problem that focuses on the potential for gain and promotes an orientation toward internal control and challenge. Through chanting Nam-myoho-renge-kyo, studying Buddhist philosophy, and receiving guidance from seniors in faith, SGI members develop the ability to cognitively reconstruct negative events in ways that reduce or eliminate stress and create a sense of psychological empowerment.

Imamura (1998) illustrates the Buddhist call for positive reframing well in the following passage.

> Life is duhkha [suffering] (like riding on a cart with badly made wheels). Life's imperfections and pain are not eradicated but are instead embraced as familiar friends and transformed into valuable lessons that show us again and again our blind self-centeredness, the result of clinging to a very limited and impoverished view of life. Suffering or unhappiness is the outcome of a failure to see that life is in constant flux and that nothing is permanent in this world, a failure to see the interconnectedness and interpenetration of things in the world, and a failure to see the illusory nature of the conceptual self or ego. Happiness requires a complete transformation of the individual's paradigms or worldviews, that is, a cessation of erroneous worldviews. (p. 231)

Implications for Research and Action

We have seen how the philosophy and practice of Nichiren Buddhism may foster psychological empowerment and develop internal psychological resources for stress resistance. Through providing a philosophy of life based upon the belief that all human beings possess a Buddha nature, Nichiren Buddhism empowers people to believe in their inherent capacity for growth and for positive impact on their environment. It fosters deep commitments to develop one's potentialities and to advance the potentialities of humanity to live in harmony. It encourages total responsibility for one's life, and a belief in personal control of one's destiny. It promotes cognitive restructuring of negative experiences as challenging opportunities for growth. This system of beliefs builds tremendous optimism, hope, courage, and confidence. It fosters a sense of self-efficacy, competence, and personal control that defines psychological empowerment. Combined with the practice of chanting Nam-myoho-renge-kyo, this system of beliefs depicts the process through which self-empowerment and hardiness may emerge.

The next step for research with the SGI-USA is to empirically test the extent to which the noted empowering and stress resistant characteristics exist and their relationship with coping behaviors, personal goal attainment, and stress and/or well-being outcomes.

Empowerment at the Organizational/Community Setting Level

The notion of religious organizations serving an empowering role for individuals is not new. A growing number of community psychologists have begun to study organizational characteristics related to the collective empowering of members (cf., Dockett, 1999a; Maton & Salem, 1995; Maton & Wells, 1995, McMillan, Florin, Stevenson, Kerman, & Mitchell, 1995; Speer, Hughey, Gensheimer, & Adams-Leavitt, 1995; Watts, 1993). Recall that an "empowering organization" involves "processes and structures that enhance members' skills and provide them with the mutual support necessary to affect community level change (Zimmerman, 1995); and enhance members' psychological sense of control as well as the resources and ability to achieve their personal goals (Maton & Salem, 1995).

Maton and Salem (1995) identified four characteristics of empowering organizations that seem to be common across diverse types of community settings, based on a multiple case study of a religious fellowship, a mutual self-help organization, and an educational program for African American students. These empowering characteristics include: (1) a belief system that inspires growth, is strengths-based, and is focused beyond the self; (2) an opportunity role structure that is pervasive, highly accessible, and multifunctional; (3) a support system that is encompassing, peer-based, and provides a sense of community; and (4) leadership that is inspiring, talented, shared, and committed to both setting and members.

Based upon 12 years of participant observation, interviews, and doctrinal analyses, the SGI-USA would appear to be an empowering setting. With a membership of over 300,000 in more than 70 community centers throughout the United States, its potential to affect positive influence is sizable and growing. Brief descriptions of the SGI-USA organizational life are provided below as evidence of its empowering potential, based on the Maton and Salem (1995) model.

Belief system

According to the Maton and Salem (1995) model, belief system includes those organizational ideologies, values, and cultural norms that shape its view of practitioners, shape practices and structures that provide opportunities for growth, and provide goals and norms that inspire and sustain members efforts toward change. Specifically, an empowering belief system is one that inspires growth (by defining challenging, motivating goals and means of achieving those goals), is strengths-based (meaning each individual is perceived to have the capability to achieve those goals and is a valuable resource), and is focused beyond the self (meaning it focuses members on a larger spiritual or humanity-based mission).

To appreciate the growth-inspiring, strengths-based, beyond-self nature of SGI-USA's belief system, it is necessary to understand something of its founding mission and guiding philosophy. Soka Gakkai means "The Society for Value-Creation." It was established in 1930 by a Japanese educator named Tsunesaburo Makiguchi for the purpose of enabling people to actualize the innate potentialities for value within their own lives and to create value within society. Innate potentialities refer to the Buddha nature – the potential for attaining enlightenment, boundless wisdom, and infinite compassion. The overarching goal of the organization, through the cultivation of humanistic values and the protection of all life, is to achieve a harmonious co-existence among all races, cultures, and nationalities of the world or, in other words, world peace. The central philosophy that guides the attainment of world peace is based on the concept of human revolution. Describing this process of inner reformation as it relates to the mission of world peace, the SGI President Daisaku Ikeda (1987) stated:

> The movement that we advocate for a human revolution does not stop at a change of personality, but extends to a change in the most basic attitudes and perceptions about the nature of life itself; it is a change of the entire human being. I know and believe as the firmest article of faith that the human revolution of a single person can change the fate of a nation, our world and all humanity. (p. 257)

These transcendent goals and the humanistic values upon which they are based, undoubtedly, are responsible for the deep sense of commitment members have toward their own development, the organization's development, and societal change. In samples of the written work of the organization's international president, we can see the translation of these humanistic values into organizational norms. Norms of respect for the uniqueness of each individual's potentialities are revealed in the Japanese concept of *o-bai-tor-i* to which Ikeda often refers. This concept expresses the idea that the blossoms of the cherry, plum, pear, and peach trees each emit their unique fragrance contributing to the beauty of the orchard. Through this metaphor which contains the concepts of values-pluralism and multiculturalism, members are encouraged to appreciate and honor the values and cultural traditions of each individual, as this not only expands our perception of reality beyond the narrow barriers of our own cultural ethos but constitutes a bridge for building unity, cooperation, and world peace. While respect for diversity is highly valued, unity is also a central norm. Encouraging members to transcend superficial differences of race and culture, SGI President Ikeda employs the Buddhist concept of unity – "many in body, one in mind" (*itai doshin*): "Without a mind of unity, neither growth nor rapid progress is possible. Without the beautiful bonds of your comrades, there can be no happiness for the individual, either" (Ikeda, 1992, p. 219). Collectively, these norms may contribute to explaining the SGI-USA's unique standing as "the largest and most racially diverse Buddhist organization in American (Chappell, 2000).

Thus, the SGI-USA belief system would appear to be tremendously empowering. It inspires growth by providing challenging, motivating goals for members to develop their own potentialities (Buddha nature) while contributing to the transformation of the society (the Bodhisattva Imperative). The belief system is strengths-based in embracing a philosophy of human equality and dignity (all human beings equally possess a Buddha nature and are worthy of respect), of values-pluralism (each person's potentialities are unique), and of the sanctity of life (each life is precious). Its focus beyond the self is apparent in its mission of attaining world peace, although the larger mission is interdependently linked to members' personal goals in that only through developing one's own humanity and that of others will the attainment of world peace be possible.

Opportunity Role Structure

An empowering opportunity role structure is one that is pervasive (has many roles for members to enter at multiple levels of the organization), highly accessible (requires "varying levels of skills, responsibility, and self-confidence" and encourages members to take on new roles and responsibilities), and multifunctional ("contains many opportunities for skill development..., for skill utilization, and for exercise of responsibility") (Maton & Salem, 1995, p. 643).

In the SGI-USA, the use of a democratic organizational structure is one mechanism through which it facilitates the social integration of members into meaningful organizational roles. Based on fundamental Buddhist egalitarianism, a circle system of organization is emphasized at the local levels, which promotes equality and solidarity. Through decentralizing authority and granting maximum autonomy to its subdivisions, the organization actively discourages authoritarian tendencies, and allows the maximum number of members to participate in organizational leadership. The opportunity role structure is pervasive and contains an immense number of highly accessible and multifunctional roles at multiple levels throughout the SGI-USA. An abundance of basic activity groups comprise the organization, from divisional groupings by gender and age, to special interest groups by, for example, vocation, parenthood, and cultural-artistic activity, to support groups of young men- and women-in-training. In addition, there is the basic organizational unit comprised of geographically organized neighborhood discussion groups, which constitutes the first-line source of social support and training in the practice of Buddhism. Enriching these basic activity groups, a host of special activity groups are established to carry out unique SGI-sponsored projects. These include such activities as the recent Women's Peace Conference at The World Bank attended by over 2,000 participants; the youth-sponsored Victory Over Violence Campaign; and worldwide and nationwide exhibitions on "Nuclear Arms: Threat to Our World," "War and Peace," "Humanity in Education: The Soka School System," "Ecology and Human Life," and "Gandhi, King, Ikeda: A Legacy of Building Peace."

All groups operate as semi-autonomous settings with social and religious functions that require substantive member input and contributions to operate successfully. Within and across groups, from the local through the national level, there are multiple opportunities for roles of functional importance to be assumed by a single individual. The roles are highly accessible in that they require skills at all levels of complexity and responsibility from, for example, stuffing envelopes, to stage crew, to overall project coordination. These abundant opportunities for meaningful role involvement not only foster a sense of empowerment but, as indicated in the social support literature, enhance psychological and physical health by providing an alternative source of meaning, activity, life satisfaction, and social identity in the lives of individuals. The multifunctional nature of roles can be seen in the on-going training and education within the SGI-USA where members might be on the provider or the recipient end of skill development.

In line with its mission to promote world peace, the fundamental purpose of all training is to enable people to polish their lives so that they can steadily establish a life of great value. The development of capable people is viewed as the foundation of everything. Toward this end, all activities within the organization are treated as arenas in which members can grow in faith, develop their potentialities for value creation, and develop their skills in the art of worthy living.

Support System

An empowering support system in the Maton and Salem (1995) model is one that is encompassing (includes many types and sources of support), is peer-based (support giving and received by peers), and provides a sense of community both within and beyond the setting.

Encompassing support is evident in the SGI-USA, which Ikeda often states exists for the sole purpose of supporting the members. Organizational norms of friendship, respect, equality, values-pluralism and unity create a highly supportive climate in which members are afforded extraordinary levels of *esteem support.*

Conveying that all are equal while beautifully unique, that all are fundamentally interdependent and therefore absolutely essential to one another's happiness, members receive constant recognition of their self-worth. Through the organization's belief system, opportunity role structure, and skill development activities, abundant opportunities exist for members to receive help in understanding a problem and how to deal with it from a Buddhist perspective (*informational support*). While *esteem* and *informational* support are prevalent throughout the organization, the primary and most fundamental source of support is the neighborhood-based discussion group that constitutes the basic unit of the organization.

Peer-based support is evident in the discussion group that serves as a support group in the traditional sense of the construct. It is a small group of peers where close bonds of friendship develop, and where *esteem, informational, instrumental* and *social companionship* forms of support are readily available. Living out the Bodhisattva imperative, members-peers reach out and help each other during times of need, serve as a feedback and guidance system to help understand problems in living, assist in the task of developing coping strategies, and generally serve as a source for intimate communication and unconditional positive regard. Recently the support function has been extended through e-mail technology to the creation of a "Circle of Compassion" established in one locale to provide collective prayer and various types of support for members, family, and friends challenged by serious health conditions and death. In the discussion groups and on-line, peers share their challenges, successes, failures, guidance, and strategies for success. In member reports, there is amply evidence that the social support they have received has been instrumental in enhancing their sense of control and ability to successfully cope with high stress challenges and achieve their goals.

A strong sense of community can be seen within and across geographical units where, for example, members report a sense of membership, mutual influence, and need satisfaction. A sense of community beyond the organization is shown, for example, in member-initiated projects aimed at improving the neighborhoods in which they live.

Leadership

Leadership, as defined in the Maton and Salem (1995) model refers to key individuals with formal or informal responsibilities. Their capacity for direct influence on members and for indirect influence through motivating other leaders can have an empowering effect when certain leadership characteristics are present. Empowering leadership is (a) inspirational (passionate, clear vision, role model capable of motivating others); (b) talented (interpersonally and organizationally in the sense of working well with others, mobilizing resources, maintaining stability, supporting change, and effectively responding to external threats); (c) shared (open to expansion as new leaders emerge), and (d) committed to both setting and members (encouraging full participation and participatory decision making) (p. 650).

Daisaku Ikeda was inaugurated in 1960 as the third President of the Soka Gakkai, the largest organization of Buddhist lay believers based in Japan. Under his leadership the organization has grown to more than 8 million households in Japan and over 4 million in 176 other countries and territories around the world. Ikeda founded the Soka Gakkai International (SGI), which he currently heads. He has established Soka (Jap. Value Creating) educational institutions from kindergartens to universities, a publishing house, a concert association, an art museum, a research institute, a global policy institute, and cultural centers, among others. His talented efforts have been recognized by the United Nations Peace Award and numerous honorary doctorates, literary awards, and citizenship awards from universities and institutions around the world. He is a distinguished author and poet laureate with myriad books translated in the major world languages including a number of published dialogues with world figures. He is an indefatigable global peace educator, traveling the world to dialogue and build bonds of friendship with world leaders in the fields of peace, education, art, and politics.

As the disciple and successor of the second Soka Gakkai President Josei Toda, Daisaku Ikeda is passionate about the notion of "human revolution," and educational reform as essential keys for fostering a spirit of human solidarity around the world. "I have decided to make education my final undertaking, and I have poured all my energy into that goal" (Ikeda, 2001, p. 1). His vision has been clear and he has role modeled the continuous achievement of that vision though the Soka educational institutions he has established and the peace proposals submitted to the United Nations each year, among other major accomplishments.

Shared leadership is evident in the many social and governmental leaders supporting his efforts around the world, as well as his passing of responsibility for leadership to the youth of the organization as successors of the legacy of the Soka Gakkai presidents. His commitment to the organization and to the members is reflected in his caring, compassion, and extraordinary efforts to develop the membership through writing, lecturing, attending meetings, traveling the globe, as well as his personalized acknowledgments of the suffering or successes of members around the globe.

Implications for Research and Action

To further the study of empowering community settings, Maton and Salem (1995) have made a set of recommendations for future research that is important for theory development, social policy, and community action: (1) Do the proposed organizational characteristics exist in other empowering community settings? (2) Is there a relationship between empowering characteristics and empowering outcomes? (3) Do empowering community settings share common characteristics that distinguish them from non-empowering settings? (4) Are there unique characteristics associated with particular types of settings? (5) Are the proposed characteristics necessary or sufficient to produce empowering outcomes. These questions need to be answered in a variety of empowering organizations.

The next step for research with the SGI-USA would be to empirically test the extent to which the noted empowering characteristics exist and their relationship with empowered outcomes. We are reminded by Rappaport (1995) of the implications for action: "mechanisms identified in empowering settings have serious implications for our roles as interventionists.... When empowering organizations already exist, we can learn a great deal about empowerment by collaborating with them to learn about and help them spread their story ... " (p. 800).

Empowerment at the Societal Level

Societal empowerment or political empowerment focuses on changing the larger social structures and institutions that maintain positions of powerlessness and poverty (Albee et al., 1988; Alinsky, 1946; Freire, 1970; Rappaport, 1986, as cited in Kroeker, 1995). This would include national and international structures that influence resources and policies. Strategies used to bring about institutional change include social action approaches such as community organizing in which large numbers and special tactics are used to gain access to needed resources, and/or social policy approaches focused on affecting political/legislative change. Engaged Buddhist organizations draw upon the same strategies.

"Engaged Buddhism," a term coined by Vietnamese Buddhist monk Thich Nhat Hanh in the 1950's, is defined as the "active involvement by Buddhists in society and its problems" (Kraft, 1996, p. 65). Contrary to the view of Buddhists as escapist, engaged Buddhists seek to actualize the ideals of wisdom and compassion in the life of society. They may function as activists applying Buddhist principles to create ethical, social, political, and economic change, or simply as citizens applying Buddhism in their everyday life and relationships (Rothberg, 1992).

Buddhist activists share commonalities with community psychology. They share the goals of promoting the well-being of individuals and their communities. Both espouse an ecological perspective of life, with the principle of interdependence being fundamental to understanding events. They embrace common phenomena of interest, including empowerment of individuals and communities, respect for diversity, human rights, social justice, nonviolence, sense of community, and community/global harmony. They employ common techniques of social action, including grass-roots activism, citizen participation, education and information dissemination, networking with organizations, community development, and public policy (Duffy & Wong, 1996; Rothberg, 1992, p. 269). However, central differences do exist in the knowledge base and principles that guide social activism in psychology compared to Buddhism. According to Buddhist scholar/activist Robert Thurman (1996), the basic principle motivating Buddhist activism is a "universal altruism of great love, great compassion, great empathy" which is manifested in the bodhisattva's "unswerving commitment to complete self-transformation and complete world-transformation" (p. 77). Alternatively, Buddhist scholar Kenneth Kraft (1996) views the ecological principle of inter-dependence as the cornerstone of engaged Buddhism. This principle, known as *engi* (Jpn), describes the dependent origination of all things – the coexistence/symbiosis of humanity, the natural world, and the cosmos. It holds that everything arises and continues to exist by virtue of its relationship with other phenomena. Awareness that everything is connected to everything else (mind to body, body to mind; self to environment, environment to self; Serbian violence against ethnic Albanians, NATO violence against Serbs), is expected to foster a sense of universal responsibility and appreciation for others. Both views acknowledge an awareness of the oneness of all phenomena as the fundamental organizing principle for Buddhist social activism.

Examples of Buddhist social action in Asia (Rothberg, 1992 p. 269) include: the Buddhist response to Sri Lanka and Cambodian violence with peace walks, dialogue, and nonviolence training; resistance and reconciliation movements in response to war and/or opposition in Vietnam, Tibet, Burma, and parts of Bangladesh; Sri Lanka's network of village-based community development activists who linked personal and social transformation; Thailand's community development monks who led a movement against ecological devastation.

Examples of socially engaged activities in North America (Rothberg, 1992) are seen in the projects and/or community centers of the Buddhist Peace Fellowship (a major socially engaged Buddhist organization in North America, founded in 1978 by Robert Aitken and Anne Aitken, Nelson Foster, and others), the Bangkok-based International Network of Engaged Buddhists, the Interracial Buddhist Council, and the SGI-USA. Illustrative activities include:

- working on human rights issues through organizing grassroots participation in the development of the Earth Charter.
- grassroots movements seeking the control and eventual abolition of nuclear weapons and frequently protesting the Nevada Test Site and the Nuclear Guardianship Project for responsible care of radioactive waste.
- public policy efforts such as running for political office, or obtaining membership status as a Nongovernmental Organization with the United Nations.
- submitting peace proposals to the United Nations.

- interfaith dialogues such as the South Carolina Partners in Dialogue group which focuses on issues of racism and other diversity issues.
- networking of other Buddhist organizations such as the Interracial Buddhist Council and the Buddhist Alliance for Social Engagement or BASE.
- interfaith networking focused on public policy initiatives regarding the freedom of religion act, school prayer, ecological sustainability, and nonviolence.
- establishing educational institutions such as SGI-USA's Soka schools and universities.
- contributing to relief and refugee programs around the world.

Implications for action

It is important for psychologists to collaborate with socially engaged Buddhist organizations to learn about Buddhist approaches to grass roots activism, community organizing, community development, and nonviolence. Activists and writers such as Sulak Sivaraksa of Thailand and the Swedish-born Helena Norberg-Hodge, based in Ladakh and England have written "penetrating critiques of Western models of "development" and globalization offering alternative Buddhist-based models (Rothberg, 1992). A cross-fertilization of our knowledge would enrich our understanding. Collaborative partnerships between Buddhism and Psychology may be helpful in designing programs of social action.

A Final Thought

Community psychologists studying Buddhism are like "new kids on the block" in what is a very old "neighborhood." Buddhism began 2600 years ago. It has a long and rich history of addressing suffering, promoting individual enlightenment, psychological empowerment, and community empowerment against social injustice. Buddhism has long known and used what psychological research is only recently beginning to validate as sound approaches to the development of psychological and community well-being. That these consistencies emerged in different contexts and from different methodologies points to the potential value of more deeply studying the wisdom of Buddhist psychology. Both psychology and Buddhism can benefit from a collaborative partnership in which our differences are used as transformative resources. Using our differences in ways that inform each discipline, through teaching and educating one another rather than simply complementing one another is what McMillan (2001) termed "transformative trades." Such an approach would reflect the highest level of maturity in community collaboration.

Author's Note

Portions of this chapter were presented in the symposium, Where Buddhism and Psychology Meet: Perspectives on Empowerment, at the 1999 American Psychological Association Convention, Boston, Massachusetts, August 19–23. A lengthy, slightly modified excerpt from *Resources for Stress Resistence: Parallels* in *Psychology and Buddhism* (1993) appears in this chapter with the permission of Saka Gakkai International-USA. I wish to thank Guy McCloskey and Greg Martin for their perceptive comments on an earlier draft of this manuscript.

References

Albee, G. W., Joffe, J. M., & Dusenbury, L. A. (Eds.) (1988). *Prevention, powerlessness and politics: Readings on social change*. Newbury Park, CA: Sage.

Alinsky, S. D. (1946). *Reveille for radicals*. Chicago: University of Chicago Press.

Beck, A. T. (1976). *Cognitive therapy and the emotional disorders*. New York: International Universities Press.

Chappell, D. (2000). Inclusive Buddhism. In. C. S. Queen (Ed.), *Engaged Buddhism in the West* (pp. 299–325) Boston: Wisdom Publications.

Cohen, E., Mobray, C. T., Gillete, V., & Thompson, E. (1992). Preventing homelessness: Religious organizations and housing development. *Prevention in Human Services, 10*, 169–185.

Dockett, K. H. (1993). *Resources for stress resistance: Parallels in psychology and Buddhism*. Santa Monica, CA: Soka Gakkai International-USA.

Dockett, K. (1999a, June). Engaged Buddhism and community psychology: Partners in social change. In J. Kress, (Chair), *Action Roundtable: Bringing together community psychology and Religion/Spirituality: Towards an action-research agenda for SCRA*. Action Roundtable conducted at the meeting of the Society for Community Research and Action, Yale University, New Haven, CT.

Dockett, K. (1999b, August). Psychological perspectives on Buddhist empowerment. In A. J. Marsella (Chair), *Where Buddhism and Psychology Meet: Perspectives on Empowerment*. Symposium conducted at the meeting of the American Psychological Association, Boston MA.

Dockeki, R. R. (1982). Liberation: Movement in theology, themes in community psychology. *Journal of community psychology, 10*, 185–196.

Duffy, K. G. & Wong, F. Y. (1996). *community psychology*. Boston: Allyn and Bacon.

Ellis, A. (1977). The basic clinical therapy of rational-emotive therapy. In A. Ellis & R. Grieger (Eds.), *Handbook of rational-emotive therapy*. New York: Springer.

Finkel, N. J. & Jacobsen, C. A. (1977). Significant life experiences in an adult sample. *American Journal of community psychology, 5*, 165–175.

Freire, P. (1970). *Pedagogy of the oppressed*. New York: Herder & Herder.

Hammond, P. & Machacek, D. (1999). *Soka Gakkai in America: Accommodation and conversion*. Oxford: Oxford University Press.

Hurst, J. (1998). Nichiren Shoshu and Soka Gakkai in America. In S. C. Prebish & K. K. Tanaka (Eds.), *The faces of Buddhism in America* (pp. 79–98). Berkeley: University of California Press.

Hood, R. W. Jr., Spilka, B., Hunsberger, B., & Gorsuch, R. (1996). *The psychology of religion*. New York: Guilford.

Ikeda, D. (1987). The human revolution: A prerequisite for lasting peace. *McGill Journal of Education, 22*(3), 257.

Ikeda, D. (1992). *Buddhism in Action*, VI, 219. Tokyo: Nichiren Shoshu International Center.

Ikeda, D. (1993, March). The sun of "Jiyu" over a new land. *Seikyo Times*, 52–56.

Ikeda, D. (1999, May). Toward a culture of peace: A cosmic view. *Living Buddhism*, 18–43.

Ikeda, D. (2001, June 22). True religion means commitment for peace. *World Tribune*, p. 1

Imamura, R. (1998). Buddhist and Western psychotherapies: An Asian American perspective. In C. S. Prebish & K. K. Tanaka (Eds.), *The faces of Buddhism in America* (pp. 228–237). Berkeley University of California Press.

Jason, L. A. (1997). *Community building: Values for a sustainable future*. Westport, CN: Praeger.

Jason, L. A. (1999, August). The role of religion and spirituality in community building. In A. Marsella (Chair), *Where Buddhism and psychology meet: Perspectives on empowerment*. Symposium conducted at the meeting of the American Psychological Association, Boston, MA.

Kloos, B. & Moore, T. (2000). The prospect and purpose of locating community research and action in religious settings. *Journal of community psychology, 28*, 119–137.

Kobasa, S. C. (1982). The hardy personality: Toward a social psychology of stress and health. In J. Suls & G. Sanders (Eds.), *Social Psychology of Health and Illness* (pp. 3–32). Hillsdale, NJ: Lawrence Erlbaum.

Kotler, A. (1996). *Engaged Buddhist reader*. Berkeley, CA: Parallax Press.

Kroeker, C. J. (1995). Individual, organizational, and societal empowerment: A study of the processes in a Nicaraguan agricultural cooperative. *American Journal of community psychology, 23*, 749–764.

Kraft, K. (1996). Engaged Buddhism. In A. Kotler (Ed.), *Engaged Buddhist reader* (pp. 64–69). Berkeley, CA: Parallax Press.

Lefcourt, H. M. & Davidson-Katz, K. (1991). Locus of control and health. In C. R. Synder & D. R. Forsyth (Eds.), *Handbook of social and clinical psychology* (pp. 246–266). Elmsford, New York: Pergamon Press.

Marsella, A. (1998). Toward a global community psychology. *American Psychologist*, 53(12), 1282–1291.

Maton, K. I. & Salem, D. A. (1995). Organizational characteristics of empowering community settings: A multiple case study approach. *American Journal of community psychology, 23*, 631–656.

Maton, K. I. & Wells, E. A. (1995). Religion as a community resource for well-being: Prevention, healing, and empowerment pathways. *Journal of Social Issues, 51*, 177–193.

Maton, K. I. (1989). Community settings as buffers of life stress? Highly supportive churches, mutual help groups, and senior centers. *American Journal of community psychology, 17*, 203–232.

McMillan, B., Florin, P., Stevenson, J., Kerman, B., & Mitchell, R. E. (1995). Empowerment praxis in community coalitions. *American Journal of community psychology, 23*, 699–728.

McMillan, D. (2001). Comments on two papers: Perkins/Long and Mahan. In J. R. Newbrough, Empirical Advances in Sense of Community: Current Issues and Applications, a poster cluster presented at the Eighth Biennial Conference on Community Research and Action, Atlanta, GA.

Moore, T. (1991). The African American church: A source of empowerment, mutual help, and social change. *Prevention in Human Services, 10*, 147–168.

Pargament, K. I. (1997). *The psychology of religion and coping: Theory, research, and practice*. New York: Guilford.

Pargament, K. I. & Park, C. L. (1995). Merely a defense? The variety of religious means and ends. *Journal of Social Issues, 51*, 13–32.

Pargament, K. I. & Maton, K. I. (2000). Religion in American life: a community psychology Prospective. In J. Rappaport & E. Seidman (Eds.), *The handbook of community psychology* (pp. 495–522). New York: Kluwer academic/Plenum Publishers.

Prebish, C. S. & Tanaka, K. K. (1998). *The faces of Buddhism in America*. Berkeley: University of California Press.

Perkins, D. D., & Zimmerman, M. A. (1995). Empowerment theory, research, and application. *American Journal of community psychology, 23*, 569–579.

Rappaport, J. (1977). *Community psychology: Values, research, and action*. New York: Holt, Rinehart and Winston.

Rappaport, J. (1981). In praise of paradox: A social policy of empowerment over prevention. *American Journal of community psychology, 9*, 1–25.

Rappaport, J. (1987). Terms of empowerment/exemplars of prevention: Toward a theory for community psychology. *American Journal of community psychology, 15*, 121–148.

Rappaport, J. (1995). Empowerment meets narrative: Listening to stories and creating settings. *American Journal of community psychology, 23*, 795–807.

Rappaport, J. & Simpkins, R. (1991). Healing and empowering through community narrative. In K. I. Maton & K. I. Pargament (Eds.), *Religion and prevention in mental health: Community intervention* (pp. 29–50). New York: Haworth.

Rothberg, D. (1992). Buddhist responses to violence and war: Resources for a socially engaged spirituality. *Journal of Humanistic Psychology, 32*(4), 41–75.

Rotter, J. B. (1966). Generalized expectancies for internal and external reinforcement. *Psychological Monographs, 89*(1 Whole No. 609).

Seikyo Times, (1988, November). The oneness of life and its environment, 18.

Seligman, M. E. P. & Maier, S. F. (1967). Failure to escape traumatic shock. *Journal of Experimental Psychology, 74*, 1–9.

Seligman, M. E. P. Greer, J., & Maier, S. F. (1968). The alleviation of learned helplessness in the dog. *Journal of Abnormal and Social Psychology, 73*, 256–262.

Solarz, A. (2000). SCRA mission statement. E-mail communication.

Speer, P. W., Hughey, J., Gensheimer, L. K., & Adams-Leavitt, W. (1995). Organizing for power: A comparative case study. *Journal of community psychology, 28*, 57–73.

The Writings of Nichiren Daishonin, (1999a). On omens, 644–648. Tokyo: Soka Gakkai.

The Writings of Nichiren Daishonin, (1999b). On attaining buddhahood in this lifetime, 3–5. Tokyo: Soka Gakkai.

The Writings of Nichiren Daishonin, (1999c). The opening of the eyes. Part Two, 251–298. Tokyo: Soka Gakkai.

The Writings of Nichiren Daishonin. (1999d). Happiness in this world, 681–682. Tokyo: Soka Gakkai.

The Writings of Nichiren Daishonin. (1999e). A ship to cross the sea of suffering, 33–34. Tokyo: Soka Gakkai.

Thurman, R. A. (1996). Nagarjuna's guidelines for Buddhist social action. In A. Kotler (Ed.), *Engaged Buddhist reader* (pp. 79–90). Berkeley, CA: Parallax Press.

Thurman, R. A. (1999). *Inner revolution*. New York: Riverhead Books.

Watts, R. J. (1993). Community action toward manhood development: A look at concepts and concerns from the frontline. *American Journal of community psychology, 21*, 747–773.

Zimmerman, M. A. (1995). Psychological empowerment: Issues and illustrations. *American Journal of community psychology, 23*, 581–601.

Zimmerman, M. A. (2000). Empowerment Theory: Psychological, Organizational, and Community Levels of Analysis. In J. Rappaport & E. Seidman (Eds.), *The handbook of community psychology*. (pp. 43–63). New York: Kluwer Academic/Plenum Publishers.

Zimmerman, M. A. & Rappaport, J. (1988). Citizen participation, perceived control, and psychological empowerment. *American Journal of community psychology, 16*, 725–750.

Chapter 9

The Role of Religion and Spirituality in Community Building

Leonard A. Jason and John Moritsugu

The purpose of this chapter is to attempt a synthesis of Buddhist values that underlie individual change and community psychology theory that provides a rationale for environmental and ecological influences on individual change. Both traditions have helped transform the world, one from a more inward spiritual framework and the other from a more action-oriented, environmental perspective. Each makes unique contributions and their combination provides the possibilities for a synergy that provides for even more comprehensive solutions to human suffering. In this chapter, we will first review briefly major characteristics of these two fields, and this will be followed with examples of how both traditions might enrich each other.

Buddhist Perspectives

Often, the lay person thinks of Buddhism as a monastic tradition, one that focuses on renunciation of the world in the hope of attaining enlightenment. This type of spiritual orientation might seem far removed from the more action-oriented approach of community psychologists. However, this school of Buddhism, which is called Theravada, in principle could have far impacting consequences on the external world, for if many individuals were to embrace these types of practices, clearly there would be less violence and conflict, and these are goals of the community psychology discipline. However, those from a Theravada perspective might see much of the work of external oriented, change-agents as being somewhat superficial, for to bring about surface change would not change the fundamental reasons for the sufferings of the masses.

In contrast to this approach, the Mahayana school is more active in their efforts to bring change into the external world. An example of the approach is Zen Buddhism. Members of the Zen school focus on practicing zazen, a form of meditation where the conscious mind is quieted and the unconscious is liberated. The mind returns to the ultimate reality of the void or emptiness that contains all (Owens, 1992). Those within the Mahayana school of Buddhism believe that our task in life is not to only achieve individual liberation but to help others achieve this state. When we discuss in this chapter the possible integration of community psychology and Buddhist philosophy, we will be referring to the Mahayana school of Buddhism.

Buddhist practice has most often focused on individual efforts at change. As Dockett (1999a) has stated, in the United States Buddhism has more often been used as a form of personal psychotherapy or quest for self-enlightenment rather than a vehicle for social change. However, it is clear that those from the Mahayana school have at times embraced more community and large-scale efforts at change, and examples of such programs will be discussed in later sections. A powerful synthesis might be possible by focusing on Buddhist values that underlie individual transformations and community psychology theory that provides a conceptual context and rationale for these changes.

The Field of Community Psychology

The field of community psychology emerged in the late 1960s. It represented an effort by some psychologists to become more active in helping to solve some of the social and community problems that confronted our country during that turbulent period (Duffy & Wong, 1996). This field has always been directed more toward external change than inner transformation, so the principles of Buddhism have rarely been considered by those espousing this community perspective.

Among the members of this field, there is much controversy about how to actually bring about community change. Cook and Shadish (1986) have suggested that there are three ways of implementing social change. They claim that the most successful model involves making incremental modifications in existing social problems. Advocates of this approach feel that few policies are approved if they call for more than marginal changes in the status quo. A bolder approach is the use of demonstration programs to test the efficacy of a planned innovation; however, detractors of this model claim that many successful demonstration programs have never been widely replicated. On the other end of the spectrum lie the interventions that change basic social structures. Albee (1986) supports this model, and believes that we will always have excessive amounts of psychopathology as long as we have exploitation, imperialism, excessive concentration of economic power, nationalism, institutions that perpetuate powerlessness, poverty, discrimination, sexism, racism, and ageism. Each of these models deals with external conditions, even though reduction in prejudice could be argued to represent an internal state. The community psychology means to accomplish these objectives has rarely been from a spiritual point of view. Even though the elimination of deplorable environmental conditions are laudable goals, it is the thesis of this chapter that only a transformation of our values such as by embracing Buddhist principles will provide us the templates to successfully work on the forces that cause unequal distribution of the world's resources.

At a more theoretical perspective, most community psychologists subscribe to either a Social Competence, Empowerment or Ecological model, and each will be described below. Some theorists focus on a Social Competence model where the goal is to prevent disorders and enhance competencies (Duffy & Wong, 1996). Examples of such approaches include the drug abuse prevention programs that focus on teaching skills to youngsters to resist being pressured into taking drugs. The social competence approach, one that is endorsed by many community psychologists, is limited by its ahistorical and philosophical tenets. For example, many interventions within this model might help individuals develop skills and competencies that allow them to gain more resources, become more independent and even self-satisfied. However, there are dangers in an approach that does not have guiding values, and behavior change in itself might reinforce tendencies to become less interconnected with one's family and community. Buddhist philosophy would perceive such interventions as possibly having second order negative consequences. While this model is the most-straight forward, at the same time, it misses many of the richer theoretical ideas of the other models to be described below.

Another community psychology model involves Empowerment, and those adopting this paradigm attempt to enhance justice and people's sense of control over their own destinies (Rappaport, 1981). Many community psychologists feel more comfortable with this type of model, as it clearly is action oriented and often goes beyond the individual-level of a Social Competence model. One difficulty for practitioners of this Empowerment model involves figuring out how to decide which groups to help empower. In many communities, there are opposing groups, and each feels that their perspectives are correct, as is evidenced by the conflict between the Jews and Arabs in the Middle East. It is sometimes unclear exactly how to enhance justice in such situations, and clearly, Buddhist principles could be used to suggest some possible ways of accomplishing this, and this will be elaborated in more detail in a later section of this chapter (see also Chapter 10 in this volume).

Another paradigm that has captured the attention of many community psychologists is the Ecological model (Kelly, 1985, 1987, 1990). Kelly's goal has been to develop and propose theories of how people become effective and adaptive in varied social environments. The ecological paradigm is a guiding framework for understanding behavior in interaction with its social and cultural contexts. In this way, it is a more theoretically rich and useful model than the ones reviewed above. Kingry-Westergaard and Kelly (1990) have suggested that a principle fundamental to ecological approaches is the need to use multiple methods to understand the complex qualities of relationships and systems. One of these methods for increasing our understanding of that which we claim to know is the collaborative relationship between the researcher and the participants. This means that concepts and hypotheses are developed and tested by both the researcher and the participants. This is a principle that would be welcomed by Buddhists, as it characterizes their values as well. This feature of the ecological model has also been espoused by many feminists, among others, who recommend that we listen to and understand people first and foremost from their points of view. When people are involved in research projects, they should be included as participants, not as subjects, and the process of being understood and represented is considered empowering.

Ecological principles could be used by professionals who join in long-term collaborative relationships with persons and settings. By involving participants actively in the planning of interventions, the recipients of the programs receive support, learn to identify resources, and become better problem-solvers who are more likely to manage future problems and issues. Interventions that have been generated from collaboratively defined, produced, and implemented change efforts are more apt to endure. By involving participants in the design of the research, investigators may gain a greater appreciation of the culture and unique needs of the community, and this may increase the possibility of the research findings being used to benefit the community. An ecological approach would analyze community traditions for responding to community problems, help evaluate or create settings that provide individuals opportunities to continue receiving support after termination of formal treatment programs, work closely with community leaders in all aspects of the health care intervention, and assess positive and negative second-order ripple effects of an intervention. An ecological perspective provides a method of conceptualizing our problems with anchor points for deeper analysis that may ultimately help us develop more appropriate health care service delivery systems.

Contextualism is a primary feature of this Ecological model, and it has been defined by Kingry-Westergaard and Kelly (1990) as our embeddedness in the world we observe. Because of this principle, knowledge is relevant only within a given frame of reference. This idea was further developed by Bry, Hirsch, Newbrough, Reischl, and Swindle (1990), who viewed knowledge as limited by its historical and cultural context. They believe that we do not simply glean knowledge from our objective observations of an objective world, but that the nature of the knower contributes to the nature of what is known, implying that science tells us as much about the investigator as it does about the phenomena being studied.

These ideas from the Ecological community model hint at a paradigm that disavows the possibility of foundational knowledge. In other words, what we learn from one setting or community group might be specific to that group, and there might not be any knowledge that is generalizable to multiple settings. Here we see a difference between advocates of the Ecological model versus adherents of Buddhism, who clearly do espouse that there are fundamental values and ways of breaking the bonds of individual suffering. If this Ecological model perspective is taken to its extreme, it can lead to the loss of all connection with foundational values, a loss exemplified in the contemporary philosophy called deconstructive postmodernism. This worldview posits that there are no universal truths, but rather that all concepts are culturally constructed and all meaning is temporary and relative. Adherents believe that this philosophy will liberate its proponents from all domination, but its critics fear that this liberation could lead to valuelessness. Spretnak (1991) suggests that this fashionable philosophy leads to a sense of groundlessness, detachment, and shallow engagement. Ragsdale (2003), in Chapter 3 of this volume, uses the term "nihilistic relativism" to refer to this loss of connection with foundational values.

The Ecological approach is a powerful model that provides its adherents new ways of understanding social and community phenomena, but in many ways it lacks a value base, which makes it also problematic to decide with which groups to collaborate. As an example, an Ecological approach could be used to provide resources and legitimacy to community groups and organizations whose missions are directed toward further control and domination of other people and of the environment. It is this value framework that is so often lacking within many of the models that we have discussed, and the thesis of this chapter is that Buddhist traditions could provide guides for energizing the visions of the field of community psychology.

Buddhism and other philosophies from the East have contributed to an alternative way of seeing the world, one that does assume the possibility of fundamental knowledge. Spretnak (1991) has coined the word ecological postmodernism, and it joins the value base of spiritual traditions with the action-oriented perspective of ecological community psychology. Such a framework might provide community psychologists a more vibrant sense of interconnectedness, one that is conscious of the unity in which we are all embedded. In the next section, we review some of the foundational values within the Buddhist school of thought.

Buddhist Values

As mentioned in the previous section, the community psychology models generally do not endorse the existence of any fundamental values that would be applicable to diverse groups, and they would argue that the task of the community psychologist is to learn of and be sensitive to the different values and traditions that exist within every community. Buddhists, in contrast, would be willing to propose fundamental values or principles that could be generalizable, and below we will sketch out some of these more universal principles.

According to Goleman (1992), Buddhism focuses on the death of the ego. Advocates of this religion believe that suffering is due to unrealistic expectations in a world of impermanence. The goal is to achieve transcendence, to be freed of desire and fear, in order to participate in this turbulent and sorrowful world with joy and rapture (Campbell, 1980). In one type of Buddhism, through 227 observances and prohibitions, followers of this religion restrain their actions in order to produce a calm and subdued mind. In order to control the mind, Buddhists employ the technique of mindfulness, a process that includes restraint of the senses. In an effort to facilitate detachment from internal thoughts and perceptions, the practitioner of Buddhism cultivates the habit of noticing sensory perceptions, but trying not to allow these perceptions to stimulate the mind into chain reactions of thoughts. Through bare awareness of the subtle sensations, without judging them as bad or good, one might eradicate patterns of response that might otherwise cause deep complexes. Beginners at this discipline often find it difficult to fix the mind on a single object without being distracted by thoughts. This is a challenging task as the mind processes 126 bits of information per second, or 7,560 per minute (Csikszentmihalyi, 1990).

As mentioned before, Buddhists believe that life is full of experiences that produce suffering. In the first of the Four Noble Truths, the Buddha taught that suffering can be experienced as a result of birth, old age, sickness, death, separation from loved ones, desire, attachment, and clinging. In the Second Noble Truth, the cause of suffering is attributed to attachment and desire, which flame anger, jealousy, grief, worry, and despair. The Third Noble Truth is that understanding the truth about life brings about the cessation of suffering. The Fourth Noble Truth is the path that leads to the cessation of suffering (Nhat Hanh, 1991). Suffering can be eliminated only through the Eightfold Noble Path: rightness in speech, action, and livelihood (morality); rightness in concentration, mindfulness, and effort (meditation); and rightness in understanding and thought (wisdom).

For Spretnak (1991), foundational values can be found in the Buddhist efforts to bring serenity to the mind or in the Native Americans' reverence for and balance with nature. Foundational values can also be seen in the bodhisattva, who according to Buddhist teaching is a person with great compassion, love, and empathy (Thurman, 1996). The bodhisattva is committed to not only personal transformation but also the transformation of others, and this sense of responsibility for others is fostered by the foundational value that involves the interdependence of all things.

The power of these ideas is that they provide a framework for those who are interested in bringing out a reduction in suffering, a goal of both Buddhists and community psychologists. The Buddhists have been clear on what the source of suffering is, and they have developed specific practices for those engaged in the effort to change the mind. The key question that a Buddhist might pose for a community psychologist is if the world were to be more equal in terms of the distribution of resources, a very real goal of community psychologists, would the individuals who no longer lived in poverty be any happier or content or satisfied with their lives. The Buddhist might respond that the real change would need to be with ways of thinking, whereas the community psychologist would respond that the world needs to be changed before people have the possibilities of a better life. In fact, both approaches are not irreconcilable, and true liberation might need to be accomplished in both the internal and external world.

In the sections below, we will examine ways that psychologists might use these types of foundational values, both in assessment and therapy. Throughout our discussion, we will review the possible implications of these ideas to broader community-level interventions. This will be followed with examples of actual Buddhist inspired community-level interventions.

Buddhist Influenced Ways to Measure Important Psychological Constructs

There has been a tendency among psychologists to focus on mental disorder or pathological traits rather than wellness or health. In contrast, Dockett (1993) has shown how issues such a stress resistance can be seen from a Buddhist point of view. Foundational ideas are a central characteristic of this approach. Some psychologists have focused more on health promoting psychological attitudes such as wisdom, and this construct stipulates that foundational values are evident.

Jason et al. (2001) recently developed the Foundational Values Scale, a test designed to measure the construct of wisdom, with ideas borrowed from eastern religions. The first component, Harmony, consisted of items assessing balance, self-love, good judgment, appreciation, and purpose in life. These are internal domains; they tap some concepts of Berry's (1988) pattern of subjectivity, Wegela's (1988) aspect of spaciousness, and Burkhardt's (1989) characteristic of finding a purpose in life. It is interesting to note that, to the extent to which one is balanced, has an appreciation of life, and can cope with uncertainty, one has a higher likelihood of being less burdened by stress. The second component of the Foundational Values Scale, Warmth, includes kindness, compassion, and animation. This domain seems to be related to Berry's (1988) pattern of communion, Wegela's (1988) aspect of warmth, and Burkhardt's (1989) characteristic of harmonious interconnectedness. The qualities of kindness and compassion seem to be related to being in the present and having a sense of humor. This dimension includes the extension of hope and happiness to others through warmth, humor, and kindness. The third component of the scale is Intelligence. It appears that it is not merely the quality of intelligence but how it is used that determines its connection to wisdom. Using one's intelligence to solve problems and help others appears to be a key feature of wisdom-related intelligence. The fourth component, Nature, includes a concern and reverence for the environment, and a sense that all life is interconnected. This domain is closely related to Berry's (1988) pattern of differentiation and Wegela's (1988) aspect of spaciousness. It appears that one component of perceived wisdom is concern for the environment. It is interesting that this component is also related to the experience of flow, for it is perhaps one's love for and appreciation of the external world that allows one to be so deeply involved in an activity that nothing else seems to matter. This dimension is reflected in foundational knowledge as practiced by Native Americans, who have revered and remained in balance with nature for thousands of years (Spretnak, 1991). The final component, Spirituality, consists of living a spiritual life and having a fellowship or union with God.

The study of wisdom and scales to measure it has important implications for those with interests in promoting community interventions, as it provides the potential for introducing vital, energizing symbols and messages that could be used to restore a sense of meaning to those who are discouraged and alienated. A better knowledge of wisdom could be potentially useful in understanding topics about which community psychologists have particular interest including the development and sustenance of community leaders, resiliency in the face of oppression, coping with uncertainty, and framing events in a larger context. As an example, wisdom among community activists might involve a strategic vision rooted in their faith and the discipline to adhere to a chosen pathway for a substantial time even when the road is very hard and full of distractions.

There are often practices and values within the settings and communities within which we work. Is it not possible that many of our interventions and change efforts are less successful because the values that are part of our interventions are not supported or even opposed by overarching values within the settings that we work. In such situations, the study of values might allow us the opportunity to find whether the interventions that we mount are value consistent or discordant with the setting values, and then we might have a better approach for how we might intervene. Before setting up a particular intervention, we might first better understand or even attempt to change those setting or community values or practices that do not support the aims of our interventions.

The first author, to provide a more concrete example of this principle, worked for many years developing youth smoking prevention programs in schools. However, he found that the majority of merchants in the community sold minors cigarettes (Jason et al., 1991). What the author learned was that often our efforts at bringing about behavior change will be hampered or compromised because of the values within the communities or the settings from which we situate our programs. If we develop smoking cessation programs and disregard the fact that the community leaders openly sell dangerous tobacco products to minors, it is clear that our preventive interventions will be less successful (Rhodes & Jason, 1988). The larger implications are clear: programs that involve Buddhist practices and principles might be best integrated into those settings that are value concordant with the overall philosophy of Buddhism. If one develops prevention programs in the schools that are geared toward helping youngsters not engage in risky behaviors such as smoking, or if we teach youngsters meditation practices, values and supports within the schools and local community need to be understood. If schools feature competition and authoritarian decision making, such values might be incompatible with Buddhist principles, whereas as those settings that support cooperation and more egalitarian values might be more value consistent with the messages within transformational interventions. When the mores and values of such contextual variables are supportive of the interventions, there is greater opportunity for the development and maintenance of transformational skills, interests and practices.

Buddhist Influenced Therapies

These foundational ideas from Buddhist thought have had their greatest influence in psychology at the more individual level, and in particular influencing several forms of therapy. One of the more popular forms in Japan is called Morita therapy (Reynolds, 1984). Practitioners of Morita therapy offer clients a variety of meditative strategies (e.g., counting the breath, mantras, prayer) that they might constantly return to an awareness of their immediate circumstances. The three key principles in this approach concern the importance of accepting one's feelings, knowing one's purpose, and doing what needs to be done. The richness of life comes from living it, not through thinking about it. Of course, such principles could easily be adapted to more community-based interventions by, for example, using the media to transmit these ideas to larger audiences or by teaching such principles in primary preventive school-based interventions.

In the mid-1970s, Ron Kurtz developed Hakomi body-centered psychotherapy, which was heavily influenced by Taoism and Buddhism (Johanson & Kurtz, 1991). Rather than analyzing and talking about life, clients are encouraged to turn their awareness toward the present moment, thus cultivating the state described in the Buddhist concept of mindfulness. Clients practice staying with an experience (e.g., feelings of anxiety); and as they report on it, the experience deepens and then one experience will lead to another and the process will move from surface experiences to core beliefs which generate and organize these experiences. (Johanson & Kurtz, 1991; p. 14). Such practices could also be extended to neighborhoods and community groups, and by doing so, these generative principles could be considered useful in community interventions.

In the West, a number of other therapies also have eastern spiritual dimensions; these are often called transpersonal therapies (Weide, 1973). In these approaches, the therapist uses traditional therapeutic techniques as well as meditation and other awareness exercises from the East (Vaughan, 1979). The goals are to develop the capacity to take responsibility for oneself; to experience the full range of emotions while remaining detached from the personal melodrama; and to meet one's physical, mental, and spiritual needs. Rather than curing ailments, the therapist's job is to allow clients to tap into their inner resources and allow natural healing to occur. Therapy is a process of awakening or becoming conscious. Such individual oriented therapies could also be used to humanize work settings, and as such, the principles could be used to bring about larger-scale changes in the community.

Wegela (1988) is another psychotherapist who has tried to bring Buddhist ideas to the practice of therapy. In her work, she identified three goals from a Buddhist point of view: spaciousness, clarity, and warmth. Spaciousness is an accommodation to whatever experiences arise within oneself. Clarity is a full apprehension of the textures, temperatures, and colors of one's experiences, without embellishment. And finally, warmth is an experience of compassion for oneself and others. Wegela adds that one can bring these qualities to any experience, and that in doing so, one experiences intrinsic health. Regardless of one's external condition or physical difficulties, health is always within us if we are open to these experiences. The purpose of the healer is to uncover what already exists.

The ideas of Wegela are so very different from many current western-oriented, health psychotherapists, who seem to be more interested in techniques that involve superficial interventions, ones which have no philosophical and spiritual foundations. Lazarus (1985) states that we often prescribe mechanical procedures best used to facilitate problem-focused coping with minor, surface aspects of problems in living. For example, therapists sometimes help clients cope with adversity by teaching them to think positively, and consider the clients who do not succeed at this technique ungrateful or resistant. This tendency to downplay the negative ends up trivializing authentic distress by denying its legitimacy. Perhaps the Buddhist notions of Wegela could be integrated into community-level interventions that help transform current practice of therapists and medical personnel to be more conscious of these unhelpful practices, and to begin a dialogue about the fundamental values that living beings are capable of experiencing.

Ecological Transformational Interventions

The first author has coined the term Ecological Transformational to describe the types of work engaged in by community psychologists with Eastern philosophical interests (Jason, 1997). Community psychologists can function as visionaries and mystics by identifying the issues that we as a society will need to face and deal with in the future. Those who are in this discipline also engage in archeological excavations to better understand the religious, historical, and philosophical issues that are contributing to our current social problems. The field of community psychology is also predicated on the assumption that some of our most complex and intransigent social and community problems can be synergistically transformed by the recognition, appreciation, and utilization of those assets and inner resources that already exist within social settings. This function represents the alchemist role of the community psychologist. And finally, the discipline espouses a commitment to public articulation of our values, and by such action, we explicitly adopt the distinct role of advocate, while many other social scientists adopt more impartial program evaluation roles.

Eco-Transformational interventions programs support Buddhist notions such as our interconnectedness with the natural world, and help us live in balance with nature, as opposed to trying to control her. This model would support those scientific and technologic investigations that help explore the mysteries of life, and re-affirm and validate the importance of rituals, traditions, and initiatory processes that help people and their communities mature and develop intimate bonds. Finally, Eco-Transformational interventions attempt to recapture the sense of community that provides responsibility, mission, and commitment to the welfare of one's community.

Families, communities, and organizations often progress through identifiable phases in their journey toward maturity, intimacy, and conscious loving. Shaffer and Anundsen (1993) suggest that these stages involve excitement (getting high on possibilities), autonomy (jockeying for power), stability (settling into roles and structures), synergy (allowing self and group to mutually unfold) and transformation (expanding, segmenting, or disbanding). Communities need to fully experience each of these stages, to learn from them, and then to move on to their next phases. When developing a social and community intervention, one needs to recognize that resolution of each of these stages provides opportunities for transformative growth. Buddhist practices could be used to help members endure the stresses that each of these phases can produce.

There are many forms of community, ranging from functional to conscious (Shaffer & Anundsen, 1993). Functional communities focus on external tasks, pay little attention to group process, and are structured according to a hierarchy of fixed roles. Examples include traditional extended families or small towns. On the other hand, there are conscious communities that focus on individual and group development, and are characterized by openness, diversity, role sharing, and regular renewal. Examples of these include intentional families and long-term neighborhood or peer groups. Buddhist principles could be used to help residential communities become more conscious and visionary, where deep trust and open group process are a part of everyday behavior.

In our daily work, we are more likely to deal with every day problems such as drug abuse. An important question involves how might the Buddhist and community perspectives enable us to develop more engaging and transforming interventions. Below, we will provide a case examples of current community-level interventions, and we will show how attending to the Eco-Transformational issues might allow an integration of Buddhist and community psychology so that our interventions are more enduring and significant.

Oxford House

Oxford House was founded by Paul Molloy and a group of men recovering from alcoholism (Jason et al., 1997). While living in a halfway house in Montgomery County, Maryland, he saw 12 fellow house members forced to leave the house because they had reached six months residency, the maximum length of stay. Of these 12 men, 11 relapsed within 30 days. Paul and the other residents then received word that the halfway house had lost its funding and would close within 30 days. After considerable confusion and exchange of ideas with members of the Alcoholics Anonymous community, the residents decided to rent the house themselves. Although they initially had wanted to hire a staff person, they were unable to do so because of the cost. They decided to run the house in a democratic fashion. They named their community Oxford House, after the Oxford Group, an organization that inspired the founders of Alcoholics Anonymous.

In discussing the way the house should operate, local A.A. members urged the residents to keep the house simple. Many had disliked the old halfway house's rules. One house member spoke about his experience in a college fraternity, which had housed 16 men without a house manager. A plan for organizing the house emerged from these discussions. Members agreed that one positive aspect of the halfway house had been its reinforcement of sobriety through the immediate eviction of residents who used alcohol or other drugs. The basic rules of conduct for Oxford House were, and remain, simple: operate democratically, with each member paying his or her rent and doing all assigned chores; and stay sober. Deviation from these rules is cause for immediate eviction. There are no professional staff members at Oxford Houses, and all costs of the program are covered by members of the Oxford Houses.

Six months after the first Oxford House was formed, it had accumulated enough resources to begin a second; members of the second house, in turn, worked to form a third. Within thirteen years the number of Oxford Houses had grown to more than twenty. In July of 1988, Congressman Edward Madigan asked residents of Oxford House for ideas for legislation that would help promote the Oxford House concept nationwide. After residents testified about their experiences, new legislation was introduced to help spread this innovation. A provision within the

Federal Anti-Drug Abuse Act of 1988 mandated that each of the 50 states establish a revolving fund of $100,000 to be used to establish group homes for substance abusers along the lines of the Oxford House model. Between 1988 and 1999, the number has increased to more than 700 houses.

After treatment for substance abuse, whether it is in hospital-based treatment programs, therapeutic communities, or recovery homes, many patients return to former high-risk environments or stressful family situations. Returning to these settings without a network of people to support abstinence increases chances of a relapse. As a consequence, substance abuse recidivism following treatment is high for both men and women. Under modern managed care, private and public sector inpatient substance abuse facilities have reduced their services dramatically. Thus, there is a tremendous need to develop, evaluate, and expand lower cost, residential, non-medical, community-based care options for substance abuse patients.

So, what might the lesson of Oxford Houses be for individuals with Buddhist philosophies? Oxford Houses are behavior settings where individuals have the support of other non-using adults to begin their path toward abstinence. If a therapist or treatment program were to offer individuals with drug and alcohol problems Buddhist principles, and not provide those individuals behavior settings and safe environments to protect themselves from temptation and drug solicitations, the probability of success would be attenuated. However, if Buddhists would also think in Eco-Transformational terms, they would provide not only Buddhist philosophy and practice opportunities, but also work toward establishing settings, where individuals have the chance to begin self-explorations and practices that might allow more opportunity for developing spiritual pursuits, like Buddhism. However, without the support and structure of these types of settings, particularly for individuals who are such high risk of relapse, it would be difficult to have the stability and support to develop the transformational internal foundational values that might provide even sturdier long-term recovery.

Today we are faced with the dilemma of thousands of people who are drug addicted, homeless, and who live in poverty. What can a Buddhist offer to such individuals? The lesson from the Oxford Houses are clear: when people become very sick with chronic illnesses or drug abuse problems, they need not only psychological strategies (which can include Buddhist meditational approaches) and medications to control symptoms, but often a setting or community to protect them so that can regain their faith and heal. At present, there are few settings in the world that affords this type of support for people. What is needed are families, Oxford Houses, or communities who are willing to take in individuals for extended periods of time. This approach represents a different way of extending services – combining strategies that (a) strengthen inner resources through instilling hope, confidence, enthusiasm and the will to live, and (b) provide a place for people to live that is protected and nourishing – represents a more comprehensive program that could be applied to many of our more recalcitrant problems. If these types of more comprehensive approaches become more common, our effectiveness in helping people will thereby be enhanced. Community psychologists and Buddhists would agree that we become a more caring and humane society when we invest resources into the establishment of decent living conditions for all our citizens.

In the section below, we will examine several individuals and Buddhist groups that have developed spiritual interventions at the community-level. These are inspiring examples of what can occur when Buddhist principles are combined with visionary leaders who are attempting to bring about structural changes in the world.

Buddhist Initiatives

Ahangamage Tudor, a Sri Lankan Buddhist born in 1931, was deeply affected and inspired by the life and teachings of both Gandhi and the Buddha (Jason et al., 2000). In 1958, Ariyaratne founded the Sarvodaya Shramadana Movement to promote community development and to work against social injustice. Buddhist philosophy suffuses Ariyaratne's work, as he sees all beings as interdependent and ultimately as striving toward "awakening." He believes that this notion of "awakening" could be a resource for social change by opening up people's capacity to work together and to experience compassion, joy, and responsibility. Ariyaratne firmly believes in a bottom-up approach, always seeking to promote the well being of the community based on needs that have been delineated by community members. There is an emphasis on fostering the competencies that are already present within each community, thereby promoting the self-esteem of all involved. The accomplishments of Sarvodaya include the building of schools, encouragement of literacy, promotion of health care and sanitation, building of roads and transportation facilities, promotion of locally produced goods, and fostering of peace between people of different races, faiths, and classes. Today, these community development programs have been initiated in over 8,600 villages. Furthermore, the Sarvodaya Shramadana Movement has become international, aiming at "world awakening" not only in Sri Lanka, but also in Africa and in other parts of Asia (Ariyaratne, 1996). The Sarvodaya movement seeks to promote social change that is aimed at comprehensive solutions to society's problems. Ariyaratne readily recognizes that there are no simple solutions to solve community difficulties and he believes that to be effective, change must occur on every level.

Mohandas Karamchand Gandhi (1869–1948) developed his philosophy by integrating ideas from different religions (including Hinduism and Buddhism) (Jason et al., 2000). He welcomed the views of the different religious and political factions within the party and advocated for the needs of each group as the movement progressed. Gandhi led civil disobedience movements that were based on taking economic power back into the hands of Indians. He promoted the social welfare of all disenfranchised groups, such as the Untouchables and other castes of lower socioeconomic/social status. Ultimately, Gandhi believed that it is only through spiritual empowerment that people can sustain change in the other areas.

Rothberg (1998) has described Buddhist resistance in response to wars in the Vietnam, Tibet, Burma, and Bangladesh. Many of these movements have borrowed from ideas developed by Gandhi. A Vietnam Buddhist monk Thich Nhat Hanh coined the term "engaged Buddhism" (Kraft, 1996), which involves the expansion of Buddhist practices as a strategy for social and community change (Rothberg, 1992; Thurman, 1999). In addition, monks in Thailand have led a community development movement against ecological devastation. In North America, community projects have been sponsored by the Buddhist Peace Fellowship, the Bangkok-based International Network of Engaged Buddhists, The Interracial Buddhist Council, and the Soka Gakkai International (Dockett, 1999, 2003). Buddhists have been in the forefront on movements to abolish nuclear weapons, to develop the Earth Charter, to develop dialogue on interfaith topics, and have contributed to relief programs.

The Need for a Road Map for Social and Community Interventions

A question central to any intervention and to intervention processes as a whole is whether or not there are fundamental developmental and psychological initiations that we as human beings need to progress through, and whether or not certain core values might underlie our efforts to help others. Without road maps or guides, it might be difficult to design interventions that address the structural issues that are predisposing so many contemporary citizens to a sense of isolation and alienation. To the extent that we are dealing with a crisis of values and a breakdown of a psychological sense of community, our methods of conceptualizing our problems might require religious and philosophical theories as anchor points for deeper analysis. In this chapter, we have argued that Buddhist values could provide one such foundation.

In earlier times, before the advent of the industrial age, colonial imperialism, and the breakdown of extended kinship groups, there were rituals, customs, and rites that helped ease the transition from the dependent status of youth to the more independent role of adulthood. Is it not possible that some of the problems within our youth represent an attempt to deal with the loss of the myths and rituals that gave previous generations a more tangible sense of meaning within society? Is it not possible that some of our efforts could be used to explore the remnants of that mythology that still reside within our youth, and to actively help them recreate myths that are meaningful to their families and communities? Buddhist practices provide a comprehensive road map for individuals that helps them imaginatively transform life's customs and routine, and gives meaning to all phases and changes that we undergo.

Many of our social interventions and conceptualizations of community problems have omitted reference to heuristic ideas within the fields of religion philosophy, and mythology. In part, some of these ideas are considered incompatible with the scientific method. However, it can be argued that a broadened conceptualization yields many rich benefits. For example, each individual life has its psychological and metaphysical themes, and their resolution greatly influences one's ability to participate in a communal or family setting. Because each person is on his or her own unique voyage, and has different shadows to contend with, it is not unusual for conflict to occur among those who are trying to create new collective settings. Even though each journey is a solo mission, a critical task along that journey is to learn to live together in community. This is an element often neglected by those describing the spiritual journey: the creation of social settings that provide a sense of community to all members, a sense of meaning to one's spiritual yearnings, and altruism that refuses to be preoccupied with one's own individual needs.

Buddhism and the other wisdom traditions speak to deep sources within our souls. Our analyses and social programs would be immeasurably enriched by learning how to honor our thoughts (through Buddhist practices). This tradition might help us return to a balance with nature, both with and within the natural world; restore and honor symbols and traditions that have provided meaning to our lives; and restore the sense of connectedness with life that people once had with their communities and their land.

The real task for community psychologists is to help each people and communities find their personal and communal mythologies. This will require that people and communities search their own experiences, and their own and other cultures, for those symbols and traditions that energize and vitalize them. It will require the blending of old and new, foreign and familiar; and a respectful primary focus on the meaning beneath the stories and symbols. We believe that foundational values, such as those that exist within Buddhist thought, might provide a sturdy road map for this journey toward individual transformation and community change.

References

Albee, G. W. (1986). Toward a just society. *American Psychologist, 41*(8), 891–898.

Ariyaratne, A. T. (1996). Waking everybody up. In A. Kotler (Ed.), *Engaged Buddhist Reader* (pp. 91–97). Berkeley, CA: Parallax Press.

Berry, T. (1988). *The dream of the earth.* San Francisco: Sierra Club Books.

Bry, B. H., Hirsch, B. J., Newbrough, J. R., Reischl, T. M., & Swindle, R.W. (1990). Criteria of excellence II. Hypothesis generation: Human science and attribute-centered social regularities. In P. Tolan, C. Keys, F. Chertok, & L. Jason (Eds.), *Researching community psychology: Issues of theory and methods* (pp. 101–108). Washington, DC: American Psychological Association.

Burkhardt, M. A. (1989). Spirituality: An analysis of the concept. *Holistic Nursing Practice, 3*(3), 69–77.

Campbell, J. (1980). *Transformation of myth through time. Volume II.* (Available from Dolphin tapes, P.O. Box 71, Big Sur, CA 93920).

Cook, T. D. & Shadish, W. R. (1986). Program evaluation: The worldly science. In M.R. Rosenzweig & L.W. Porter (Eds.), *Annual Review of Psychology* (pp. 193–232). Palo Alto, CA: Annual Reviews.

Csikszentmihalyi, M. (1990). *Flow: The psychology of optimal experience.* New York: HarperCollins.

Dockett, K. H. (1993). *Resources for stress resistance: Parallels in psychology and buddhism.* Santa Monica, CA: Soka Gakkai International-USA.

Dockett, K. H. (1999a, June). Engaged Buddhism and community psychology: Partners in social change. In J. Kress (Chair), *Action Roundtable: Bringing together community psychology and Religion/Spirituality: Towards an action-research agenda for SCRA.* Action Roundtable conducted at the biennial meeting of the Society for Community Research and Action, Yale University, New Haven, CN.

Dockett, K. H. (1999b, August). *Psychological perspectives on Buddhist empowerment.* In A. J. Marsella, (Chair), *Where Buddhism and Psychology Meet: Perspectives on Empowerment.* Symposium conducted at the 106th Annual Convention of the American Psychological Association, Boston.

Dockett, K. H. (2003). Buddhist empowerment: Individual, organizational, and societal transformation. In K. H. Dockett, G. R. Dudley-Grant, & C. Peter Bankart (Eds.), *Psychology and Buddhism: From Individual to global community.* (pp. 173–196) New York: Kluwer Academic/Plenum Publishers.

Duffy, K.G. & Wong, F. Y. (1996). *community psychology.* Boston: Allyn and Bacon.

Goleman, D. (1992). The buddha on meditation and states of consciousness. In C. T. Tart (Ed.), *Transpersonal Psychologies* (pp. 203–230). New York: HarperCollins.

Jason, L. A. (1997). *Community building: Values for a sustainable future.* Westport, CT: Praeger.

Jason, L. A., Ferrari, J. R., Smith, B., Marsh, P., Dvorchak, P. A., Groessl, E. J., Pechota, M. E., Curtin, M., Bishop, P. D., Kot, E., & Bowden, B.S. (1997). An exploratory study of male recovering substance abusers living in a self-help, self-governed setting. *Journal of Mental Health Administration 24*, 332–339.

Jason, L. A., Ji. P. Y., Anes, M. D., & Birkhead, S. H. (1991). Active enforcement of cigarette control laws in the prevention of cigarette sales to minors. *Journal of the American Medical Association, 266*, 3159–3161.

Jason, L. A., Ji, P. Y., Birkhead, S. H., Anes, M. D., & Xaverious (1992). Assessing cigarette sales rates to minors. *Evaluation and the Health Professions, 15*(4), 375–384.

Jason, L.A., Pratt, T., Ware, C., Chimata, R., Bangi, A., & Johnson, D. (2000). Social activists: Lesson for community psychologists. Paper submitted for publication.

Jason, L. A., Reichler, A., King, C., Madsen, D., Camacho, J., & Marchese, W. (2001). The measurement of wisdom: A preliminary effort. *Journal of community psychology, 29*(5), 585–598.

Johanson, G. & Kurtz, R. (1991). *Grace unfolding. Psychotherapy in the spirit of the Tao-te-Ching.* New York: Bell Tower.

Kelly, J. G. (1985). The concept of primary prevention: Creating new paradigms. *Journal of Primary Prevention, 5*, 269–272.

Kelly, J. G. (1987, April). Beyond prevention techniques: Generating social settings for a public's health. Paper presented at the Tenth Erich Lindemann Memorial Lecture. Harvard Medical School, Boston, MA.

Kelly, J. G. (1990). Changing contexts and the field of community psychology. *American Journal of community psychology, 18*, 769–792.

Kingry-Westergaard, C. & Kelly, J. G. (1990). A contextualist epistemology for ecological psychology. In P. Tolan, C. Keys, F. Chertok, & L. Jason (Eds.), *Researching community psychology: Issues of theory and methods* (pp. 23–31). Washington, DC: American Psychological Association.

Kraft, K. (1996). Engaged Buddhism. In A. Kotler (Ed.). *Engaged Buddhist reader*. Berkeley, CA: Parallax Press.

Lazarus, R. C. (1985). The trivialization of distress. In J. C. Rosen & L. J. Solomon (Eds.), *Prevention in health psychology* (pp. 279–298). Hanover, VT: University Press of New England.

Nhat Hanh, T. (1991). *Old Path White Clouds: Walking in the footsteps of the Buddha*. Berkeley, CA: Parallax Press.

Owens, C.M. (1992). Zen buddhism. In C. T. Tart (Ed.), *Transpersonal psychologies* (pp. 155–202). New York: HarperCollins.

Ragsdale, E. (2003). Value and meaning in Gestalt psychology and Mahayana Buddhism. In K. H. Dockett, G. R. Dudley-Grant, & C. P. Bankart (Eds.), *Psychology and Buddhism: From individual to global community* (pp. 71–101). New York: Kluwer Academic/Plenum Publishers.

Rappaport, J. (1981). In praise of paradox: A social policy of empowerment over prevention. *American Journal of community psychology, 9*, 1–25.

Reynolds, D. K. (1984). *Playing ball on running water*. New York: Quill.

Rhodes, J. E. & Jason, L. A. (1988). *Preventing Substance Abuse Among Children & Adolescents*. New York: Pergamon Press.

Rothberg, D. (1992). Buddhist responses to violence and war: Resources for a socially engaged spirituality. *Journal of Humanistic Psychology, 32*, 41–75.

Rothberg, D. (1998). Responding to the cries of the world. Socially engaged Buddhism in North America. In S. C. Prebish & K. K. Tanaka (Eds.), *The faces of Buddhism in America*. Berkeley, CA: University of California Press.

Shaffer, C.R. & Anundsen, K. (1993). *Creating community anywhere. Finding support and connection in a fragmented world*. New York: G. P. Putnam's Sons.

Spretnak, C. (1991). *States of grace*. New York: HarperCollins.

Thurman, R. A. (1996). Nagarjuna's guidelines for Buddhist social action. In A. Kotler (Ed.), *Engaged Buddhist reader*. Berkeley, CA: Parallax Press.

Thurman, R. A. (1999). *Inner revolution*. New York: Riverhead Books.

Vaughan, F. (1979). Transpersonal psychotherapy: Context, content, and process. *The Journal of Transpersonal Psychology, 11*(2), 101–110.

Wegela, K. K. (1988). "Touch and go" in clinical practice. Some implications of the view of intrinsic health for psychotherapy. *Journal of Contemplative Psychotherapy, 5*, 3–23.

Weide, T. N. (1973). Varieties of transpersonal therapy. *The Journal of Transpersonal Psychology, 5*(1), 7–14.

Chapter 10

Transcending Self and Other

Mahayana Principles of Integration

Kathleen H. Dockett and Doris North-Schulte

If a worldwide consciousness could arise that all division and all antagonism are due to the splitting of opposites in the psyche, then one would really know where to attack.

JUNG, 1958, p. 101

The key to resolving all forms of conflict among ethnic groups lies in discovering and revealing a kind of universal humanity that transcends differences within the self.

IKEDA, 2000a, p. 25

At the threshold of the Third Millennium, humanity is faced with the challenges of globalization and living harmoniously within a multicultural, multinational, and multiethnic global village. To meet these challenges will require that we view ourselves as global neighbors sharing a common future that transcends national and ethnic boundaries. Yet, if history is any teacher, we will need new principles to guide our efforts. This century and the last reflect a complex set of interrelated crises including global warming, environmental degradation, discrimination, poverty, terrorism, and divisions among people based on differences of race, ethnicity, religion, language, and nationality. Too often, these divisions among people lead to violent conflict.

Ethnopolitical conflict, war, and genocide are particularly devastating. In today's world, we see all levels of ethnopolitical conflict, including: outright genocides (e.g., Rwanda and Cambodia), wars short of genocide (e.g., Turkey, Yugoslav, Guatemala, Sri Lanka), "more than 30 low-intensity wars (e.g., Afghanistan, Kashmir, Kosovo, Israel, Angola); ... governmental repression of autonomy movements (e.g., Tibet, Kurds, Rwanda, Burundi, Northern Ireland); ... the destruction of indigenous peoples (e.g., Amazon, Borneo, Pacific Islands); and ... over 40 million refugees and displaced persons ..." (Marsella, 1998, p. 1283).

The question for our collective survival is how can we transition from this era of darkness and killing into an era of light and peace? Upon what values can we create a global culture of peace? What are the principles by which we can live in harmony with persons from different backgrounds, respecting and valuing our differences? This is the problem to be solved in the 21st Century if society is to survive.

This chapter describes the special contributions Buddhist psychology can make to the understanding and prevention of ethnic conflict. We present a Buddhist view of the root causes of ethnic conflict and how Buddhist values and principles may be applied to the prevention of these all too prevalent occurrences. Four Mahayana principles of integration are discussed: *True Self*, the *Eternity of Life*, compassion for all or the *Bodhisattva Way*, and global interdependence or *Dependent Origination*. We begin by framing the magnitude, nature, and causes of ethnopolitical conflict.

Ethnopolitical Conflict

Magnitude and Nature

Ethnopolitical conflict is defined as "conflicts between ethnic, religious, linguistic, and national groups within states" (Connor as cited in Rouhana & Bar-Tal, 1998). In its extreme form, it is defined as genocide (*genos* [Greek] = race or tribe, and *cide* (Latin) = annihilation or killing), which is an attempt to kill many or all members of an ethnic group. Genocide "might well be identified as Public Health Problem Number One on Planet Earth, for it is the major cause of unnatural deaths of human beings" (Carny, 1985, p. 448).

The global nature of the problem is evident in the brutal ethnic wars in Cambodia, Rwanda, Yugoslavia, Guatemala, Sri Lanka, and the Israel-occupied West Bank/Gaza. Within our national borders as well, the increasing racial and ethnic hate crimes and civil unrest for example in Los Angeles, Birmingham, and New York, and the lawlessness of some 800 militias and paramilitary groups across America, have been labeled by Carl Rowan (1966) as ominous signs that portend the coming of race wars in America. Certainly, as psychologist Vickie Mays has observed, "No continent is immune" (Mays, Bulock, Rosenzweig, & Wessells, 1998, p. 737).

Ethnic conflicts are tremendously diverse. They are "often rooted in histories of colonialism, ethnocentrism, racism, political oppression, human rights abuse, social injustice, poverty, and environmental degradation" (Mays et al., 1998, p. 737).

The following statistics only begin to highlight the magnitude of the problem:

- Violent ethnic conflict between 1945 and 1990 involved an estimated 100 national and minority groups (Gurr as cited in Mays et al., 1998).

- "In the 1990's alone, two dozen ethnic conflicts have *each* resulted in at least a thousand deaths, and some have killed hundreds of thousands" (Mays et al., 1998, p. 738).
- Post-Cold War conflicts, mostly intrastate, have caused an estimated six million deaths (Takamura, 2000).
- Over 80% of the casualties are civilians because these conflicts often take place in and around communities rather than in designated "battlefields" (Garfield & Neugut as cited in Mays et al., 1998, p. 738).
- Over 40 million are refugees and displaced persons (Marsella, 1998, p. 1283).
- Up to 300,000 children under 18 years of age have served as "child soldiers" in ongoing conflicts. Daily, some 800 are killed or wounded. Between 1987 and 1997, 2 million were killed, 6 million disabled or injured, and 10 million psychologically traumatized (Ikeda, 1999, p. 31).

Unlike the technologically managed violence in political and economic wars, ethnic conflicts are bloody internal wars, saturated by cruel, vicious, and personal violence (Emminghaus, Kimmel, & Steward as cited in Kimmel, 1999). The horrible atrocities, mass rapes, and ethnic cleansing of the wars in the former Yugoslavia, Rwanda, Bosnia, and Guatemala are exemplary of the primal violence that characterizes cultural wars.

Tragic examples of the destruction of human life and human rights throughout our history include the following:

- Nazi Holocaust and genocide of 6.5 million Jews.
- genocide of Native Americans.
- enslavement, lynching, and mass murders of African Americans.
- genocide of half a million Sinti-Roma peoples during World War II.
- apartheid in South Africa.
- genocide of one million Rwandans in the Spring of 1994.
- slaughter in Sierre Leone.
- massive killing in the Congo.
- genocide of two million Cambodians between 1975–1979.
- genocide of Armenians.
- wars just short of genocide in Guatemala, Sri Lanka, and Turkey.
- religious and ethnic warfare in the former Yugoslavia, mass killing in Bosnia.
- 30 years of bloodshed in Northern Ireland.
- 23 years of ethnic conflict in Afghanistan.
- Israeli-Palestinian conflict which has escalated beyond a low-level ethnic war.
- ethnic conflicts in Burma, Tibet, Thailand, Vietnam, Iraq, Lebanon, and Sudan.

In spite of all the efforts of organizations such as the United Nations and the Peace Institute, the continued prevalence of national ethnic conflicts and violent attacks on individuals around the world based on ethnic affiliation, "race," or religion has created an urgent need to seek "new" ways to lessen ethnic conflict and to promote harmony among peoples of the world. Since World War II, there have been numerous attempts to analyze the psychology of hatred, ethnic conflict, wars, genocide, and their effects on the individual and the group, beginning with the Holocaust studies (Arendt, 1963) and continuing to the present day (Chirot & Seligman, 2001). Chirot (2001) suggests that psychology's contribution to understanding ethnopolitical conflict has been modest, growing largely out of theories of group conflict, with issues surrounding identity formation being little understood.

Causes of Ethnopolitical Conflict, War, and Genocide

Staub's (1998, 2001) empirically based theory of group violence has identified patterns of events that instigate and predispose a culture toward genocidal or group violence. Conditions that instigate genocide include: (a) difficult conditions of life in a society such as economic problems, political conflict, and/or great social change; (b) conflicts involving vital interests such as territory needed for living; (c) conflict between dominant and subordinate groups, and (d) a history of conflict and antagonisms between groups. Other factors include scapegoating of a group as responsible for the difficult life conditions, and the escalation of harmful acts along the continuum of destruction, depending on the behavior of community leaders, elites, and bystanders internal and external to the community. Staub (1998) also identified a set of predisposing cultural factors that when present in combination make genocidal or group violence more likely. These include (a) a history of devaluation of some group that is part of the culture, for example as unintelligent or lazy, (b) monolithic versus pluralistic society, (c) authority orientation, and (d) unhealed group trauma of previously persecuted groups who are more likely to react to new threats with violence.

Central to both instigating and precipitating factors is the existence of group-based identities and conflict involving those identities. One can observe this in the aftermath of the Cold War in 1989, when the genesis of wars shifted from national states toward groupings of people that Kimmel (1999) calls "cultural states." According to Fukuyama (as cited in Kimmel, 1999, p. 57), "The emergence of 'cultural states' is related to a decline in the power of national states, both internally (a loss of patriotism) and externally (a breakdown of international relations)." "As a national state is superceded by cultural movements of peoples whose identities are anchored in existential feelings, called primordial sentiments (Geertz as cited in Kimmel, 1999), the individual's sense of being a state citizen (civic identity) diminishes (Kaplan as cited in Kimmel, 1999, p. 57)." As a consequence, subgroups of people emerged with strong cultural identities that glorify their group and demonize others. This is exemplified in the conflicts of Bosnia, Rwanda, Guatemala, Sri Lanka, Afghanistan, Lebanon, and Sudan where a resurgence of cultural identities had occurred based on primordial sentiments of ethnicity, language, race, tradition, religion, and region. According to Chirot (2001), "with the fall of communism, there were few if any alternative ways for people to find support groups or identities except through their ethnic memberships" (p. 13), and feeling threatened, people withdrew back into their primal identity groups (Staub, 2001). Thus, as national identities have been shaken, cultural identities have become more central, and as primal cultural identities have become more central, universal and cosmic identities have become more remote.

Contributions of Buddhism to Understanding the Causes of Ethnic Conflict

A Crisis of Identity

This brings us to the question of how Buddhism explains the cause of ethnopolitical conflict, and what contributions it might make in this regard. Buddhist leader Daisaku Ikeda (2000b) asserts: "The severance of relationships within human society, coupled with the processes of economic, communications, and political globalization, has generated fissures between cultures, races, religions, and civilizations, giving rise to conflicts of various kinds at the interstices" (p. 2). This severing of relationships, he asserts, is caused by *people's failure to understand the nature of our existence, our identity, and our relationships with each other and with other life in the universe*. Similarly, the root cause of genocide is viewed as a failure to recognize the magnificence of a single human life – one's own or that of another. In essence, a crisis of identity lies at the core of much of the ethnic violence around the globe (Ikeda, 2000b; Takamura, 2000).

In the Lotus Sutra, the major work of Mahayana Buddhism, a more fundamental explanation of the cause of ethnic conflict may be found (as cited in Ikeda, 2000b, p. 2).

> The Lotus Sutra expounds the principle of the five defilements of the present world: ["Defilements" as used here refers to corruption or distortion.]
>
> (1) *defilement of the age*, such as war or other disruptions of the social or natural environment;
> (2) *defilements of desires*, the tendency to be ruled by emotions such as greed or anger;
> (3) *defilement of living beings*, the physical and spiritual decline of human beings;

(4) *defilement of thoughts*, deriving from mistaken views or values; and
(5) *defilement of life span*, the distortion of life itself, which leads to a disordered and shortened life span.

> The Chinese Buddhist teacher T'ien-t'ai (538–597) explained this theory as follows: First, the human spirit is polluted with the "defilement of desires" – specifically greed, violence and ignorance of the true nature of life – together with misplaced values that are described as the "defilement of thought." It becomes polluted with violence, greed and egoism, as well as extreme ideas such as fundamentalism. This impact is collectively known as the "defilement of living beings." If each level of human society – the family, local society, the nation or the state – comes under the sway of these negative influences, this will be passed on over generations and continue into the future, becoming the "defilement of life span." At this stage, historical grudges and violence become embedded in the depths of the consciousness of a people or country. If this negative cycle continues, humanity as a whole will fall prey to the "defilement of the age."

Elements of all five of the defilements can be seen in the ethnic conflicts of today. "Ignorance of the true nature of life" signifies the failure of human beings to understand our true identity, the spiritual equality of all life, and the mutual interdependence of all life. "Misplaced values" include attachment to transient identities of ethnicity and nationality as though they are permanent. "Historical grudges and violence in the consciousness of a people" (also identified by Staub [1998, 2001] as a factor that instigates group violence) are exemplified in the long-standing intergenerational conflicts of Northern Ireland, Rwanda, Afghanistan, and the Israel-Palestine states. Finally, the defilement of the life span is reflected in outright genocide, mass killings, and lesser violence that Staub (2001) notes have become widespread in the second half of the 20th Century, and show evidence of escalation in the 21st Century.

Attachment to Difference

The very process of enculturation and social identity formation is a breeding ground for disharmony between ethnic groups because it encourages attachment to difference. In the process of social identity formation (Turner as cited in Myers, 1999), we classify people into categories, identify with our own in-group, and compare our group with other groups, with a favorable bias toward our own group. Enculturation processes can lead to ethnocentrism or the belief that one's own culture is superior. It can also predispose one group to scapegoating others (where one group is blamed for some difficult condition of life), stereotyping and demonizing others, and discriminatory behavior. In Rwanda for example, "in-group bias was the cause of the murder of half the minority Tutsi population and the huge refugee movements when the Hutus were defeated" (Myers, 1999, p. 354).

Attachment to difference is a central cause of conflict between ethnic groups, from a Buddhist perspective (Ikeda, 1995, 2000a; Martin, 1995).

> Human beings have tended to emphasize one another's differences, classifying people into categories and practicing discrimination. History has seen members of the same human family divided again and again and led into one endless conflict after another, because of their stubborn attachment to difference in race, ethnicity, nationality, gender, sexual orientation, and religion. Each group emphasizes its uniqueness; each group knows and draws upon its own history for its justification. The result is the deadly crisis we see today – the savage brutality and destruction of human life and human rights on a global scale. (Ikeda, 1995, p. 148)

The historical Buddha, Shakyamuni, is quoted as having described the root cause of conflict and war in India to lie in an attachment to distinctions in ethnic and other differences emanating from the heart. Hall (1979) wrote that it is in the heart that true kindness lives and that this kindness serves to "bridge all that lives" (p. 27). At the age of 80, Shakyamuni Buddha is quoted as saying "I perceive a single, invisible arrow piercing the hearts of the people" (Takakusu as cited in Ikeda, 2001, p. 44). The "arrow" is symbolic of a prejudicial mindset, with an unreasonable emphasis on individual differences (Ikeda, 2001). Accordingly, Ikeda states:

> The "invisible arrow" of evil is not to be found in the existence of races and classes external to ourselves but is embedded in our hearts. The conquest of our own prejudicial thinking, our own attachment to difference, is the necessary precondition for open dialogue. Such discussion in turn is essential for the establishment of peace and respect for human rights. (p. 45)

Overcoming these attachments is essential to peace. Ikeda (2000a) believes that the "key to resolving all forms of conflict between ethnic groups lies in discovering and revealing a kind of universal humanity that transcends differences within the self" (p. 25). Similarly, McCauley (as cited in Chirot, 2001) holds that "some sort of identity larger than the individual and longer lasting than single lives may be necessary for all of us" (p. 25).

The Buddhist worldview embodies a unifying set of values and principles that if embraced could enable us to transcend our differences. These include a belief in the:

- spiritual equality, inherent dignity, and sanctity of all life – that all people possess an innate goodness called the Buddha nature, and because of this inherent greatness, every human being is worthy of respect and every life is precious.
- mutually interdependent nature of our relationships with one another.

- impermanence of life and the concept of non-self, non-attachment.
- eternity of life based on the law of cause and effect over many lifetimes.

Failure to understand these fundamental identities and relationships along with the resulting delusional attachment to difference is the source of the current crisis of identity and the ethnic conflict of today, from a Buddhist perspective.

Consequently, Buddhist solutions to the crisis of identity call for embracing broader concepts of:

- self-identity, as one with the universe.
- social identity, as mutually interdependent with others.
- universal identity, as a global citizen with the wisdom, courage, and compassion to foster relationships of harmony and peace.

The concept of using broader boundaries of identity is consistent with the social psychology strategy of altering the social categories we use through the re-categorization model. Based on social identity theory (Tajfel & Fraser, 1978) and self-categorization theory (cf., Turner et al., 1987), we understand that social categorization can cause intergroup discrimination (Tajfel & Fraser, 1978; Tajfel & Turner, 1979 as cited in Hewstone & Cairns, 2001). Consequently, interventions have been focused on three strategies for change: (1) eliminating categorization (de-categorization), (2) altering which categorizations are used (re-categorization), and (3) crossed categorization (Wilder as cited in Hewstone & Cairns, 2001, p. 331). In the re-categorization approach according to Hewstone and Cairns (2001), by transforming group member's perceptions of boundaries from "us" and "them" to "we," a "common-in-group identity" may be established that according to Gaertner, Dovidio, Anastasio, Bachman, and Rust (as cited in Hewstone & Cairns, 2001) can result in reduced intergroup bias (in-group favoritism). The "common-in-group identity" model resolves in-group versus out-group conflict by changing group boundaries and creating a superordinate identity. Re-categorization of self and other into a common-in-group identity "should reduce bias by increasing the attractiveness of former out-group members once they are included within a superordinate group structure" (Hewstone & Cairns, 2001, p. 333).

How one goes about achieving this re-categorization is the focus of this chapter. We discuss four Mahayana Buddhist principles of integration that provide an alternative understanding of who we are, and our relationship with ourselves and other life in the universe (Dockett, 1997, 1999a, 2000; Ikeda, 1993; Martin, 1995). These are the integrating principles that offer a possible solution for the prevention of ethnic conflict.

Mahayana Buddhist Principles of Integration

This chapter contends that a strong case can be made for integrating Buddhist psychology into Western psychological approaches to understanding and preventing ethnic conflict. "The Buddhist tradition offers rich resources for peacemaking and the cultivation of non-violence" (Queen, 1998, p. 25). Buddhism holds that it is the "attachment to difference" (Ikeda, 1995, 2001; Martin, 1995) that creates ethnic conflicts and therefore Mahayana Buddhist principles of integration could serve as guidelines to implement a change that would lead to the cessation of ethnic conflicts and the creation of a sustainable peace. Mahayana Buddhism could easily contribute to the psychological dimensions of the causes of ethnic conflict.

The challenge will be to create a coherent set of integrative principles that can provide individuals and groups with the knowledge and skills to empower themselves to create a sustainable peace. To achieve this change, Buddhist principles suggest there must first be a change within the individual heart and thus the mind. Ikeda (2001) calls this inner change a "Human Revolution." Ouspensky (1979) refers to it as an awareness of a higher knowledge. Whatever the definition, this change involves the development of a clear understanding of the true self and thus gaining the knowledge to empower oneself to constructively create peace and happiness in one's life and in one's environment. Empowerment is described as a "construct that links individual strengths and competencies, natural helping systems, and proactive behaviors to social policy and social change" (Perkins & Zimmerman, 1995, p. 569). This kind of self-control or empowerment is, Egendorf (1986) tells us, "... not a matter of interpretation (the Freudian revision of foreign policy thinking) or of a set of procedures for working out agreements (the conflict resolution approach). It grows out of a way of being" (p. 274).

In using the concept of integrative principles, we are referring to ideologies capable of fostering unity among people of different backgrounds. These are principles upon which people can live side by side and enjoy their differences while working to create a harmonious society.

Psychology, in applying its theories to everything in life from child rearing (Erikson) to dreams (Freud), to racism (Poussaint), and even to religion (Jung) itself, and their relation to the individual, the groups, and "the other," has thousands of direct observation cases connected to various theories and approaches. Over the past fifty years, there have been numerous studies and books written about ethnic conflict, racism, genocide, its treatment, and its effects on individuals and groups, ethnic minorities, and ethnic majorities. Buddhism, however, as a theoretical approach dealing with such issues, lacks such substantial empirical validation of its application. Where psychological theories have been extensively explored in relation to ways of understanding and changing the racist behavior of individuals or groups, Buddhist principles have been largely ignored. Buddhist principles are only beginning to be examined by psychology for their possible contributions to psychological approaches to "the self" and "the other" in creating peace initiatives.

Modern studies on physical healing have shown religion to be helpful in shaping the unconscious to control all forms of the healing process in physical illness (Atkins, 1996; Bedard, 1999; Chopra, 1989; Siegel, 1986), and in mind and stress (Dockett, 1993; Maslow, 1986). These studies have shown a relationship between the integration of "the self" in mind and in body based on religious belief and drastic outcomes in the form of healing. Why not then, explore the use of Buddhist principles of integration in shaping a process towards preventing ethnic conflict and creating universal peace.

Incorporating the Mahayana Buddhist concepts of *True Self*, the *Eternity of Life*, compassion for all or *Bodhisattva Imperative*, and global interdependence or *Dependent Origination* as guiding principles to create peaceful societies would be the beginning of an earnest effort to create the synthesis between Buddhist Psychology and Western psychology, in a *new* way, not ignoring the great efforts of the Peace Psychology approach. In using these Mahayana teachings as integrative principles for the prevention of ethnic conflicts one could address the illusion of significant differences among human beings as what it is, a distortion of truth. It is this distortion that keeps the cycle of conflict going. Mahayana Buddhism views world change as centered in the individual human change (Ikeda, 1993) or the internalizing of the locus of control (Dockett, 1993).

Mahayana Buddhism

Mahayana Buddhism contains principles that provide the individual with a new understanding about the nature of the individual identity, our human existence on this planet, our relationships with others, and our relationship to the universe (DeBary, 1972; Ikeda, 1993; Kalupahana, 1976) and thus lends itself as an ideal model for ethnic conflict prevention.

Mahayana Buddhism has been attributed to a reaction against the teachings of Theravada Buddhism (DeBary, 1972; Dhammananda, 1987; Suzuki, 1972). The Theravada School stresses the individual attainment of Nirvana, while "Mahayana Buddhism rejects sole, personal enlightenment for the enlightenment of all human society" (Mizuno, 1987, p. 114).

The principles of Mahayana Buddhism are concerned with the empowerment of the individual (Dockett, 1999b) as the most important component for creating a social change towards a just society (Kotler, 1996). This empowerment is based on the knowledge and acquired wisdom the individual gains from these principles dealing with the self, our interdependence with others, and our place in the universe. Based on the Mahayana worldview, each individual possesses the potential to actively contribute to creating a society of peace void of ethnic conflict. In that process, the individual would learn to appreciate life and the necessity of diversity or difference in sustaining life. The individual comes to understand the sanctity of all human life; "for if my life is sacred, so is yours." Egendorf (1986), in his book *Healing from the War*, poses the question

"What does it mean to be human?" He continues:

> Asking this question is a powerful act, for it opens the possibility that each of us can contribute to humanity by the way we respond, by the way we go about our lives. By asking this question of ourselves we become better prepared to ask it of each other, and when we clarify together what we offer to the world, rather than what we expect from it, then we will appreciate anew our contribution as a people. (p. 4)

Mahayana Buddhist principles offer the means to create unity on the individual, group, community, and global levels and thus could effectively contribute much to preventing ethnic conflict.

True Self or Buddha Nature

> That all beings have the nature of Buddha shows the true meaning of self or ego; the Self is Tathagata. In the Buddha's teaching the ego is nothing but Buddha-nature, and the meaning of no-self is equivalent to the great self, i.e., Buddha. (Mahaparinirvana –Sutra –Daihatsunehan-gyo (Jpn.) (Suzuki, 1972, p. 115)

In the present world of seemingly universal ethnic conflict, identity has emerged again as a determinate factor in who lives or who dies. The color of one's skin, religion, nationality, and ethnic membership are tied to our individual and collective identity. Even though this accepted identity is only a part of the self, more often than not, it becomes the focal point of our own and of others' feelings about us (Weinreich, 1991). As Allport (1954) tells us, "people adhere to their own families, clans, ethnic groups (because) the self could not be itself without them" (p. 29).

Yet, who are we, individually and collectively? Do we define our own selves or are we what and how others define us? Are we defined by what our society wants or demands of us as a member of the minority or majority group? Is our identity defined by labels placed from outside ourselves? Are we limited in our choices based on what others want or expect of us? Both Buddhism and psychology address these questions. There have been various attempts among psychologists and psychoanalysts to define the identity of the "self." Fromm (1941) in *Escape from Freedom* talked about the "real self" as opposed to the "pseudo self," while Erikson (1964) in *Childhood and Society* favored describing it as a symbiosis between "self and ego."

Our attitude towards "the self" has far reaching implications. In the normal process of learning about ourselves we often take on images and ideas that have been imposed from outside by others, which in turn become internalized as a fixed identity (Schachtel, 1961). These ideas and images then become fixed in our minds as our true selves. Depending on one's status or place in society, these ideas and images become fixed as either positive or negative attributes (Schachtel, 1961). These fixed defining attributes appear then as unchangeable parts of our character and our identity. Not only do these fixed attributes become permanent and unchangeable parts of our identity, but also become a part of the attributes of a family, ethnic group, societal group, or "race." These characteristics of our self-perception will then constantly surface in everything we do.

Negative characteristics become obstacles to our finding happiness and peace and can lead to various forms of paranoia and delusion, stress and self-destruction (Poussaint, 1969; Poussaint & Alexandar, 2000), and aggression towards others in the form of dehumanization as a means to alleviate self-hatred. Montague and Matson (1984) even speak of self-dehumanization that reaches such a point of virulence that it feeds on the dehumanization of others.

Misconceptions about the true self exist among ethnic minorities and ethnic majorities. Arrogance and vanity can likewise become parts of a fixed identity supported by misconceptions about one's true identity. Around the world, ethnic majority members may suffer from this form of delusion, viewing themselves to be better or superior to others outside their group. Unfortunately, those who suffer from the delusion of superiority rely on the *truth* of the delusion to maintain their self and their group identity. The delusion that one is superior to another is even more insidious because, one's identity is then solely based on an imagined attribute that then needs continuously, time and time again, to be defended in order to be maintained as the status quo and thereby maintain one's self-identity. Such people are always faced with the threat of losing their status and thus, constantly create negative causes that usually involve subjugating and misusing others, even to the point of murder or genocide (Schachtel, 1961). Blumberg (1998) questions whether psychology could actually have an effect in treating ethnic conflicts that are usually based on ethnocentric attitudes. He suggests that maybe psychology, like the other sciences, should just offer advice.

Buddhism does not suggest treatment or offer advice; it offers values and principles that may contribute to prevention. This prevention begins with the discovery of the true self and establishes it as the basis for an internal revolution or the cause that gives rise to a peaceful effect in the external world. Mahayana Buddhism addresses the means to the discovery of the true self. Mahayana Buddhism advocates the discovery of the individual's true self as a prerequisite for understanding the interdependency of all life. Takayama (1978) tells us that Buddhism, like psychoanalysis, seeks to uncover the identity of the true self, but unlike psychoanalysis, in Buddhism the true self identity is aware of and acknowledges the equality and interdependence of all life rather than being concerned about the identity of the individual ego. In fact, in Buddhism it is in the overcoming of one's ego or *lesser self* that one begins to understand the self (Dhammananda, 1987).

In Mahayana Buddhism attachment to the so-called lesser self or ego consciousness results in ignorance and delusions that cloud the true self or Buddha nature. The most fundamental ignorance is that of turning away from the reality of one's interconnectedness with all beings (Kawada, 2001). Describing the lesser self, Kawada states:

> It is this sense of one's self as separate and isolated from others that gives rise to discrimination against others, to destructive arrogance and acquisitiveness. The lesser self is deeply insecure, and vacillates between feelings of superiority and inferiority with regard to others; in the pursuit of its own fulfillment, the lesser self will unthinkingly harm or wound others ... the *mano* [ego] consciousness functions to create a strong sense of disjunction between self and others and to generate discriminatory attitudes toward those we experience as "other." (p. 20)

It is this ego or the lesser self that attaches great importance to difference resulting in ignorance and delusion and eventually conflict with others. It is the lesser self that most psychological theories address. "One's grief arises from positing an enduring self where no self endures, from seeking to protect it from change, when one's very law is change" (Macy, 1991, p 124).

In Mahayana Buddhism, the principle of true self or Buddha nature offers the individual an opportunity to become aware of his or her *true* identity, or potential for Buddhahood. As an integrating principle for creating peaceful societies, *true self* teaches that gaining awareness of our true identity will help the individual not only to accept him- or herself as a person of immeasurable value, but would open the individual to realizing that this potential for Buddhahood is shared by every other person on the planet. At the core of that awareness is the realization that if I, the individual, have a true self or Buddha nature, then perhaps so does everyone else. If I possess a Buddha nature this means that I have the possibility of becoming a Buddha; if I possess this nature, then so do my child, my neighbor, and even my enemy. Therefore one must bow to a potential Buddha, not slay him. Since I would want the respect due to a Buddha, I must give that respect to all others, because they possess the same nature as I do.

In Chapter Twenty of *The Lotus Sutra*, there is the story of Bodhisattva Never Disparaging who honors every human being, even to the point of being physically and mentally abused for his respectful behavior.

> For what reason was he named Never Disparaging. This monk, whatever persons he happened to meet, whether monks, nuns, laymen, or laywomen, would bow in obeisance to all of them and speak words of praise, saying, "I have profound reverence for you, I would never dare treat you with disparagement or arrogance. Why? Because you are all practicing the bodhisattva way and are certain to attain Buddhahood".... Many years passed in this way, during which this monk was constantly subjected to curses and abuse. He did not give way to anger, however, but each time spoke the same words, "You are certain to attain Buddhahood." When he spoke in this manner, some of the group would take sticks of wood or tiles and stones and beat and pelt him. But even as he ran away and took up his stance at a distance, he continued to call out in a loud voice, "I would never dare disparage you, for you are all certain to attain Buddhahood." (The Lotus Sutra, 1993, pp. 226–227)

The Christian saying "Do unto others as you would have them do unto you" likewise describes how this recognition works. Since each person is "the other" to all other persons, accepting and upholding the principle of true self would mean realizing and acknowledging the error and futility of hating one's self and others based solely on the superficial differences of ethnicity, culture, "race," or religion. This principle would be a major step in enabling individuals to transcend all differences of the temporary, transient self. This integrative principle would be a necessary step in learning to appreciate the diversity and dignity of all life.

In Mahayana Buddhism there are three "evils" of the mind under which other negative attributes can be designated. These three evils or delusions of the mind are: greed, anger, and ignorance. Under the heading of ignorance falls the symptom of apathy or the Christian "sin" of sloth. In psychology, a major symptom of sloth or apathy or *acedia* is the lack of feeling about self and others. This lack of feeling is accentuated by a lack of knowledge or ignorance of the true self. Apathy is also void of all compassion and any feeling of obligations to self and others (Montagu & Matson, 1984) thus allowing for the destruction of self and others.

Buddhists believe that ethnic conflicts will not disappear by instituting laws to forbid them. They will cease when each individual becomes aware of his or her true self and the shared Buddha nature of all humankind. Mahayana Buddhism also negates a fixed identity, based on the principle of the consistency of life and death. As Takamura (2000) states in his analysis of Buddhist values and conflict resolution: "Buddhism takes a very flexible view of identity" (p. 23). Each individual life is a multilayered, constantly evolving scheme of identity and self-definition. For example, one maybe an African American (a category of identity that did not exist when in my teen years), a woman, a wife, a daughter, a psychologist, and a Nichiren Buddhist. The significance of each of these layers of identity (or social roles) varies depending upon the setting and the specific individuals with whom one interacts. Buddhism acknowledges the great diversity of identity within each individual. Our identities, like all phenomena, are in a constant state of flux from moment to moment, from setting to setting, from birth to death, and from lifetime to lifetime throughout eternity.

Takamura (2000) continues:

> What we experience as personality, or identity, are in fact profoundly engraved tendencies or patterns of behavior. The technical term is karma. But this is not fixed or immutable. Likewise, what we know as national character or culture is the sum or accrual of these individual tendencies, reinforced through a shared history. But again, these group identities are not fixed, eternal, or unchanging. They are relative, contingent, and evolving.
>
> And they are undergirded by our most fundamental identity – that is, our genuine humanity. The technical term is Buddha nature, which might be described as our inherent capacity to sense our oneness with the entirety of being. (p. 23)

An expanded consciousness that can awaken to this principle of the true self or Buddha nature would empower the individual to take action to improve his or her own life and the lives of all humankind and would lead to the establishment of universal harmony and peace. The awareness of our true self or Buddha nature may be the single greatest attribute towards the abolishment of ethnic conflict in the world.

Just as Shakyamuni gained insight or *enlightenment* into his true self – Buddha nature or the consciousness of being a vital part of the universe, a Buddha – both as cause and effect, so must each individual first begin by becoming aware of this same relation within one's self if peace is to be created in the world. Once the nature of one's life is understood then one can begin to understand the relationship of the self to others, and the self to the universe. This is the difference between an enlightened person who seeks peace and one who gropes and stumbles in the darkness creating havoc and chaos all around. Acting on this consciousness the individual is far removed from learned helplessness (Seligman, 1991), scapegoating, and conflict.

Eternity of Life

> Thereupon the Buddha addressed all those bodhisattva-mahasattvas: Good sons! Now I must clearly announce and declare to you. Suppose you take as atomized all those worlds where an atom has been deposited or where it has not been deposited, and (count) an atom as a kalpa, [the time] since I became Buddha still surpasses these by hundreds of thousands of myriads of kotis… From that time forward I have constantly been preaching and teaching in this saha-world, and also leading benefiting all living beings… (The Threefold Lotus Sutra, 1975, p. 250)

The person, who acknowledges the value of self and others, must also come to understand the second of our principles: th*e* eternity of life. On the simplest level, it can be explained thusly; we have come into this world with the history and genes of past generations, not only from our parents and grand parents, but also from countless generations in the past, and we carry the genes of the future. Whether we like it or not, we also carry and create negative and positive causes, termed karma in Buddhism, as well. Our true self is eternal, reflecting the continuous procession of life with its causes and effects. Our present lives reflect the past and what we do now will affect the future.

Shakyamuni (Gautama) Buddha says in the sixteenth chapter of the *Lotus Sutra* (*Saddharmapundarika-Sutra, Myo Ho Renge Kyo*), the major work of Mahayana Buddhism, that his life is limitless. He shares for the first time, that he did not attain enlightenment under the Bodhi tree, but actually attained enlightenment in an unlimited time in the past in another manifestation. "The time is limitless and boundless – a hundred, thousand, ten thousand, hundred thousand, nayuta aeons – since I in fact attained Buddhahood" (*The Major Writings of*

Nichiren Daishonin, 1981, p.103). He continues to tell his listeners that his physical existence in the world, as well as that of all other Buddhas in the past and for those to come in the future, is for the sole purpose of helping human beings to understand their *true identity*, which is the same as his (i.e., a potential for Buddhahood). By declaring the equality of all human life, he tells us that, just as his true self is eternal, so is every individual's life. The first of the five incorrect views about life is "belief that the perceivable self, which is only a temporary aggregation of elements determined by cause and effect, is a true, persistent entity" (Mizuno, 1987, p. 118). Change is a part of nature. Everyone and everything changes. Change is a part of the eternity of life (Ohnishi, 1993).

Buddhism rejects the concept of an eternal soul. Buddhism views a soul as a temporary ego-identity that would become extinct at death (Dhammananda, 1987); however, the concept of eternal life, which first is mentioned in the Lotus Sutra, Chapter 16, is neither created nor dies.

> The Buddha teaches that what we call ego, self, soul, personality, etc., are merely conventional terms that do not refer to any real, independent entity .... To children, a rainbow is something vivid and real; but the grown ups know that it is merely an illusion caused by certain rays of light and drops of water. The light is only a series of waves or undulations that have no more reality than the rainbow itself. (Dhammananda, 1987, p. 115)

Within the framework of the principle of the eternity of life, the awareness and acceptance of the self and others throughout time and space is a pillar of Mahayana Buddhist practice. Buddhism tells us that the eternity of life, no matter, how we might want to reject it, is within us. We are not new in this universe. To deny the concept of eternity of life, not only denies the past, but also denies the future (Ohnishi, 1993) and creates a world of delusion.

When one thinks about Buddhism and the concept of the eternity of life, one thinks about the word "reincarnation." This word, says Richard Causton (1995), congers up a caricature of what the eternity of life really means in Buddhist philosophy. The eternity of life

> is also not to be confused with the Christian concept of an individual's soul living eternally after death in either Heaven or Hell; rather, the Buddhist concept of the eternity of life places the life of the individual in the context of the universe as a whole, asserting that since the entire universe exists in one form or another throughout eternity, so must all the living things contained within it exist eternally in one form or another. (Causton, 1995, p. 137)

It is necessary in talking about the eternity of life, to also talk about death. Life and death are two sides of the same coin and the consistency of life and death can be compared to waking time and sleeping time. Buddhism believes that one can go to bed (die) a Bosnian and wake up (be reborn) a Serb, thus recreating the historical cycle of violence unless one becomes aware or "Awakened" to his or her individual true self or Buddha nature and that nature in others. Equally important is the awareness that this individual life is transient and changeable. The Buddhist principle of the eternity of life affords each individual a new view about her or his personal life and its relationship to others. If one could die and then be reborn into a group of people one might hate or abuse in this life, one might think twice about mistreating others, because to harm others would be to harm oneself.

Mahayana Buddhism tells us that the eternity of life means we have had more mothers and fathers than we can imagine and have been a member of all known ethnic groups on this planet; more important, however, is that we will continue to experience these memberships among all peoples in the universe. To reject anyone is to reject one's true self. This means you have been a Zulu warrior, a medieval European craftsperson, a thief in Baghdad, an inventor in China, a shaman among the Maori, a child soldier in the United States Civil War and all of these live within the present you as a result of the causes you made in the past. You were then and you are now, but one thing is sure, you are and never have been alone on this planet. You share these manifestations and lifetimes with millions of others, not as the you reflected in the mirror, but as the eternal true self. This is a simplified version of the Mahayana Buddhist concept of the eternity of life.

The Bodhisattva Way

> The Bodhisattva is enlightened in his own mind, which is also the mind of all beings. When his mind is pure the mind of all beings is also pure, for the substance of one Mind is that of all beings. When the dust of one's own Mind is thoroughly wiped off, all beings also have their minds free from dust. When one's mind is freed from greed, anger, and folly, all beings are also freed from greed, anger, and folly. Such a Bodhisattva is known as the All-knowing One. (Manjusri-vikridita-sutra Daishogonhomon-gyo) (Suzuki, 1972, p. 124)

While Theravada Buddhism stresses individual personal enlightenment, Mahayana Buddhism advocates enlightenment for all; therefore, Mahayana Buddhism is considered to contain the "true spirit of Buddhism," which is compassion towards all living things. It is the bodhisattva who delays his or her own Nirvana in order to help others toward enlightenment who plays the most important role in Mahayana Buddhism (Dhammananda, 1987). The bodhisattva is not only dedicated to his or her own attainment of wisdom, but simultaneously is dedicated to helping others achieve the same wisdom and happiness (Dockett, 1993). This motivation is manifested in the "magnificent bodhisattva's unswerving commitment to complete self-transformation and complete world transformation" (Thurman, 1996). Thus Mahayana Buddhism could be considered a prescription for peace (Galtung, 1990).

It is the compassionate bodhisattva, as exemplified by the example of the very human Shakyamuni Buddha, whose actions of compassion for others serves as the model of the Bodhisattva Way and distinguishes Mahayana from Theravada Buddhism. In the final chapter of The Lotus Sutra, Shakyamuni vows to make all human beings aware of their Buddha nature. The *raison d'etre* of Mahayana Buddhism is compassion as exemplified in the principle of the Bodhisattva Imperative, or the universal attainment of enlightenment.

Another important part of Mahayana Buddhism is in its intent of equality among all practitioners. In Mahayana Buddhism, and in particular The Lotus Sutra, the lay person is viewed as equal in practice to monks and nuns.

> Mahayana ... wished to make the Buddhist life open to all, priest and layman alike. With it the ideal became, not the Arhat bent upon his own salvation, but the bodhisattva to which all may aspire. This was and remains the most important of many important points in Mahayana. (Suzuki, 1972, p. 33)

Mahayana Buddhism, especially as practiced by Nichiren's followers based on the Lotus Sutra, teaches that it is through one's daily life struggles and the interactions between human beings, including all ones' desires, struggles, and sorrows, that happiness and enlightenment can be achieved. Mahayana Buddhism teaches that the common person is or can achieve Buddha status through the Bodhisattva Way or compassionate action for others. A bodhisattva is a person motivated by a "universal altruism of great compassion, great love, and great empathy" (Thurman, 1996). The compassion of the Bodhisattva necessitates action.

Contained within the principle of the Bodhisattva Imperative are various actions and characteristics attributed to the bodhisattva such as: (1) generosity towards all; (2) patience; (3) working towards achieving wisdom and teaching it to others; (4) helping to lead all humans toward Buddhahood; and (5) great compassion (De Bary, 1972; Suzuki, 1972). Added to these traditional attributes are: (6) taking 100% responsibility for the events of one's life and for changing those events; (7) accepting responsibility for changing negative events within one's environment into positive experiences; (8) realizing that difficulties are a natural part of existence, and those difficulties have value and meaning in helping the individual attain wisdom (enlightenment) (Dockett, 1999b).

David Chappell (1999a) writes that the pressing issue of peace "requires an organized bodhisattva practice that unites and harmonizes the desire of individuals to contribute to society." For the individual to be able to contribute to society, the individual – the bodhisattva or would-be Buddha – would need to develop courage and self-control that would enable him or her to become empowered and use that empowerment to help others. "A Bodhisattva is a future Buddha, and we are all future Bodhisattvas, while those who have already taken the Bodhisattva vows are already on the first rung of the ladder of Bodhisattvaship. This thought gives a great impetus to leading the Buddhist life" (Suzuki, 1972, p. 000).

With a strong "sense of mission and responsibility," the bodhisattva strives for peace in all realms of life and is a contributing participant in the creation of happiness (Kawada, 2001). Mahayana Buddhism seeks to help the individual transcend difference and dissolve the dichotomy between the self and others by actualizing the principle of the bodhisattva. Thus, the Bodhisattva Imperative provides a blueprint for ethnic conflict prevention since the Bodhisattva seeks harmony within his or her own life and within the environment he or she lives thus striving to create a land of peace, void of ethnic conflict.

Dependent Origination

Dependent origination is a major principle of Mahayana Buddhism. This principle could serve as a universal guideline for peace as it explains the fundamental doctrine of the interdependence of all things. Describing dependent origination as "the web of life that binds all people," Daisaku Ikeda (1993) states the most important implication of this teaching is that we do not exist alone. The meaning of our lives and our happiness arises through our interconnectedness with those around us, our community, and our world. According to this concept all entities exist because of mutually interdependent relationships, and without other entities, one's own existence would not be. When people awaken to the interdependent nature of their existence, they would naturally develop a sense of responsibility and appreciation for others, and compassionate, altruistic behavior would naturally follow (Martin, 1995).

At a profound level, the principle of dependent origination undergrids the imperative of the bodhisattva to care for others. Given the interconnectedness of all life, to help others is to help oneself. It is from this worldview that the truly altruistic behavior of the bodhisattva arises.

The principle of dependent origination is not limited to human beings, but encompasses everything within our universe, sentient and insentient beings, which include animals and nature (see Chapter 11 in this volume).

Western religion has emphasized the dominance of "man" over animal and environment. There is a duality that first talks of man as having "dominion" over animals and earth, (kjv. Genesis: 1:26) and second, talks of establishing an equal covenant to man and animal, alike (kjv: Genesis: 9:12). In the Old Testament Noah is clearly instructed to gather up the animals "two by two" and to place them on board the ship so that they would be saved, along with him and his family (Allen, 1963). When one thinks about this incident, whether real or imaged, it is a clear indication of the equality and interdependence of all life on the planet. It could be viewed in terms of the Buddhist principle of dependent origination. All elements of the phenomena were interdependent; nature in the form of the storm, could be said to represent the obstacles of existence that both humans and animals encounter living on the planet; Noah and his family, using their human skills and knowledge, built the boat for the animals and themselves; the animals in turn, nourished the humans with cheese and eggs to eat and wool to keep them warm, while the forests of the land supplied the material for the boat and fruits, berries, and herbs from its trees and bushes to nourish them during the storm. The story shows that because one existed, the others existed. If you remove one component of the story, it loses its meaning. The story is a clear case of mutual interdependence. "Man" did not dominate over the animal or nature, but was a part of the whole event carrying out his mission in the phenomena. That awareness created peace on the ship.

Mahayana Buddhism teaches that attachment to difference brings about suffering rather than joy; however, suffering is conducive to helping individuals reflect on their lives and the causes they have made. Transcending difference does not negate developing an awareness and acceptance of the diversity in our universe. It warns us, however, of attaching too much attention to trying to prove that one individual or group is better or worse than another or that one group has "dominion" over another. Mahayana Buddhism contends that diversity is, in fact, an essential part of nature and is required for continued life on the planet. Mahayana Buddhism teaches that within our difference, every human being can develop the true self, as one is, not by changing ethnicity, race, gender, occupation, or nationality, but through the awareness and practice of these basic philosophical principles. In Buddhism, there is the parable of the two bundles of reeds tied together in a field. The wind surrounds them buffeting them here and there, but they are able to maintain an upright position, sometimes swaying one way and sometimes the other way; but because they are tied together, they are able to maintain their upright position. The sun shines down on them equally and the rain gets them both wet. If the cord, however, is severed and one is removed, the other will fall or be blown away. Buddhism contends that this is the *true* existence of all life on this planet; one can exist because the other exists. The basic Buddhist principle of dependent origination serves as one of the major integrating principles for uniting self and other. If realized and practiced it would lead to the development of a sense of responsibility and appreciation for others and to compassionate actions to live in harmony. In this way, the principle of dependent origination could contribute to the prevention of future ethno-political conflicts.

The further one gets away from understanding the interconnectedness and interdependence of all life on this planet, the more one becomes alienated from self and others and the more one is willing to kill others and wage a war to create some kind of supposed superior status and exclusive place in society. Such actions are based on delusionary and distorted views. To deny the interdependence and value of the entire human race is to deny one's own humanity and ultimately, one's individual Buddha nature.

Four Buddhist principles have emerged in this paper that could serve as potential resources for the development of individuals. In carrying out the will of the Mahayana Sutras and especially the Lotus Sutra which teaches respect of difference, by performing bodhisattva deeds, with a developed consciousness of the true self, the eternity of life, and the interdependence of life over time and space, individuals would become hopeful, self-empowered citizens who would actively work to create peaceful societies. Imbued with a feeling of control over their lives, these individuals would feel compelled to actively engage in creating cultures of peace for themselves and all of humanity. A life based on Mahayana Buddhist principles could provide the individual with a profound sense of purpose and meaning to the activities of life. These Mahayana principles teach the transcendence of difference based on an inner knowledge and wisdom, not a transformation of difference to fit anyone else's distorted illusions. When these approaches become accepted as "common sense" in society, then harmony and creative coexistence in our global human society will be natural and inevitable.

The most important implication of these Mahayana principles of integration is that we as human beings can create and sustain peaceful societies, but it begins with our own individual internalized peaceful change based on the knowledge of who we truly are. These principles teach us that we do not exist alone. Our difference is a natural part of our existence and is needed to help us create meaning and value in our lives as well as to live up to our potential as compassionate human beings. Human happiness arises through our interconnectedness with those around us and with our environment.

Some scholars (Chappell, 1999b; Kimmel, 1999) have argued that Buddhist compassion and caring is not enough. It does not address the special problems of organized society's structural violence, social oppression, and environmental degradation. While we concur that legal safeguards are a necessary condition for creating the context for peace, the challenge as history has shown time and again is that we cannot legislate change in the minds and hearts of the people. Thus, this chapter contends that the integration of these basic Mahayana Buddhist principles into our global consciousness provides a beginning for a new way of thinking about the self and the other that would eventually address the global issues and lead to local, national, and global peace.

Author's Note

Portions of this paper were presented in the symposium, Healing for the Millennium II: Buddhist Applications to Social Problems, at the annual meeting of the American Psychological Association Convention, Washington, DC, August 4–8, 2000. We wish to express our appreciation to Guy McCloskey and Greg Martin for their generosity of time and wisdom in commenting of earlier versions of this chapter.

References

Allen, D. C. (1963). *The legend of Noah: Renaissance in art, science, and letters.* Urbana: University of Illinois Press.

Allport, G. W. (1954). *The nature of prejudice.* Reading, MA: Addison Wesley.

Arendt, H. (1963). *Eichman in Jerusalem: A report on the banality of evil.* New York: Viking.

Atkins, C. R. (1996, July). *Modern Buddhist healing.* Paper presented at The Society for Buddhist-Christian Studies Conference on Socially Engaged Buddhism and Christianity. Chicago: DePaul University.

Bedard, J. (1999). *Lotus in the fire: The healing power of Zen.* Boston: Shambala.

Blumberg, H. H. (1998). Peace psychology after the cold war: A selective review, *Genetic, Social and General Psychology Monograph, 124*(1), 5–37.

Causton, R. (1995). *The Buddha in daily life: An introduction to the Buddhism of Nichiren Daishonin.* London: Rider Books.

Chappell, D. W. (1999a, June). The global significance of the Lotus Sutra. *Living Buddhism, 3*(6), 11–19.

Chappell, D. W. (1999b). *Buddhist peacework.* Boston: Wisdom Publications.

Charny, I. W. (1985, September). Genocide: The ultimate human rights problem, *Social Education: Human Rights Education: Issues, Approaches, Resources, 49*(6), 448–452.

Chirot, D. (2001). Introduction. In D. Chirot & M. E. P. Seligman (Eds), *Ethnopolitical warfare: Causes, consequences, and possible solutions* (pp. 3–26). Washington, DC: American Psychological Association.

Chirot, D. & Seligman, M. E. P. (2001). *Ethnopolitical warfare: Causes, consequences, and possible solutions.* Washington, DC: American Psychological Association.

Chopra, D. (1989). *Quantum healing.* New York: Bantam Books.

DeBary, W. T. (1972). *The Buddhist tradition.* New York: Vintage.

Dhammananda, K. Sri. (1987). *What Buddhists believe.* Kuala Lumpur, Malaysia: The Buddhist Missionary Society.

Dockett, K. H. (1993). *Resources for stress resistance: Parallels in Psychology and Buddhism.* Santa Monica, CA: Soka Gakkai International-USA.

Dockett, K. H. (1997, November). *A Buddhist perspective on diversity: Principles by which we can promote harmony and unity in diversity.* Paper presented at annual meeting of the Culture Department, Soka Gakkai International-USA, Fort Lauderdale, FL.

Dockett, K. H. (1999a, August). Principles of integration: A Buddhist perspective on diversity. In D. Pryor (Chair), *Buddhism and psychology: Reflections in personal transformation and global responsiveness.* Symposium conducted at the annual meeting of the American Psychological Association, Boston, MA.

Dockett, K. (1999b, August). Psychological perspectives on Buddhist empowerment. In A. J. Marsella, (Chair), *Where Buddhism and psychology meet: Perspectives on empowerment.* Symposium conducted at annual meeting of the American Psychological Association, Boston, MA.

Dockett, K. H. (2000, August). Ethnopolitical conflict, genocide, war: Buddhist alternatives for integration. In A. J. Marsella & K. H. Dockett (Co-Chairs), *Healing for the Millennium II: Buddhist applications to social problems.* Symposium conducted at the annual meeting of the American Psychological Association, Washington, DC.

Egendorf, A. (1986). *Healing from the war: Trauma and transformation after Vietnam.* Boston, MA: Shambala.

Erikson, E. (1964). *Childhood and society.* New York: W.W. Norton.

Fromm, E. (1941). *Escape from freedom.* New York: Farrar & Rinehart.

Galtung, J. (1990, July). The path toward peace lies in dialogue and action. *Seikyo Times, 348*, 43–46.

Hall, M. P. (1979). *Buddhism and psychotherapy: The healing of heart doctrine*. Los Angeles: The Philosophical Research Society.

Hewstone, M. & Cairns, E. (2001). Social psychology and intergroup conflict. In D. Chirot & M. E. P. Seligman (Eds.), *Ethnopolitical warfare: Causes, consequences, and possible solutions* (pp. 319–342). Washington, DC: American Psychological Association.

Ikeda, D. (1993, March). In search of new principles of integration. *Seikyo Times*, 33–39.

Ikeda, D. (1995, January). *The New Human Revolution*, Vol. 1, 148–158. Santa Monica, CA: Soka Gakkai International-USA.

Ikeda, D. (1999, May). Toward a culture of peace: A cosmic view. *Living Buddhism*, 18–43.

Ikeda, D. (2000a, May). Peace through dialogue: A time to talk: Thoughts on a culture of peace. *Living Buddhism*, pp. 17–43.

Ikeda, D. (2000b). Message to the 108th Convention of the American Psychological Association. Unpublished manuscript. Tokyo: Soka Gakkai International.

Ikeda, D. (2001). *For the sake of peace: Seven paths to global harmony. A Buddhist perspective*. Santa Monica, CA: Middleway Press.

Jung, C. G. (1958). *The undiscovered self* (R. F. C. Hull, Trans.). Boston: Little, Brown.

Kalupahana, D. J. (1976). *Buddhist philosophy: A historical analysis*. Honolulu, HI: University of Hawaii Press.

Kawada, Y. (2001). Nichiren Buddhism and empowerment. *Living Buddhism, 5*(9), 18–23.

Kimmel, P. R. (1999). Cultural and ethnic issues of conflict and peacekeeping. In H. J. Langholtz (Ed.), *The psychology of peacekeeping*. Westport, CT: Greenwood.

Kotler, A. (Ed.). (1996). *Engaged Buddhist reader*. Berkeley, CA: Parallax Press.

Macy, J. R. (1991, July). *Mutual causation in Buddhism and general systems theory: The dharma of natural systems* (Buddhist Study Series). State University of New York Press.

Marsella, A. J. (1998). Toward a global community: Meeting the needs of a changing world. *American Psychologist, 53*, 1282–1291.

Martin, G. (1995, July). A Buddhist perspective on diversity. *Seikyo Times*, 20–31.

Maslow, A. (1986). *Toward a psychology of being*. New York: Wiley & Sons.

Mays, V. M., Bulock, M., Rosenzweig, M. R., & Wessells, M. (1998). Ethnic conflict: Global challenges and psychological perspectives. *American Psychologist, 53*, 737–742.

Mizuno, K. (1987). *Basic Buddhist concepts*. (C. S. Terry & R. Gage, Trans.). Tokyo: Kosei.

Montagu, A. & Matson, F. (1984). *The dehumanization of man*. New York: McGraw-Hill.

Myers, D. G. (1999). *Social psychology*. (6th ed.). Boston: McGraw-Hill.

Ohnishi, S. (1993). The eternity of life and karma, *Seikyo Times, 9*, 2–29.

Ouspensky, P. D. (1979). *A new of the universe: Principles of the psychological method in its application to problems of science, religion, and art*. New York: Vintage.

Perkins, D. D. & Zimmerman, M. A. (1995). Empowerment theory, research, and application. *American Journal of community psychology, 23*(5), 569–579.

Poussaint, A. (1969). A Negro psychiatrist explains the Negro psyche. In N. E. Hoopes (Ed.), *Who Am I? Essays on the alienated.* (pp. 84–106). New York: Dell.

Poussaint, A. & Alexander, A. (2000). *Lay my burden down: Unraveling suicide and the mental health crisis among African-Americans*. Boston: Beacon Press.

Queen, C. S. (1998). The peace wheel: Nonviolent activism in the Buddhist tradition. In D. L. Smith-Christopher, (Ed.). *Subverting hatred: The challenge of nonviolence in religious traditions*. Cambridge, MA: Boston Research Center for the 21st Century.

Rouhana, N. N. & Bar-Tal, D. (1998). Psychological dynamics of intractable ethnonational conflicts: The Israeli-Palestinian Case. *American Psychologist, 53*, 761–770.

Rowan, C. T. (1996). *The coming race war in America*. Boston: Little, Brown.

Schachtel, E. G. (1961). On alienated concepts of identity. *The American Journal of Psychoanalysis, XXI* (2), 120–127.

Seligman, M. E. B. (1991). *Learned optimism*. New York: Knopf.

Siegel, B. (1986). *Love, laughter, and miracles*. New York: Harper and Row.

Staub, E. (1998). Early intervention: Prediction and action. In H. J. Langholtz (Ed.), *The psychology of peacekeeping* (pp. 31–39). Westport, CT: Greenwood.

Staub, E. (2001). Ethnopolitical and other group violence: Origins and prevention. In D. Chirot & M. E. P. Seligman (Eds), *Ethnopolitical warfare: Causes, consequences, and possible solutions* (pp. 289–304). Washington, DC: American Psychological Association.

Suzuki, B. L. (1972). *Mahayana Buddhism: A brief outline*. New York: Macmillan.

Takamura, T. (2000, June). Buddhist values and conflict resolution. *Living Buddhism*, 21–24.

Takayama, N. (1978, October). Defining the human identity. *Seikyo Times*, 26–34.

Tajfel, H. & Fraser, C. (Eds). (1978). *Introducing social psychology: Analysis of individual reaction and response*. New York: Penguin Books.

The Lotus Sutra (1993). (B. Watson, Trans.). NY: Columbia University Press. (Original work published 406 BC)

The Three Fold Lotus Sutra. The Sutra of Innumerable Meanings. The Sutra of the Lotus Flowers of the Wonderful Law. The Sutra of Meditation on the Bodhisattva Universal Virtue. (1975). (B. Kato, Y. Tamura, & K. Miyasaka, Trans.). (W. E. Soothill, W. Scheiffer, & P. P. Del Campana, Rev. ed.) New York: Weatherhill/Toyko: Kosei.

The major writings of Nichiren Daishonin. (1981). Vol. II. (The Gosho Translation Committee, Ed. and Trans.). Tokyo: Nichiren Shoshu International Center.

Thurman, R. A. F. (1996). Nagarjuna's guidelines for Buddhist social action. In A. Kotler (Ed.), *Engaged Buddhist reader* (pp. 79–90). Berkeley, CA: Parallax Press.

Turner, J. C. (1987). *Rediscovering the social group: A self-categorization theory*. New York: Basil Backwell.

Weinreich, P. (1991). Ethnic identities and indigenous psychologies in pluralist societies, *Psychology and Developing Societies, 3*(1), 73–92.

Yamamoto, S. (2003). Environmental Problems and Buddhist Ethics: From the Perspective of the Consciousness-Only Doctrine. In K. H. Dockett, G. R. Dudley-Grant, & C. Peter Bankart, *Psychology and Buddhism: From individual to global community* (pp. 239–257). New York: Kluwer Academic Plenum Publishers.

Chapter 11

Environmental Problems and Buddhist Ethics

From the Perspective of the Consciousness-Only Doctrine

Shuichi Yamamoto

In this chapter, I describe Buddhist views of nature and environment, and the contribution of the Consciousness-Only doctrine of Buddhist psychology to solving environmental problems. In particular, I emphasize an important role of the *alaya*-consciousness in the deeper layer of our minds from the perspective of the Consciousness-Only doctrine. The *alaya*-consciousness is the root entity that forms the framework of all existences, i.e., our own bodies, our minds, and our environments. To put its important role concretely, the concept of *alaya*-consciousness is able to give accounts of the enlargement of human desires as the cause of environmental problems, responsibility as environmental ethics, and the effects of products of science and technology on our minds. Finally, I discuss a methodology for reforming the *alaya*-consciousness through social movements and the bodhisattva way, and the solution of environmental problems at its most basic source.

Introduction

For the last two millennia, human beings never faced a truly serious threat to their existence as a species. But now, as we start the third millennium, the ever-deepening crisis in the global environment raises the real possibility of human extinction. If environmental destruction cannot be reversed, it is more than likely that the earth will degenerate, leaving the global ecosystem in ruins and making it impossible for our species to survive.

Tremendous efforts have been made over the past fifty years to try to control problems in the environment, and some of those problems, e.g., Minamata disease and ouch-ouch disease are the local problems in Japan, have been solved or at least alleviated. The irony is, however, irrespective of such efforts that we have created new problems, e.g., destruction of ozone layer and exogenous endocrine disrupters, one after another, so that now the environmental picture is, on balance, worse than ever before. Together, environmental problems such as the green house effect, marine pollution, and destruction of rainforest are expanding in scale and growing more serious in nature. How are we ever to break the hold of this vicious circle? One thing is clear, and that is the need for a fundamental reappraisal of the material civilization that has been propelled onward by science and technology. Buddhism has much to offer in the quest for answers to the environmental crisis. It's approach is gradualist, through a human revolution. Like reform through education, the Buddhist method may seem circuitous, but it seeks to get to the heart of the problem.

Recently, I described Buddhist views of nature and the environmental and summarized several points addressing Buddhist issues on environmental problems (Yamamoto, 1998a,b, 1999). In addition, Kawada (1994), Harvey (2000) and Keown (2000) have discussed generally Buddhist thought and Buddhist ethics in relation to global problems. The relation of Buddhism to ecological ethics has been discussed in detail by Schmithausen (1991a,b, 1997, 2000).

In this article, alongside summarizing several points dealing with Buddhist perspectives on the environment, I would like to examine some of the ways Buddhism can contribute to solving the environmental problem by focusing on the doctrine of Consciousness-Only (*yui-siki*) (italicized terms are Buddhist terms in Japanese) by Vasubandhu (*Sesin*), which is often referred to as the Buddhist version of psychology. The Consciousness-Only teachings that were expounded by Asanga (*Mujaku*) and Vasubandhu in fourth or fifth century of India are called the Yogacara School (*Yugagyo-ha*) (Harvey, 1990).

Principles of Buddhism: Views of Nature and the Environment

How nature is perceived in Buddhism depends on how truth is recognized, which is an important factor in making judgment in values and ethics. I would first like to itemize how Buddhism perceives nature and the environment.

Concept of Relationships Based in the Doctrine of Dependent Origination

One characteristic of Buddhist thought in recognizing the occurrence of phenomena is found in the doctrine of dependent origination or conditioned arising (*engi*), which is derived from the Four Holy Truth (*Shitai*) (Harvey, 1990). The following are phrases often used as fundamental definitions of this doctrine which was set forth in Early Buddhism. "When this exists, that exists. When this is born, that is born. When this does not exist, that does not exist. When this disappears, that disappears." These phrases mean that an entity does not exist and generate independently, but that every entity exists only because of its relations with or the conditions of other entities. Buddhism teaches that an entity cannot exist independently because of the fundamental interdependence and interconnectedness of all phenomena. The relation of ontology (relation of space) and relation of formation (relation of time) are included in the doctrine of dependent origination.

The above-mentioned concept of nature and environment seen in the doctrine of dependent origination is similar to concepts of ecology. Everything is somehow connected. Therefore, the very principles of bio-diversity and symbiosis of nature and living things are primary in maintaining our world. This doctrine of dependent origination underlies everything in Buddhism.

Fundamental Biospheric Egalitarianism in Humans, Living Things, and Nonliving Things

An important aspect in environmental ethics is how human beings, living things, and nonliving things are perceived. In Buddhism, humans, living things, and nonliving things are fundamentally recognized to be equal in life levels. The term "life levels" does not refer to the common meaning of life, but refers to the fundamental power, which supports living beings. Buddhism teaches that this fundamental power, which can be called life potentially, also exists in nonliving things.

According to Nakamura (1988), since ancient times, the people of India did not consider there to be a distinction between animals and humans. The term "living beings" (*shorui*) included humans and animals as quite the same existence. In Indian ethical systems, there was not only a mutuality between humans but also a mutuality between humans and animals. Moreover, Nakamura points out that as a unique characteristic of Buddhism there are scriptures that treat many species of animals as heroes in stories.

Similarly, in Chinese and Japanese Buddhism there is a thought that "even plants, mountains, and rivers have "Buddha-Nature" (*bussho*). This thought is called *Somoku-jobutsu, Somoku-kokudo-sikkai-jobutsu, or Hijo-jobutsu* in

Japanese. These Japanese terms respectively mean that grass and trees attain Buddhahood (*jobutsu*); plants and earth can become Buddhas (*hotoke*); and nonsentient beings (*hi-jo*) can become Buddhas. There is no difference between sentient beings (*u-jo*) and nonsentient beings, because all beings have Buddha-Nature (Schmithausen, 1991a).

This reflects the fact that China and Japan had an origin in an evergreen forest civilization abundant with nature. Japanese and Chinese Buddhism teach that not only humans and animals but also even nonliving things such as plants, mountains, and rivers have Buddha-Nature, and that all existences can attain enlightenment. Since all living things and nonliving things have this Buddha-Nature, they are regarded as having an equal dignity. Indian Buddhism, however, explains that plants and nonliving things cannot become Buddhas, and that only humans and animals, as sentient beings, can attain enlightenment. In the modern edition *Nanden-Daizokyo* (1935) of the Buddhist scriptures edited by Tripitakas (*Sanzo*) et al., on the other hand, it is written that the Buddhist monk Gotama refrained from harming any kind of seed and plant life. From this it seems that the dignity of plants and their seeds were accepted.

What appear in the phenomenal world naturally appear as different phases of objects, e.g., people, animal, plant, mountain, and river. Buddhism recognizes the differences of the phenomenal world with a pair of concepts called sentient beings and nonsentient beings. These concepts could be expressed in the difference of whether the entity is sentient (*jo*), has feelings or consciousness. As seen in ancient India, it was thought that sentient beings indicated humans and animals, and nonsentient beings indicated plants, organisms, and nonliving things. Looking at this from the standpoint of modern ecology, it is probably better to look at these things, including animals, plants, and simple organisms, as sequential from one to the other, rather than separating these things into simplistic categories.

Another concept that recognizes living things and nonliving things is the Buddhist doctrine of the three realms of existence (*san-seken*). This concept breaks down the differences of all phenomena. The three realms of existence consist of the realm of the five aggregates (components; *go-un-seken*), the realm of sentient beings (living beings; *shujo-seken*), and the realm of nonsentient beings (environment; *kokudo-seken*). The realm of the five aggregates consists of matter (form; *shiki-un*), perception (*ju-un*), conception (*sou-un*), volition (*gyo-un*) and consciousness (*shiki-un*). Matter shows a material side where life is composed and perception, conception, volition, and consciousness shows mental sides. Perception means the function of receiving or apprehending external information through one's sense organs. Conception indicates the function by which life grasps and forms some idea or concept about what has been perceived. Volition means the will to initiate some sort of action following the creation of conceptions about perceived objects. Consciousness indicates the subjective entity supporting and integrating the other four aggregates, as well as the discerning function of life which makes value judgments. The realm of sentient beings means that the five aggregates of life unite temporarily to form an individual living being. Therefore, differences of life will be caused in how the five aggregates are temporarily united. For instance, though all of the five aggregates appear in humans, only matter appears and the other four aggregates are latent in nonliving things. For animals, matter of the five aggregates is actualized in all animals. Different functions of the other four mental sides appear according to each animal. Moreover, for plants, there may be some mental actions being actualized other than just matter. This is the diversity of life that Buddhism recognizes.

An Environmental View in the Concepts of the Nonduality of Life and Its Environment and the Three Realms of Existence

The relationship between life, as the subject, and its environment is significant when thinking about the problems of environmental crisis. An "environment" can only be defined when there is a corresponding subject. In Buddhism there is a concept that is congruent with this way of thinking called the nonduality of life and its environment (*e-sho-funi*). The non-duality of life and its environment is one of ten kinds of non-dualities (*jippuni-mon*) taken from the *Fa-hua-hsuan-i-shih-ch'i* (*Hokkegengi-shakusen*) in *Taisho-Shinshu-Daizokyo* (1963). It is the work of Chan-jan (*Tannen*) of the T'ien-t'ai (*Tendai-chigi*) sect. The ten kinds of non-dualities are the oneness of body and mind (*shiki-shin-funi*), the oneness of internal and external (*nai-ge-funi*), the oneness of the goal of practice and the true nature of phenomena (*shu-sho-funi*), the oneness of cause and effect (*in-ga-funi*), the oneness of the impure and the pure (*zen-jo-funi*), the oneness of life and its environment (*e-sho-funi*), the oneness of self and others (*ji-ta-funi*), the oneness of thought, word, and deed (*sango-funi*), the oneness of the provisional and true teachings (*gon-jitsu-funi*), and the oneness of the ten endurances for Bodhisattvas to practice (*ju-nin-funi*).

The nonduality of life and its environment explains the relation between subject and its environment. *E-sho* is a contraction of the Japanese terms *e-ho* and *sho-ho*. The syllable *ho* here means manifest effect, or results of karma (*go*). *Sho-ho* indicates the living self or subjective world, and *e-ho* indicates the insentient environment or the objective world. Though *sho-ho* indicates the subjective world, this Japanese term is also expressed as the proper reward. And in the same manner, *e-ho* as the objective world is also expressed as the dependent reward. The objective world (*e-ho*) and the subjective world (*sho-ho*) are relative concepts. That is, the environment as objective world differs depending upon the subjective world.

The effects of an individual living being's past karma manifest themselves in both its subjective life and its objective environment. Since the syllable *funi* means "two in phenomena but not two in essence," *e-sho-funi* means "life and its environment are two distinct phenomena but nondual in their fundamental essence." Both the subject and its environment coexist or are nondual in a situation that is a result of karma. That is, this concept means that the subject is born into an environment suitable to it and the environment becomes suitable for the subject.

The third of the three realms of existence, in addition to the realm of the five aggregates and the realm of sentient beings is the realm of nonsentient beings. This realm indicates that which supports the existence of life. Thus, living beings are inseparable from their environments, having a close relation with the environment.

In the field of ecology, the act that one makes on its environment is expressed as the environmental formation effect and the effect that the environment has on one is expressed as the environmental effect. From a physical viewpoint, the environmental formation effect and the environmental effect can be considered to have the same meaning as the following quote from a Japanese Buddhist teacher, Nichiren (*The Major Writings*, 1275/1999): "To illustrate, environment (objective world) is like the shadow, and life (subjective world), the body. Without the body, no shadow can exist, and without life, no environment. In the same way, life is shaped by its environment." In other words, the state of life of an individual is reflected in the world around him or her, and the world itself corresponds to the individual. The concept of the possession of the nonduality of life and its environment are fundamental to the view that change in the subject or individual can effect change in the environment.

One of the important points in the life-centric environmental view is that we should grasp the subject and its environment as inseparable and the other is that we should consider the meaning of the environment for the subject. When we consider the environment from the Buddhist view, the destruction of the environment means not only the destruction of a physical base for humans and living things, but also the destruction of the mind and life itself.

The Japanese term *ho* of the subjective world (*sho-ho*) or the objective world (*e-ho*) corresponds to manifest effect in the Ten Factors of life or existence. That is, it is the resulting effect from past karma (cause and effect). The Ten Factors of life (existence) is equipped in the three realms of existence, that is, the realm of the five aggregates, the realm of sentient beings, and the realm of nonsentient beings. The manifest effect means that the cause and effect of karma (*goin-gouka*) in the mind area of the subjective world appear in the material area. Therefore, if the cause and effect of karma in the subjective world or the realm of the five aggregates and the realm of sentient beings are changed for the better, the manifest effect of the subject can also be improved.

In the same way, if the cause and effect of karma in its environment, i.e., the objective world and the realm of nonsentient beings, are improved, the manifest effect of its environment can be improved. Because the objective world and the subjective world are nondual, one's improvement enables the improvement of its environment. Here, a principle of environmental improvement in Buddhism is recognized. This is the principle in the dimension of life that one's improvement causes a change in its environment. Humans and the environment, therefore, progress each mutually influencing the other, in a relation of continuous action and reaction, such as: human activity → environmental formation action → environmental change → environmental action → human reaction → human adjustment. Both humans and the environment are historical in existence and change mutually, biologically, culturally, socially, and in other life dimensions as well.

Viewing the Five Defilements from the Perspective of Time

The five defilements consist of the defilement of period (*ko-joku*), the defilement of view (*ken-joku*), the defilement of evil passions (*bonno-joku*), the defilement of sentient beings (*shujo-joku*), and the defilement of life (*myo-joku*). The defilement of period is impurity in age and society. The defilement of view and the defilement of evil passions, which relate to individual humans, mean impurity of thought and impurity in greed (*ton*), anger (*jin*) and stupidity (*chi*) such as so-called instinct, respectively. The defilement of sentient beings means increasing of sufferings as a result of the defilement of view and the defilement of evil passions. The defilement of life means that the longevity of living beings shortens. In the *Fa-hua-wen-chu* (*Hokke-mongu*) by T'ien-t'ai (in the modern edition of *Taisho-Shinshu-Daizokyo* (1966b)), he describes that the defilement of period is caused in the following order: first, from the defilement of evil passions, the defilement of view, and the defilement of life which are immanent in the life of humans; second, to the defilement of sentient beings; and finally, to the defilement of period where darkness overwhelms the spirit of that time. Here, the darkness means that the spirit of age itself becomes ignorant of the true nature of existence (*mumyo*).

According to the theories of the three realms of existence and the five defilements in Buddhism, we could refer to the cause of the environmental crisis from three areas as follows the self, others versus the self, the natural ecosystem versus the human race. These three areas correspond to the realm of the five aggregates, the realm of sentient beings, and the realm of nonsentient beings in the three realms of existence of Buddhism, respectively. And also, these areas respectively correspond to areas of behavior, thought, morality, ethics, values, and desire, areas of the social environment such as culture, education, and religion, and areas of the natural environment such as animals, plants, microorganisms, mountains, rivers, and seas. We consider that while the occurrence of the environmental crisis is caused by the sequential process of effect from the area of the self to the area of nature via the area of others (society), the effect rebounds from the area of nature to the area of the self via the area of others (society).

Therefore the way to solve the problem of the environmental crisis is to reverse the process of this effect: i.e., the area of the self → the area of others (society) → the area of nature. In this way, Buddhism immediately aims at the change in the way of life for humans, especially in view of ethics, values, and life style, to solve the problem of the environmental crisis. Moreover, indirectly, the influence of Buddhism could affect revolution of cultures and social systems, such as science, technology, politics, economy, law, and so on.

Humanity, Society, and the Natural Environment from the Perspective of the Consciousness-Only Doctrine

Environmental Thoughts of Buddhism and the Doctrine of Consciousness-Only

As described above, the essences of Buddhist environmental thoughts and their meanings for solving environmental problems are summarized as follows.

1. *Principle of Symbiosis.* Concepts of nature and environment that are seen in the Buddhist doctrine of dependent origination are similar to concepts of ecology. Everything is somehow connected. Therefore, the very principles of bio-diversity and symbiosis of nature and living things are primary in maintaining our world.
2. *Principle of Circulation.* The concept of cycles or cycling that birth and death is repeating in the universe is important for considering the system of cycling in society. Moreover, the concept of transmigration of life and rebirth of life is significant for cultivating views of environmental ethics, because oneself in the future is determined by behaviors of oneself at the present.
3. *Perspective of recognition of the world.* In Buddhism, all phenomena are understood basically in terms of dependent origination, the idea of the interdependence and interaction among all existences. Perception of them takes place in the context of the three areas set forth by the doctrine of the three realms of existence: the area of mind vs. body; the area of the self vs. others (i.e., human society); and the area of human race vs. natural ecosystem.
4. *Relationships of Subject and the Environment.* The environmental view of Buddhism is a life-centric one, and is life-independent or anthropo-independent too. Both subject and its environment have a mutually interdependent and an interconnected relationship.
5. *Intrinsic Value of Nature.* The doctrine of dependent origination shows that everything in the ecosystem is equal in value. Because all living and

nonliving things have the Buddha-Nature, they are regarded as having an equal dignity and an intrinsic value.

6. *The Rights of Nature*. Though environmental ethics will be expanding the concept of rights from human rights into the rights of nature, the doctrine of dependent origination in Buddhism argues that human rights are based upon the rights of nature.

Buddhism holds, however, that if we grasp the above concepts at the superficial level of consciousness, we lose sight of their essence, for underneath consciousness is a vast realm of unconsciousness, and essence lies in that deeper layer, according to the doctrine of Consciousness-Only. This Buddhist idea is the doctrine of Consciousness-Only, which had been expounded by Vasubandhu (Taisho-Shinshu-Daizokyo, 1935) and others in the Consciousness-Only school (*yuishiki-ha*) of Mahayana. Therefore, I think that the doctrine has a significant meaning for understanding Buddhist thoughts.

The Consciousness Only doctrine holds that the consciousness which appears on the surface always affects the depths on the basis of dependent origination and the surface consciousness and the subsurface consciousness are always changing fluidly. In the same way, subject and its environment have a close relation still more at the depths as well as a relation which appears as phenomenon at the surface. Therefore, the phenomenon and the consciousness, which appear at the surface, are only the tip of the iceberg floating on the water. There is a vast world that extends under the surface of the water, a world that is developed with the depths of the consciousness and the phenomenon in Buddhist thought.

Characteristics of the Consciousness-Only Doctrine

First-Five Consciousness, the Mind-Consciousness, and the Manas-*Consciousness.* According to the Consciousness-Only doctrine, the uppermost stratum of human consciousness (*shiki*) is composed of the first-five consciousness (*zen-go-shiki*) that correspond to the five sensory organs (eyes, ears, nose, tongue, and body), plus the sixth (*roku-shiki*), which is mind-consciousness (*i-shiki*). The first-five consciousness means discernment of the human sense organs, i.e., the eye consciousness (*gen-shiki*), the ear consciousness (*ni-shiki*), the nose consciousness (*bi-shiki*), the tongue consciousness (*ze-sshiki*), and the body consciousness (*shin-shiki*). The mind-consciousness includes reason and integrates the perceptions of the five senses into coherent images. In contrast to these six layers of consciousness, or six consciousnesses, that deal with the external world, the seventh (*nana-shiki*) or *manas*-consciousness (*mana-shiki*) discerns the inner spiritual world. Basic awareness of self originates at this level. The passionate attachment (*shuuchaku*) to the ego (*ga*), which functions to create evil karma (*aku-go*), is also the working of this seventh consciousness. These karma include self-stupidity (*ga-chi*), which leads to ignorance of true nature; self-pride (*ga-man*), which can turn into arrogance; self-biased views (*ga-ken*), which more often than not are false views; and self-love (*ga-ai*), which is the source of greed. The *manas*-consciousness is, indeed, the root ego that sustains self-consciousness.

Then, the *manas*-consciousness is also called consideration-consciousness (*siryo-shiki*). The object that is considered is the *alaya*-consciousness (*araya-shiki*) in the depths of the *manas*-consciousness, and the *alaya*-consciousness is regarded as an entity. Buddhism understands that various suffering and evil passions (*bon-no*) are caused there. Attachment to the entity results in clinging to the thought of the existence of the self.

The Alaya-*Consciousness.* Located in the layer deeper than the *manas*-consciousness is the eighth (*hachi-shiki*) or *alaya*-consciousness. This is also known as the immortal consciousness, as it is regarded as that which undergoes the cycle of birth and death. It is the root entity of individual existence that underscores the Buddhist idea of transmigration of life, that is, eternal, continuous change of life.

According to Yokoyama (1976), the *alaya*-consciousness has two distinct characteristics. First, it is the root entity that forms the framework of all existences. It generates and influences the workings of the first seven consciousnesses (*zen-nana-shiki*). One's own body and its environment, as well as the first seven consciousnesses, all arise from what the *alaya*-consciousness is transformed.

Second, all the experiences of life that take place through the first seven consciousnesses – both physical and mental activities – are accumulated as *seeds* (*shuji*) in the *alaya*-consciousness. The seeds thus imprinted and stored there grow and mature to give birth to new existences (the environment, body, and the various consciousnesses). The seeds registered in the eighth consciousness through the three kinds of human acts (*san-go*) – bodily (*shin*), verbal (*ku*), and mental (*i*)—are together called the name and word seed (*myogon-shuji*), because those that are conceptualized through language leave especially strong imprints. There are morally good (*zen*), evil (*aku*), and neutral (*muki*) seeds, and of these, good and evil ones are called karma seeds (*go-shuji*). Buddhism attaches particular importance to the conscious acts of the first six of consciousness (*zen-roku-shiki*); hence, whether such physical and mental acts are good or evil is clearly imprinted in the *alaya*-consciousness as karma seeds. Therefore, the eighth consciousness, *alaya*-consciousness, is called the store-consciousness (*zo-shiki*), because this consciousness stores the karma seeds of all consequences of karma action.

Moreover, the *alaya*-consciousness is dyed with good or evil karma seeds though the *alaya*-consciousness is originally ethically neutral, as a blank sheet of paper. The good and evil karma seeds will decide a condition of the *alaya*-consciousness in the future world.

Common Karma and Individual Karma. Two kinds of karma seeds are imprinted in the *alaya*-consciousness: those that are common among members of a family, an ethnic group, or a society and those that are specific to individuals. The former are called common karma seeds (*gugo-shuji*), and the latter, individual karma seeds (*fu-gugo-shuji*). A person's body and mental activities are by nature individual; hence, they are formed by individual karma (*fu-gugo*). By contrast, the natural environment and social milieu do not belong to one person but are common to the members of a group or an area; hence, they are formed by common karma (*gu-go*). The text of Abhidharma-nyayanusara (*Abidaruma-Junshori-ron*) by Hsuantsang (*Genjo*) (in the modern edition of Taisho-Shinshu-Daizokyo, 1962) describes that "mountains, rivers, the earth, and so on are born from common karma, and sentient beings are born from individual karma."

Common karma applies at different levels. The common karma of a family, for example, informs its family consciousness and a particular familial environment, while that of an ethnic group informs the ethnic consciousness and a particular ethnic environment. Thus, common karma informs not only the outer layer of the social consciousness of a family, an ethnic group, a nation, and humankind as a whole, but their subconsciousness as well. Common karma also extends vertically, affecting both our ancestors and future generations. In this point of view, the relations between an individual and his or her mind, between an individual and society, and between human and nature, which relations are aspects of the Buddhist worldview, will be supported by the standpoint of the doctrine of Consciousness-Only.

Parenthetically, I would like to note the remarkable congruence between Buddhist psychology's theory of consciousness and Carl Jung's theory of the ego, the personal unconscious, and the collective unconscious (cf., Kawada, 2001; Stacks, 1996). To briefly explain, the seventh (*manas*) level of consciousness corresponds directly to Jung's concept of the personal unconscious, which consists of once-conscious elements that have been repressed or forgotten. Both theories agree as Jung stated, "Consciousness succumbs all too easily to unconscious influences. The fate of the individual is largely dependent on unconscious factors" (as cited in Stacks, 1996, p. 9). Buddhism attributes this to the functions of the karmic storehouse of the *alaya* consciousness. In addition, "Jung's concept of the archetype, which lies at the root of his theory of the collective unconscious, mirrors the Buddhist view of karma, which is the foundation of the eighth level of consciousness" (Stacks, 1996, p. 13). Both theories assert that, "people share a common and inborn pool of experience, reaching back to prehistory and beyond." Jung calls them archetypes while Buddhism calls them common karma. Both espouse "the belief that people are intimately connected to their own past and that of humanity as a whole ... because, in Buddhist terms, we all possess the 'storehouse' of the eighth consciousness that is forever recording deep within our lives the experiences registered by our first seven consciousnesses" (Stacks, 1996, p. 12). In fact, Jung (1954) equated enlightenment to an awareness of the collective unconscious. (See Bankart's discussion in Chapter 2 of this volume on the Five Manifestations of the Buddha in the West.)

Dependent Origination of the Alaya-*Consciousness.* Like the first five consciousnesses that correspond to the five sensory organs, the *alaya*-consciousness has its own objects of cognition. Whereas the eye consciousness discerns form, among other things, and the ear consciousness discerns sound, among others, the *alaya*-consciousness discerns the seeds, the environment, and the fifth through the seventh consciousnesses that are its own making. The *alaya*-consciousness has its own unique mental functions by which to discern them. Its discernments are reflected in bodily, verbal, and mental acts, which are in turn imprinted as seeds in the *alaya*-consciousness. This is called the dependent origination of the *alaya*-consciousness (*araya-shiki-engi*). According to the Wei-shih-san-shih-lun (*Yuisiki-sanju-ronju*) by Vasubandhu, he expressed that the *alaya*-consciousness is always changing and is like a torrent. In applying this concept of dependent origination to the environmental problem, we must keep in mind that the *alaya*-consciousness functions to affect the individual, society, and the natural environment.

As the individual karma seed imprinted to the *alaya*-consciousness makes an individual body and the first seven consciousnesses, the perception, discernment, and conception by the first five consciousnesses and the mind-consciousness always imprint new seeds to the *alaya*-consciousness in the individual. As a result, when three kinds of bodily, verbal, and mental acts (*shin-ku-i-no-sangou*) newly express themselves, individual karma seeds will be accumulated again. The *alaya*-consciousness always changes by thus accumulating new individual karma seeds. A feedback loop of the individual karma of the *alaya*-consciousness in the individual will be formed here.

The concept shows that the common karma imprinted in the *alaya*-consciousness always maintain dynamic relationships with society and the natural environment, and undergo constant change, thereby leading to the accumulation of new common karma, which eventually manifest themselves, becoming phenomena. In other words, a feedback loop of common karma of the *alaya*-consciousness is formed involving society and the natural environment. It is understood that individual karma, too, when shared by many members of the group or area, can potentially become common karma. Hence, the feedback loop at the individual level and the one formed involving society and the natural environment can be closely interconnected.

Perspective of the Consciousness-Only Doctrine to Environmental Problems

Enlargement of Human Desires and Responsibility to the Environment

It will be possible to create an environment conducive to the symbiosis of all living things, including human beings, by recognizing that the world is governed by the principle of dependent origination and by creating a feedback loop of merciful, good common karma. Until now, human refashioning of the environment, it seems, has been singlemindedly directed toward the fulfillment of human desires.

Human desires vis-à-vis the environment have manifested themselves in automobiles, chemicals, and other industrial products and material substances, as well as in the transformation and destruction of nature through deforestation, depletion of natural resources, and development projects. What is important to note here is that the consequences of unbridled human desires appear in concrete form in the environment. As mentioned earlier, the Consciousness-Only doctrine holds that whatever is manifested in the environment and what kind of environment is created reflect the common karma. In other words, what is internal in humans, such as desires, transform themselves into components of the external environment. These products of externalized desires stimulate not only human responses to the objects of perception by the five sensory organs – form, sound, smell, taste, and texture – but also stimulate the evil passions lurking in the seventh consciousness, the *manas*-consciousness.

Initially, the common karma as a totality was small in scale, but through the feedback loop of the *alaya*-consciousness involving society and the environment, the products of human desires further stimulated popular craving for more, and they amplified the common karma over time until it has grown to constitute the common karma of humankind as a whole. In our world today we see greed expanding apparently boundlessly via the feedback loop that originates in the *alaya*-consciousness. And we see the environment saturated with things to satisfy human desires, an environment changing into the kind that corresponds with the common karma of our time.

The Consciousness-Only doctrine thus sheds light on how humans have formed the environment and how the environment has affected humans. Particularly relevant here is the idea that the nature of the environment depends on the common karma of the people who make up the particular society, for it nurtures awareness that their environment is something of their own making. That awareness in turn enables people to realize that their environment is an enlarged projection of themselves; hence, they must work hard to protect the health of their environment just as they take care to protect their own health. Also relevant is the contention that products of human desires keep amplifying through the feedback loop of the *alaya*-consciousness. By the same logic, human destruction of the environment ultimately leads to the destruction of the human spirit in its deeper layers.

Products of Science and Technology from the Perspective of the Consciousness-Only Doctrine

Let us examine more closely the destructive impact on the environment by science and technology and their products. From the perspective of the Consciousness-Only doctrine, gigantic machines that destroy nature, chemical substances that contaminate many forms of life and nature itself, and pesticides and herbicides designed to kill plants and animals are all functions of the common karma. Products of science and technology may be divided into two categories in terms of the Consciousness-Only doctrine.

Machines used to destroy nature and agricultural chemicals applied to kill pests and weeds fall in the first category – products made for purposes of destruction and/or killing, which are evil acts. In Buddhism, producing things with the conscious purpose of evil acts is considered especially conducive to the accumulation of evil karma seeds. Put another way, the science-technology products of the first category are none other than manifestations of the evil common karma. Thus, products of evil common karma seeds lead through the feedback loop to further accumulation of those seeds in society. As evil common karma seeds pile up in the *alaya*-consciousness of people, good common karma seeds diminish and become less powerful, and at some point the margin opens for unmerciful acts to be committed unconsciously. When that point is crossed, people are no longer aware that it is evil to kill life and destroy nature. That is why it is so critically important not to manufacture products of science and technology whose intended purpose is to destroy and kill.

Most products of modern science and technology fall in the second category; they are not originally intended to kill or accomplish other evil objectives. In fact, they are made to serve some useful purposes in human society. Yet it is quite possible for many of these products to end up destroying nature, contaminating or even killing living things, or harming human health. In terms of the Consciousness-Only doctrine, this bespeaks the human inability to accurately forecast the effects of certain products on the environment and failure to understand the relationship of dependent origination. Those human failings can be attributed to the state of the *manas*-consciousness. As long as the seventh consciousness is obsessed with the root ego, it is exceedingly difficult for a person to understand that this world is governed by the principle of dependent origination and that all existences in it are mutually dependent and in constant interaction. Failure to carefully consider in advance the possible effects of scientific-technological products on other beings makes people realize later that even those intended to serve human society and fulfill human desires can in the end bring about the destruction of nature, contamination of plants and animals, and have hazardous effects on human health. The examples are the earth warming by the emission of green house gases as carbon dioxide, the destruction of ozone layer by chloroflurocarbon, contamination and harming health of living things and people by agricultural chemicals, polychlorobiphenyl and exogenous endocrine disrupters.

Human knowledge of nature is still inadequate, hence it is perfectly understandable how difficult it may be to prevent beforehand all adverse effects of scientific-technological products. Precisely because of that, it is all the more important for us to understand clearly that human beings are not really capable of perceiving this world as one of dependent origination insofar as greed thoroughly permeates the root ego in the *manas*-consciousness. Once we grasp that condition, we will be aware that we have been making many scientific-technological products primarily to fulfill our desires to satisfy our five senses and part of our mind. Meanwhile, we have not thought hard enough or been wise enough about the possible consequences of our productive activities on the natural ecosystem.

Meanings of the Environmental Movement and the Way of Bodhisattva

As I described above, the *alaya*-consciousness is a root entity that comprises the surface and subsurface human mind and plays an important role in the formation of a sense of social responsibility, too. The *alaya*-consciousness is in constant flux and is always changing. But the changeable nature itself of the eighth consciousness also makes reforms possible. The question now is how to change the *alaya*-consciousness.

Let me discuss the methodology of reform from two different angles. One approaches the reform of the deeper layers (*manas*- and *alaya*-consciousness) by starting at the dimension of the first five consciousnesses and the sixth (mind). The other seeks to get at the deeper layers directly. I will call the former "reform from the social dimension," and the latter, "reform from the religious dimension."

Reform from the Social Dimension

This approach corresponds to what is known as environmentalism or the environmental movement. The movement focuses on the reform of consciousness, which, from the perspective of the Consciousness-Only doctrine, can be interpreted in the following way.

The environmental movement consists of programs in environmental education and ethics, as well as exhibitions, publishing, lectures, dialogues, and other practical activities. In terms of the Consciousness-Only doctrine, these can all be received via the first five consciousnesses, especially those of the eyes, ears, and body. The significance of the environmental movement carried out through the surface layers of consciousness is internalized in the sixth, or the mind consciousness. The more deeply imprinted in the mind, the greater the impetus for further action. From the Buddhist point of view, also, this kind of movement has great significance, for the *alaya*-consciousness is the source of these six consciousnesses, which are, in turn, objects of cognition for the eighth consciousness. Thus, whatever is perceived by the five sensory organs and is integrated in the mind (the sixth consciousness) is also discerned by the *alaya*-consciousness.

Most representative of the seeds imprinted in the *alaya*-consciousness is the name and word seed. As explained earlier, many seeds are formed and imprinted through language. Environmental education, dialogue, lectures, publishing, exhibitions, and so forth are conducted through the medium of language; hence, everything one has learned in the environmental movement is imprinted as the name and word seed in the *alaya*-consciousness. Because seeds relating to moral goodness and evil are imprinted as karma seeds, one's wishes for solutions to the environmental problem, symbiosis with other forms of life, coexistence with other nations and ethnic groups, a feeling of gratitude toward nature are all registered as good karma seeds. The seeds thus imprinted are eventually reflected as karmic effects in actions via the feedback loop of the individual. If these karma seeds are imprinted through the feedback loop of society as good common karma, then, vertically, they will affect future generations, and horizontally, the whole human race in all its ethnic, racial, and national diversity, as well as all other forms of life. Thus, the environmental movement is truly meaningful in the context of Buddhist philosophy.

Reform from the Religious Dimension

Evil passions of an individual spring up from the deeper layer of unconsciousness, hence it is extremely difficult to control them on the level of the sixth, mind consciousness. Similarly, the common karma that forms the environment and social consciousness cannot be so easily elevated to the level of mind consciousness. For these reasons, Buddhism seeks solutions to the environmental problem through religious practices aimed at direct reforms of evil passions and common karma themselves. How, then, does Buddhism suggest going about it?

The *alaya*-consciousness is sometimes called bodhisattva-consciousness (*bosatsu-shiki*), and the way of reforming the *alaya*-consciousness itself is the way of bodhisattva (*bosatsu-do*). The basic spirit of the bodhisattva way is expressed as compassion (*jihi*), maintaining patience (*nin-niku*), and emptiness (*kuu*). Compassion is extended equally to all human beings, animals, plants, and even non-life matter, regardless of whether they are good or evil. By maintaining patience one can develop the true strength with which to withstand any and all difficulties, and also put the principle of satisfaction with little desire and a little gain into practice, thereby exercising moral control over greed. Finally, the view of emptiness (*kuu-gan*) nurtures global life consciousness that stresses the relationship of dependent origination among all forms of life and seeks human coexistence with other living creatures. It also enhances the sense of gratitude and the spirit of repayment for the entire ecosystem, which is by nature interdependent. The way of bodhisattva refers to actions based on these spiritual qualities. Wisdom (*chie*) inherent in the bodhisattva-consciousness is capable of not only discerning the feedback loop formed by dependent origination of the *alaya*-consciousness, but also directing all the individual and common karma toward solution of problems confronting society as a whole.

By injecting the energies of wisdom and compassion that comprise the way of bodhisattva into the layers of consciousness, from the eighth to the first, it is possible to equip each layer with wisdom. In Buddhism, there is a term pravrtti-vijnana (*tenjiki-tokuchi*), meaning "transform the four layers of consciousness into the four-fold wisdom." This is the approach of the bodhisattva way to reform of the *alaya*-consciousness. Whereas the social approach to reform discussed earlier starts out from the upper layers of consciousness, the bodhisattva way goes directly to the deeper layers, hence it is more fundamental.

Accumulation of the energies of wisdom and compassion through practicing the way of the bodhisattva leads to accumulation in the *alaya*-consciousness of good common karma. As more and more good karma (*zen-go*) is imprinted there, the *alaya*-consciousness evolves into the great, perfect teaching-wisdom (*dai-enkyo-chi*), wisdom which reflects all phenomenal things clearly, as if in a bright mirror. Springing forth from this wisdom of dependent origination is the sense of gratitude and repayment for all phenomena and existences that have had a part in its birth. Also arising naturally therefrom is global consciousness for symbiosis and coexistence.

The other seven layers of consciousness that derive from the *alaya*-consciousness each are transformed into wisdom. The seventh *manas*-consciousness turns into the wisdom of equality of all things (*byodo-sho-chi*), the sixth mind-consciousness into the wisdom of wondrous observation (*myo-kanzat-chi*), and the first five layers of consciousness become the wisdom of accomplishing what is to be done to benefit sentient beings (*josho-sa-chi*). The wisdom of equality of all things makes it possible for the *manas*-consciousness to free itself from the obsession (*shu-uchaku*) that it embodied the *alaya*-consciousness and that it was the seat of the root ego. Liberation from an obsession with the small self (*sho-ga*), hence from self-love (*ga-ai*) and other evil passions that generate human desires, will be achieved. The wisdom of equality of all things also enables people to understand all phenomena in terms of dependent origination and to embrace all existences as equal in their intrinsic value. The Buddhist idea of compassion comes into play here. Then the wisdom of wondrous observation and the wisdom of accomplishing what is to be done for the benefit of sentient beings enable people to free themselves from evil passions, act according to the dictates of reason, and make correct judgments and accurate inferences. As a result, they can display their physical abilities as their consciousness commands. By virtue of all this, people will finally be able to overcome their inordinate material desires now dominating their first layers of consciousness and the mind-consciousness.

The two approaches to the reform of the *alaya*-consciousness – religious and social – combine to bring about changes in both individual and common karma. Eventually, these changes will lead to the solution of the environmental problem at its most basic source.

Author Note

Portions of this paper were presented in the symposium, Healing for the Millennium II: Buddhist Applications to Social Problems, at the American Psychological Association Convention, Washington, DC, August 4–7, 2000. I wish to express my gratitude to Dr. Kathleen Dockett for correcting English expressions in my chapter.

References

Harvey, P. (1990). *An introduction to Buddhism: Teaching, history and practices*. Cambridge: Cambridge University Press.

Harvey, P. (2000). *An introduction to Buddhist ethics*. Cambridge: Cambridge University Press.

Jung, C. G. (1954). *The development of personality*. New York: Pantheon Books.

Kawada, Y. (1994). *Chikyu Kankyo to Bukkyo Shiso* [The global environment and Buddhist thoughts]. Tokyo: Daisan Bunmei-sha.

Kawada, Y. (2001). Nichren Buddhism and empowerment. *Living Buddhism*, *5*(9), 18–23.

Keown, D. (Ed.). (2000). *Contemporary Buddhist ethics*. Great Britain: Curzon.

Nakamura, H. (1988). *Bukkyo Doubutsu Sansaku* [Exploring animals in Buddhism]. Tokyo: Tokyo Shoseki.

Nanden-Daizokyo. (1935). *Chobu-kyoten 1, Bonmou-kyo*, by Tripitakas (*Sanzo*) et al., p. 6. (1st ed., Vol. 6). Tokyo: Daizo-Shuppan.

Schmithausen L. (1991a). *Buddhism and nature*. A lecture delivered on the occasion of the EXPO 1990. An enlarged version with notes. Tokyo: The International Institute for Buddhist Studies.

Schmithausen L. (1991b). *The problem of the sentience of plants in earliest Buddhism*. Tokyo: The International Institute for Buddhist Studies.

Schmithausen L. (1997). The early Buddhist tradition and ecological ethics. *Journal of Buddhist Ethics*. *4*, 1–74.

Schmithausen L. (2000). *Buddhism and the ethics of nature: Some remarks*.

Stacks, T. N. (1996, December). The nine consciousnesses and Jung's theory of the collective unconscious. *Seikyo Times*, 6–13.

Taisho-shinshu-daizo-kyo. (1962). Takakusu, J., & Watanabe, K. (Eds), (Vol. 29, p. 529). Tokyo: Daizo-Shuppan. (Original work published 1926, Reprinted 1962, Abhidharma-nyayanusara (*Abidaruma- Junshori-ron*), Vol. 33, Hsuantsang [*Genjo*; Trans.]).

Taisho-Shinshu-Daizokyo. (1963). Takakusu, J., & Watanabe, K. (Eds.), (Vol. 33, pp. 918–919). Tokyo: Daizo-Shuppan. (Original work published 1926, Reprinted 1963, *Fa-hua-hsuan-I-shih-ch'i* (*Hokkegengi-shakusen*) by Chan-jan [*Tannen*; Trans.]).

Taisho-Shinshu-Daizokyo (1966a). Takakusu, J. & Watanabe, K. (Vol. 46, p. 54). Tokyo: Daizo-Shuppan. (Original work published 1926, Reprinted 1966, *Mo-ho-chih-kuan* (*Makashikan*) by T'en-t'ai [*Tendai-chigi*].

Taisho-Shinshu-Daizokyo. (1966b). Takakusu, J. & Watanabe, K. (Vol. 34). Tokyo: Daizo-Shuppan. (Original work published 1926, Reprinted 1966, Fa-hua-wen-chu (*Hokke-mongu*), (Vol. 4, Section 2) by T'ien-t'ai [*Tendai-chigi*].

The Major Writings of Nichiren Daishonin (1999). The object of devotion for observing the mind established in the first-hundred-year period after the thus come one's passing. (p. 354). Tokyo: Soka Gakkai (Original work published 1273).

The Major Writings of Nichiren Daishonin (1999). On omens. (p. 644). Tokyo: Soka Gakkai (Original work published 1275).

Vasubandhu [*Seshin*]. Wei-shih-san-shih-lun [*Yuisiki-sanju-ronju*]. *Taisho-shinshu-daizo-kyo*, (Vol. 31, pp. 60–61). Tokyo: Daizo-Shuppan (Original work published 1926, Reprinted 1970).

Yokoyama, K. (1976). *Yuishiki-Shisou Nyumon* [Introduction to the doctrine of Consciousness-Only]. Tokyo: Daisan Bunmeisha.

Yamamoto, S. (1998a). Contribution of Buddhism to environmental thoughts. *The Journal of Oriental Studies, 8*, 144–173.

Yamamoto, S. (1998b). Kankyo-rinri to bukkyou no kadai I [Environmental ethics and issues of Buddhism I.]. *Nihon Indo-gaku Bukkyo-gaku Gakkai-shi* [The Journal of India and Buddhist Studies], *47*(2), 78–84.

Yamamoto, S. (1999). Kankyo-rinri to bukkyou no kadai II [Environmental ethics and issues of Buddhism II]). *Nihon Indo-gaku Bukkyo-gaku Gakkai-shi* [The Journal of India and Buddhist Studies], *48*(1), 250–256.

Chapter 12

Buddhist Social Principles

David W. Chappell

Gotama Buddha has been called the world's first psychotherapist, but he was also socially active and spent much of his teaching career on the road engaging all elements of society in dialogue and reform rather than remaining isolated in meditation. Buddhist practice is not primarily a solitary quest, and only at times did the Buddha wander lonely as a rhinoceros. We have heard about, and some may have tried, practicing alone, living in caves or as forest renunciants. This is a special vocation, or for special times, or for unusual people. Most Buddhists most of the time lived socially, as either monastics or laity (Ray, 1994).

The institutionalized forms of Buddhism that spread across Asia were similar to Western psychotherapy in giving priority to the goal of achieving individual happiness through purity and meditation in the isolation of a monastery. Governments provided support to monastics as a symbol of social harmony as long as monastics avoided secular activities and did not constitute a danger to their political power. Even though the Mahayana Buddhist reform movement challenged monastic isolationism, it also became quickly co-opted by monastic elites. Today, however, with the increased protection of constitutional governments in Asia and the spread of Buddhism to the West, a new form of "socially engaged" Buddhism has arisen that affirms that happiness cannot be attained alone. The most satisfying and lasting happiness involves a life not only free of hatred and fear, but lived in compassion and action for others. Based on an earlier study in *Buddhist Peacework: Creating Cultures of Peace*, this article will explore the social principles of Buddhism as a dimension of Buddhist mindfulness practice.

The inner dialogue taught by the Buddha to his disciples was also expressed in a social dialogue – not unlike that of Socrates and Confucius – and evolved into an enduring social movement that became the only major cultural tradition that permeated all of Asia. The inner dialogue that is mindfulness training involved stopping or calming (*samatha*) our normal thought responses and seeing (*vipassana*) the various factors in our consciousness and world that could awaken our capacity to develop clearer understanding and non-addictive responses. It is the thesis of this article that this same mindfulness process also functions socially by taking regular and frequent "time outs" from daily pressures for mindful dialogue to discover the diversity, common ground, and variety of interpretations and responses in any social nexus we find ourselves. The patterns of this social mindfulness work, and its presence in earlier forms of Buddhism, will now be sketched.

Traditional Buddhist Social Principles

In ancient India, the Buddha discovered that individual human happiness and misery were determined not primarily by physical abundance, but by inner mindfulness. Buddhist practice focuses on the mind, on mindfulness training, on noticing the different parts within ourselves and their interactions which include cognitive, affective, and behavioral patterns. A single soul does not exist, said the Buddha, since each person is the integration of a multitude of factors. Freedom and peace come when we recognize the many voices within us, and discover their willingness to try new tunes, to forge new harmonies, or to wait their turn. The inner dialogue that constitutes mindfulness work was a new discovery by the Buddha that paralleled the discovery in other cultures by Socrates, Confucius, and Second Isaiah that the good life was more dependent on inner attitudes and awareness than the product of external events.

Buddhism began in history when the Buddha taught both personal and group practices to a community of followers. While right mindfulness and wisdom could be cultivated in private, social checks and balances occurred twice a month on the new moon and the full moon days when his disciples gathered to recite the social rules of practice (*uposatha*). If problems arose concerning practice, the disciples were to resolve them by unanimous agreement. This pattern of regular and frequent meetings to monitor moral actions, and the process of resolving problems by discussion and consensus, was the Buddhist social model of dialogue and accountability in its earliest days.

Moral Principles

While *dhyana* and *prajna* (meditation and wisdom), or *samatha* and *vipassana* (calming and insight), are two legs of the Buddhist chair, it cannot stand without social action. Traditional Buddhist morality (*sila*) was codified in the vinaya scriptures and included several hundred prohibitions, but four applied to all Buddhists: no killing, stealing, lying, or sexual misconduct. While these are universal moral values, additional rules – including voluntary poverty and chastity – were foundational to the Buddhist monastic order and marked its distinctive identity, vision, and constancy of purpose through time and across cultures. The monastic community became identified as the primary arena for cultivating meditation and wisdom and it survives as one of the world's oldest religious orders.

Buddhist morality was exceptional also because the Buddha's definition of purity was universal: the rules applied equally to everyone regardless of caste and social distinctions. The Buddha insisted that these moral standards were more important social criteria than birth or power or knowledge, that character counted more than caste. Although the Buddha did not overtly challenge the idea of caste as a social hierarchy, he did challenge its membership criteria based on birth and ritual performance. While accepting all followers regardless of caste, he did spend much of his time reforming brahmin priests by emphasizing character, and claimed that his followers were the "true brahmin" (Masefield, 1986, pp. 1–36, 147–161, 164–170).

The classic anthology of his early teachings in the *Dhammapada* begins by stating that the "Mind is the forerunner of all states," and mental attitudes lead inevitably to misery or happiness depending on whether one speaks and acts with a pure or defiled mind. However, another early *Dhammapada* text from Gandhara that survives in Prakrit has a different arrangement of its verses (Brough, 1962, p. 290) and does not begin with a focus on psychology, but with a social critique:

> Not by matted hair, nor by family, nor by birth does one become a brahmana; but in whom there exist both truth and righteousness, pure is he, a brahmana is he.
>
> What is the use of your matted hair, O witless man! What is the use of your antelope garment? Within you are full (of passions), without you embellish.
>
> If from anybody one should understand the Doctrine preached by the Fully Enlightened One, devoutly should one reverence him, as a brahmana reveres the sacrificial fire.

These verses are equivalent to verses 393, 394, and 392 respectively in the Pali Dhammapada. The implication of placing these verses first in the Gandhara text is that the social impact of Buddhist cultivation was equally as consequential as its influence on personal happiness. These verses express a social revolution in ancient India by rejecting the criteria of social status based on religious posturing and birth. Instead, the new measures of worthiness, the new criteria for respect and sanctity, were inner understanding and purity based on the Buddhist morality of non-injury and nonattachment. This same effort to rank people by their moral quality and understanding rather than by their birth or posturing was taught by Socrates in the West and by Confucius in China, who also challenged the established criteria for their social structures. The emphasis on universal morality, instead of family and clan connections, was an important new development in human culture. However, because of the Buddhist idea of rebirth in various levels of existence, from animals to gods, Buddhism even went beyond a social focus by including all people and animals alike. As a result, vegetarianism has become a mark of Chinese and Korean Buddhists with the result that temple lands often served as wildlife preserves.

Social Activism

The Buddha was also a social activist beyond his community of monastics. In the first years of his teaching career, the Buddha made a point of visiting the kings of the two most powerful states in his region, Bimbisara and Pasenadi. These kings became the Buddha's disciples, and as a result influenced thousands of their citizens toward the Buddha's path (Schumann, 1989, pp. 88–93, 105–112). While enjoying the privacy of forest retreats, the Buddha also traveled into outlaw territory to pacify the most notorious mass murderer of the day, Angulimala. If we rely on the surviving historical records, the Buddha's encounter with Angulimala was one of the most popular stories of early Buddhism since it survives in more versions that almost any other single early text (Akanuma, 1958, p.168). Also, it is well known that when the Sakya clan and the Koliyas were about to go to war over the use of water from the Rohini River, the Buddha intervened on the battlefield to avoid conflict (McConnell, 1990). While the fortnightly meeting of the Buddhist community (*sangha*) dealt mostly with internal matters, the forty-five year teaching career of the Buddha was filled with other kinds of social interaction at all levels of society. The Buddha taught kings and untouchables, brahmins and bandits.

The basic principle underlying Buddhist social activism is dependent origination, meaning the recognition that we are all interdependent and share an inescapable responsibility for the well-being of the entire world. The sangha not only was open to all castes, but also actively went out into society to help others. In the first year of his teaching when the Buddhist community was just beginning and consisted of only 60 monks, the Buddha sent them forth: "Go forth, monks, for the good of the many, for the happiness of the many, out of compassion for the world, for the benefit, for the good, for the happiness of gods and men." (Mahavagga, Vinaya 1.11.1) And the Buddhist community (*sangha*) was held up as the ideal for all society (Payutto, 1993, p. 276).

Group Procedures

Benefits for others involved more options than leaving society to join the monastic community. The Buddha not only tried to enhance the quality of life for individual laity through morality, meditation, and wisdom, but he also gave principles for social organization. The Mahaparinibbana Sutta (Digha-nikaya 16.1) records that the Buddha used seven criteria to evaluate the social strength of the Vajjian state by asking if they:

1. held regular and frequent assemblies;
2. met, dispersed, and conducted their business in harmony;
3. did not authorise what had not been authorized by their ancient tradition;
4. respected, revered, and saluted the elders among them and valued their words;
5. didn't forcibly abduct wives and daughters of others nor take them captive;
6. respected, revered, and saluted the shrines at home and abroad, and didn't withdraw the proper support given before;
7. gave proper provisions for the safety of Buddhist Arhats so that they could live in comfort, and so that other Arhats might come to live there in the future.[1]

Certain of these rules are to be expected – such as, support for the sangha, respect for elders, and respect for women in other families – but there is a remarkable insistence on maintaining traditions, both secular and religious. This principle reinforces the exceptional nonsectarian nature of early Buddhist teaching (Chappell, 1990, 1999b). In addition, there is the insistence on regular and frequent assemblies conducted in harmony and leading to harmonious settlements. A similar norm was applied to sangha meetings that used the rule of consensus for all decisions, making the sangha the epitome of democracy since everyone had a voice and everyone had to agree on all decisions.

The monastic order was innovative in providing a religious and social community that served as an alternative to people in a variety of cultures. For over a millennium in East Asia the Buddhist nunnery was the only escape for women from a male-dominated social order. In addition, most of the time monastics were excused from being drafted into the army because political leaders came to recognize the monastic rule of nonviolence for monks. This is not the place to do an institutional analysis of nonmonastic Buddhist organizations (NMBOs), or to discuss priorities of Buddhist institutional reform (Chappell, 1999b). Instead, more attention will be given to Buddhist social psychology.

[1] The sutta then reports that the Buddha recommended the first four principles to his monks, but replaced the last three with the following:

5. Do not fall prey to desires.
6. Be devoted to forest-lodgings.
7. Preserve personal mindfulness so that good companions will be attracted and will remain.

This discourse then gives several other lists focused on maintaining positive individual mental habits. Since the oral texts were preserved by monastics, it is natural that they would remember advice on their personal practices, while it is striking to see a list to prevent the decline of the Vajjin state.

Dialogue as the Practice of Social Mindfulness

Dialogue takes Buddhist mindfulness practices into the social sphere. It is a way to become aware of the different social factors involved in our shared world to develop a more inclusive understanding and to create new choices for action.

The Buddha's meditation methods consisted of recognizing a plurality of forces that shape our expectations, our habits, and our decisions. He challenged his culture's emphasis on a permanent, controlling ego (*atman*) that should be in charge. Rather, he demonstrated how our inner self was constructed through many factors in the learning processes, but that these processes inevitably lead to conflict and misery when a single factor becomes dominant. This conflict can be dissolved, however, through noticing the different elements shaping our consciousness and recognizing the inevitable misery that arises from fixation on a single interpretation as ultimate.

The good news is that by developing an inner transparency and inner dialogue about our perceptions, we discover that there are choices about how to construct our awareness, and that there are peaceful and nonpeaceful ways to perceive and respond to our world. Mindfulness training is a method to defuse our ego, our hurts, and our attachments, and a way to find sympathy and compassion with others, and an arena for discovering creative new options.

In the twofold act of calming one's mind (*samatha*) and seeing the interdependent nature of all things (*vipassana*), meditators create a psychic space in which they can see the role of their mental and emotional habits in shaping their perception and can experiment with alternative ways of viewing and reacting to the world. Balanced meditation must involve *vipassana*, namely, recognizing the interconnectedness and impermanence of experience that naturally leads to a sense nonattachment and an increased awareness of the common ground shared with others. Out of this ground, empathy and compassion arise.

Just as mindfulness training requires stopping normal activities (*samatha*) to see the factors that make up our awareness (*vipassana*), so developing compassion requires taking time out to become aware of beings other than oneself. To be effective rather than indulgent, compassion needs to be facilitated, nurtured, and guided by "regular and frequent" dialogue. This psychological change requires social activity.

Today in business management, the old command model of top-down management has been replaced by an emphasis on teamwork and nurturing horizontal relationships. When a group has a controlling person, inevitably conflict will arise. In the political sphere, dictatorships in the twentieth century have killed more people than all the killing in previous human history (Rummel, 1994). Peace requires checks and balances, participation in decision-making, and the recognition of diversity. Social peace requires recognizing and collaborating with the diversity of people, just as inner peace requires acknowledging the pluralism within.

The mindfulness practices of Buddhism remain the major form of peacework, but they involve both inner and outer dialogue. One reason that the Dalai Lama received the Nobel Peace Prize was his unusual reaction to the brutalization of Tibetans by the Chinese. Instead of expressing anger and violence, the Dalai Lama found common ground with the Chinese. He emphasized that the Chinese are just like him, they want to get rid of suffering and they want to find happiness. His capacity to find alternative ways of understanding and responding to the hurts of the world have convinced him that all people can develop a heart of compassion.

Dialogue is mindfulness training at the social level. It is not a discussion about external issues, but a sharing and hearing the personal experiences of other people that opens awareness to the range of human factors involved in social behavior. In that way, dialogue involves an exploration of one's motivations and the motivations of others.

Robert Aitken (1999) says that "enlightenment is an accident, but meditation helps one to be accident prone." Similarly, compassion is a gift, but dialogue is the process of receiving gift certificates.

Building Consensus as a Buddhist Imperative

The Buddha taught universal moral principles as the basis for society, but within his own community of monastics he added the instructions that decisions were to be based on consensus and equality, not on authority or tradition, nor on lineage or even spiritual attainment. The procedures for the Buddhist community (*sangha*) represent one of the earliest examples of radical democracy in which decisions were final only when everyone agreed (De, 1955; Khongchina, 1993). As a result, the Buddha with his disciples formed a new kind of society, an alternative community, that transcended cultural and social distinctions and that recognized minority opinion by giving it veto power. The Buddhist community was to live by consensus: everyone was to go together, or not go at all.

Consensus is not easy. The requirement of biweekly uposatha meetings of the sangha where decisions are to be made by consensus implies transforming dialogue. Only through careful and penetrating discussion, sharing of motivations, and mutual adjustment of participants to the values and needs of each other, can consensus arise and harmony result for the benefit of the common good.

There are different kinds of dialogue. Eric Sharpe, writing out of a Hindu-Christian context, has distinguished four kinds: discursive, human, secular, and interior/spiritual dialogue (Sharpe, 1975, 1987). Discursive dialogue is largely theological, whereas human and secular dialogue is limited to interchange between individuals as individuals or between religious people about secular problems. In contrast, interior/spiritual dialogue primarily involves religious contemplation, and is more experiential and less verbal than discursive dialogue. In Buddhist-Christian encounter beginning in the 1940s with the Jesuit leader, Father Hugo Enomiya-Lassalle, and continuing with Thomas Merton, Don Graham, William Johnston, Yamada Koun, Robert Aitken, and Manao Abe, contemplatives of both traditions immediately found kinship with each other.

However, consensus in the *sangha* must be more than dialogue among like-minded people, since the sangha included many kinds of different temperaments, some meditative and others less so. Rather, to find common ground among people of such diversity requires both a strong commitment to social harmony and a process of mutual sharing that can go beyond differences to discover common ground in the midst of differences. This harmony rarely happens in theological, human, or secular dialogue, whereas interior/spiritual dialogue involves a restricted group of people and themes that do not include moral or secular issues. However, the consensus of early Buddhist monastics had to deal with exactly those social and external issues.

Very few people have as much experience with interreligious dialogue as Hans Ucko who has been responsible for facilitating and overseeing Jewish-Christian-Muslim dialogue for the World Council of Churches in Geneva in the 1980s and 1990s. Yet the Buddhist-Christian Symposium held in July 1994 in Switzerland (Chappell, 1995) came as a big surprise to him. I have described his response as follows:

> He commented to me that in most dialogue meetings between Christians and Jews, or between Christians and Muslims, the partners came with clearly articulated theological positions and attempted to persuade the others of the validity of their viewpoints. In contrast, the technique used by the directors of the 1994 Symposium, Pia Gyger and Niklaus Brantschen, was to break the Symposium into small groups that began with personal sharing by each person of their inner thoughts on that day. Instead of being challenged by the others, the response invariably was an empathetic sharing of similar or complementary inner experiences by others in our group that clarified and expanded the inner experience by placing it in an interfaith context. Hans Ucko found this group of interfaith seekers and sharers to be in profound dialogue, but unusual because of its mutual sympathy and support. (Chappell, 1999a, p. 58)

It is no accident that the conference directors, Sister Pia Gyger and Father Niklaus Brantschen, are ordained Catholics, but also Zen practitioners and teachers. The process of dialogue did not focus on comparing doctrine, but was a sharing of the concerns of people. Dialogue in this Buddhistic mode requires mindfulness of internal motivating factors, the influence of bodily needs, emotions, memories of past experiences, unresolved conflicts, and behavioral patterns that are almost never raised or even inwardly acknowledged in the kinds of dialogue outlined by Eric Sharpe (1987). As the factors and relationships behind personal reflections are revealed, conceptual absolutes are left behind, new interpersonal connections become possible, shared ground is found, and integration in the midst of diversity can arise.

Mindfulness training was the method developed by the Buddha to develop inner peace, but regular and frequent dialogue leading to consensus was his method for social well-being. How this was achieved, we do not know. My proposal is that there are three crucial factors: first is constant mindfulness of the interdependent and impermanent factors in one's own consciousness that leads to nonattachment to any inner agenda; second is an appreciation of the factors in the lives of others that are similarly interdependent and impermanent; and third is a sense of compassion for others and moral commitment to social harmony. It is said that on the night that the Buddha attained enlightenment, he passed through three stages of awareness that are parallel to these three elements that I propose for achieving social consensus. First was seeing how he came to be over many lifetimes, second was understanding how others had come to be, and third was his awareness that inner obstructions and defilements (*asavas*) had fallen away and enlightenment had been attained.

In an earlier review of Buddhist interreligious dialogue by many contemporary Buddhists, I was struck that the central motive seemed to be a moral commitment to heal the suffering of others and build a peaceful world by bridging differences (Chappell, 1999a). The motive may have been cultivated by an interior/spiritual experience, but it clearly involved compassion for others. Thich Nhat Hanh (1955) begins his book *Living Buddha, Living Christ* by recalling an inter-religious meeting in Sri Lanka where participants were assured: "We are going to hear about the beauties of several traditions, but that does not mean that we are going to make a fruit salad." When it came time for Nhat Hanh to speak, he commented: "Fruit salad can be delicious! I have shared the Eucharist with Father Daniel Berrigan, and our worship became possible because of the sufferings we Vietnamese and Americans shared over many years" (Nhat Hanh, 1955, pp. 1–2). He went on to observe that many participants were shocked by his statements, but his stance is a recurring theme among such outstanding contemporary Buddhist leaders as the Dalai Lama, Robert Aitken, Daisaku Ikeda, Sulak Sivaraksa, Bhikshu Buddhadasa, and A. T. Ariyaratne.

The practice of suffusing the four directions with compassion was an early and central Buddhist practice. Kindness arises not just through inner mindfulness, but requires human interaction. Empathy develops first in the family, then among friends, and then with a wider range of humans and other beings. Empathy does not depend on organizations, but it does depend on the processes of our interactions. Compassion arises when the ego boundaries are softened in trust and sharing, when others trust their pain to you and you are open and able to feel it. This process is not a solitary event.

Compassion is a gift of the human heart and cannot be manufactured. However, social processes are a necessary condition, and some are better than others, in helping people evolve a sense of trust, caring, and universal responsibility. The Buddha recommended "regular and frequent meetings" that are convened, conducted, and concluded with consensus. The modern code words for this activity are nurturing diversity and dialogue.

Based on Buddhist principles, violence is not an option for Buddhists. In 1967, after a four-month period in which six members of the School of Youth for Social Service (founded by Thich Nhat Hanh) were killed and others wounded, the staff and students read this pledge at a funeral:

> Now, once again, we solemnly promise never to hate those who kill us, above all never to use violence to answer violence, even if the antagonists see us as enemies and kill until they annihilate us. We recall our pledge that people, no matter what their origins, never are our enemies.... Help us to keep steadily this non-violent mind in our social work by love that asks nothing in return. (Forest, 1987, p. 7; Chan, 1993)

Thich Nhat Hanh emphasizes that the enemies of Buddhists are not other people. The enemies are greed, anger, and ignorance. The enemies are patterns of denial and structures of privilege. The enemies are silence and fear. The enemies are not other people, but cognitive, psychological, and social processes.

Human Rights and Buddhist Social Morality

Dialogue is not enough. Dialogue requires mutual respect, equality, and willing partners. As long as governments or corporations control the media, communication technology will not bring peace, parity, and freedom. Modern technology in this century has facilitated the brutality of dictators as well as the compassion of peacemakers. Dialogue is a practice that needs a suitable context. Note, for example, that Jiang Zemin has refused to meet with the Dalai Lama. Aung San Suu Kyi is still under police restrictions in Myanmar (Burma). Willing dialogue partners are not there.

Buddhist morality is not enough. The Buddhist precepts apply to individual purity and the Mahayana bodhisattva precepts offer only general encouragement for universal compassion, caring for the sick, and treating all people, including enemies, as family relatives. However, the special problems of organized society, of structural violence, of social oppression and environmental degradation, are not adequately addressed (Chappell, 1996, 1999c). In his acceptance speech for the 1989 Nobel Peace Prize (as cited in Piburn, 1990, pp. 17–18), the Dalai Lama said:

> Peace, in the sense of the absence of war, is of little value to someone who is dying of hunger or cold. It will not remove the pain of torture inflicted on a prisoner of conscience. It does not comfort those who have lost their loved ones in floods caused by senseless deforestation in a neighboring country. Peace can only last where human rights are respected, where the people are fed, and where individuals and nations are free....

> Responsibility does not only lie with the leaders of our countries or with those who have been appointed or elected to do a particular job. It lies with each of us individually.... What is important is that we each make a sincere effort to take seriously our responsibility for each other and for the natural environment.

The Dalai Lama is very aware of the complex problems of our globe and urges each person to develop a sense of universal responsibility. Daisaku Ikeda similarly encourages and tries to prepare members of Soka Gakkai to be world citizens. But both the Dalai Lama and Daisaku Ikeda do much more. They offer concrete proposals and guidelines for governments to adopt. And they both appeal to and support the United Nations and the Declaration of Human Rights.

Scholars have argued that Buddhism has no doctrine of human rights, and, technically, they are right. At a metaphysical level, Buddhist teaching has always rejected the concept of an unchanging, substantial self. But the Buddha warned not to take doctrines too seriously. At a practical level, human rights have been strongly affirmed by contemporary Buddhists such as the Dalai Lama, Sulak Sivaraksa, Maha Ghosananda, Daisaku Ikeda, and others. Human rights were not written in the heavens by gods, but constructed in history by mortals. They have no more, and no less, authority than the growing consensus of the human community about political limits to protect each of us, and social goals for all of us. As a metaphysical doctrine they are inadequate, but as social norms they are an invaluable and necessary tool for Buddhist peacework.

Most Buddhists in Asian countries have suffered invasion, civil war, or oppressive political regimes in recent times. The Buddhist traditional social teaching emphasizes the inherent dignity and spiritual equality of all people, the importance of having compassion for the suffering of others, and the necessity of including all people in the decision-making process. Human rights may not be inherent in people in a metaphysical sense, but they are strongly supported by Buddhist leaders as a negotiated social contract (Modsen, 1996) based on fairness and respect since everyone wants freedom from arbitrary arrest and imprisonment, health, food, self-esteem, and education.

Human progress has not been biological, but technological and institutional. While as consumers we are well aware of technological advances, it is legal safeguards for people in this century that have given new freedom to Buddhists to develop social programs, legal safeguards that have recently been withdrawn from the Falun Gong folk Buddhist movement in China. Although Buddhist thinkers have been critical of all absolutes, including legal ones, the practical benefits of law as social contract are an important part of peacework by stabilizing social compromise. Although the Buddhist tradition has been very good in its prohibitions, and very idealistic in its emphasis on universal responsibility, it has been rather weak in the intermediate steps of social responsibility – education, health, employment, welfare, and cultural development. This "middle path" needs much more attention by Buddhists. Fortunately, it is in this middle area where many of the new contributions of Buddhist social activism are taking place.

The thirty articles of the Declaration of Human Rights have a remarkable parallel to the threefold morality of Mahayana Buddhism: do no evil, cultivate good, and save all beings. The French jurist Karel Vasak (1982) saw the three values of the French Revolution (liberty, equality, and fraternity) as representing three levels or "generations" of human rights. The human rights articles consist of prohibitions that protect individuals from governments (2-21), those that nurture individuals in their economic, social, and cultural relationships (22-27), and those that affirm the need for a global order (28-30). This structural affinity with Mahayana ethics, as well as the importance of human rights in Buddhist liberation movements and peacework, and the global spread of human rights as a shared standard, is making the Declaration of Human Rights an essential new pillar of social ethics for contemporary Buddhists.

When the Diem regime outlawed public celebration of Wesak in Vietnam in 1963, thousands of Buddhists publicly resisted nonviolently in public gatherings. The resulting arrests, torture, and killing of practitioners were detailed in a forty-five-page report on human rights violations submitted to the government by a Buddhist delegation. The appeal to human rights as a standard that is recognized worldwide has been a major advance of human civilization in the twentieth century. But it is the picture of Thich Quang Duc enveloped in flames at a Saigon intersection in 1963 that has seared itself into our collective global consciousness. Nonviolent political protest reported widely by the media has transformed our cultures. Legal protection of individuals is the first level of human rights and Buddhist morality.

But the second and third levels of human rights and Buddhist morality require mutual responsibility and global awareness that involve personal and cultural transformation. Many of these efforts are illustrated in detail in *Buddhist Peacework* (Chappell, 1999b). But for our purposes, some reflection is needed to consider the role of social responsibility within the field of Buddhist psychology.

Contemporary Buddhist Social Principles

The Buddhist tradition has always affirmed that practitioners were at different levels of maturity, and that different practices were appropriate for people at different stages of spiritual growth. The variety of paths to salvation, and their different levels, are elaborate and extensive (Buswell & Gimello, 1992), just as the American Psychological Association now lists fifty-five major divisions on its website (www.apa.org).

The diversity of Buddhist practice also reflects cultural patterns. Even though "socially engaged Buddhism" is a term that was coined in Vietnam by

Thich Nhat Hanh in the 1960s, some suggest that the social emphasis of modern Buddhism is a byproduct of Western influence, a kind of "Protestant Buddhism" (Gombrich & Obeyesekere, 1992, pp. 202–240). Even though Buddhists in the past usually emphasized the contemplative life of the monastic, in modern Asian Buddhist practice social activism is increasing (Chappell, 1999b; Queen & King, 1996). I suggest that this social role was part of Buddhism from the beginning, but became muted under traditional Asian political and cultural conditions.

Biologically there are different forms of intelligence (Gardiner, 1983) that have found various opportunities for expression based on historical and cultural factors. I am suggesting that socially engaged Buddhism is not only in imitation of Protestant missions – which was an important influence – but also is the product of new social opportunities, such as those based on new legal protections. In the past, governments restricted Buddhist public roles and social reform was rare. However, Asian Buddhists have increased independence based on church-state separation under constitutional governments. In addition, modern education has given new organizational opportunities to socially active lay Buddhist leaders, such as A. T. Ariyaratne (1999), Sulak Sivaraksa (1999), and Daisaku Ikeda (1999). Information technology also challenges Buddhists to respond to social and ecological crises. The global economy has brought affluence for some, but a population explosion and depletion of resources for most. Finding more harmonious and constructive ways to live requires a heightened awareness of our actions and their consequences, and a constant openness to possible alternatives, to avoid driving headlong and at high speed into the devastation of our world. Many modern Buddhists who have keen social sensibilities are agreeing with the Lotus Sutra, a foundational text for Mahayana Buddhism, by asserting that self-absorption is not enough and some form of social responsibility is an important part of Buddhist happiness.

Buddhist practice has traditionally been divided into three areas: morality, meditation, and wisdom. Buddhist psychology has usually been identified with cultivating meditation and wisdom, but in Buddhist practice the social dimensions of morality are always assumed. Mahayana Buddhist morality is based on three principles – avoiding harm, cultivating good, and taking responsibility for freeing all beings – but also advocates decision-making by consensus. The Dalai Lama writes that people cannot be fully happy until they have compassion for others. (Dalai Lama, 1998) The policies that have recently developed for creating a peaceful world are transparency, mutual accountability, dialogue, democracy, and human rights. Integrating Buddhist psychology and social imperatives with these policies, we might compose the following principles:

1. The foundational Buddhist rule of not harming means not hurting the well-being of oneself or others in society and the ecosystem guided by the Declaration of Human Rights and the Earth Charter.

2. Cultivating good means creating inner peace and outer compassion by seeing the diversity within ourselves and our interdependence with others that defuses the individual ego and extends our social identity to include the common ground among us.
3. Freeing all beings includes actively protecting the integrity, diversity, and creativity of others based on ecological and social mindfulness:
   a. by holding "regular and frequent" meetings conducted fairly and harmoniously where all beings, human and nonhuman, are included and given a voice, where authority is shared, responsibility is distributed, participation is balanced, decisions are democratic, and legal structures of checks-and-balances avoid favoritism;
   b. by nurturing social harmony and justice by small group dialogue where diversity can be expressed and common ground found by sharing the psychological factors and conditions that lead to decisions and actions, not by primarily focusing on the decisions and actions themselves;
   c. by building a just world by a fair and sustainable distribution of goods for the well-being of all, based on collaborative decisions informed by education, dialogue, and information about social, financial, and ecological resources.

The importance of the social dimension for Buddhist psychology is illustrated by a modern encounter in the 1930s in India. Mahatma Gandhi had worked to eradicate the caste system through "a change of heart," but the former untouchable, B. R. Ambedkar, argued for legal safeguards to ensure social change. Ambedkar publicly burned those parts of the Hindu *Code of Manu* that mandated the caste system and vowed: "I was born a Hindu, but I won't die a Hindu." Later Ambedkar was chairman of the drafting committee for the constitution of India (1947–1948) and as a member of Nehru's cabinet, he proposed that the Buddhist *dharmacakra* (wheel of the law) be on the Indian flag. In 1956, he publicly converted to Buddhism, followed by several million others. Ambedkar's social revolution is continuing in the Trailokya Bauddha Mahasangha Sahayaka Gana (TBMSG) founded in 1978 by millions of former "untouchables". Based on the Buddha's example, TBMSG members are seeking equality, but are using new social instruments: legal protection, education, social development, and international support. (Lokamitra, 1999)

Yes, Gandhi was right, the caste system will not disappear without a "change of heart". But Ambedkar was also right: new legal safeguards and specific social processes are needed to encourage opportunities to support positive inclusion. For an increasing number of Buddhists, social mindfulness and social activism is being seen as a necessary part of Buddhist psychology to achieve peace both for oneself and "for the good of the many, for the happiness of the many, out of compassion for the world, for the benefit, for the good, for the happiness of gods and humans".

References

Aitken, R. (1999). The Net of Vows. In D. W. Chappell (Ed.), *Buddhist peacework: Creating cultures of peace* (pp. 93–102). Boston: Wisdom Publications.

Akanuma, C. (1958). *The Comparative catalogue of Chinese Agamas and Pali Ikayas*. Tokyo: Hajinkaku-shobo.

Ariyaratne, A. T. (1999). Sarvodaya Shramadana's approach to peace building. In D. W. Chappell (Ed.), *Buddhist peacework: Creating cultures of peace* (pp. 69–77). Boston: Wisdom Publications.

Brough, J. (1962). *The Gandhari Dharmapada*. London: Oxford University Press.

Buswell, R. B. & Gimello, R. M. (Eds.) (1992). *Paths to liberation: The Mmarga and its transformation in Buddhist thought*. Honolulu: University of Hawaii Press.

Chan K. (Cao Ngoc Phuong). (1993). *Learning true love: How I learned and practiced social change in Vietnam*. Berkeley: Parallax Press.

Chappell, D. W. (1990). Six Buddhist attitudes toward other religions. In S. Sivaraksa et al. (Eds.) *Radical conservatism: Buddhism in the contemporary world* (pp. 443–458). Bangkok: Thai Inter-Religious Commission for Development.

Chappell, D. W. (1995). The 1994 European Buddhist-Christian Symposium. *Buddhist-Christian Studies*, *15*, 239–240.

Chappell, D. W. (1996). Searching for a Mahayana social ethic. *Journal of Religious Ethics, 24*(2), 351–376.

Chappell, D. W. (1999a). Buddhist interreligious dialogue: To build a global community. In P. Ingram & S. King (Eds.), *The sound of liberating truth: Buddhist-Christian dialogues in honor of Frederick J. Streng* (pp. 3–35). Surrey, UK: Curzon.

Chappell, D. W. (Ed.), (1999b). *Buddhist peacework: Creating cultures of peace*. Boston: Wisdom Publications.

Chappell, D. W. (1999c). Universal bodhisattva social ethics. In Bulgyohak Nonchong (Ed.), *Essays on Buddhist studies: Commemoration of the sixtieth birthday of President Jeon Chong-yoon*. (1343–1388). Sixtieth Birthday Commemorative Committee, Seoul: Chontae Bulgyo Moonhwa Yon-goowon.

Cobb, J. (1982). *Beyond dialogue: Toward a mutual transformation of Christianity and Buddhism*. Philadelphia: Fortress Press.

Dalai Lama, His Holiness the Fourteenth. (1990). The Nobel peace prize lecture, Oslo, Norway. In S. Piburn (Ed.), *The Dalai Lama: A policy of kindness*. Ithaca, NY: Snow Lion.

Dalai Lama, His Holiness the Fourteenth. (1998). *The Art of Happiness*. New York: Riverhead Books.

Dalai Lama, His Holiness the Fourteenth & Ouaki, F. (1999). *Imagine all the people*. Boston: Wisdom Publications.

De, G. (1955). *Democracy in early Buddhist sangha*. Calcutta: University Press.

Forest, J. H. (1987). *The unified Buddhist church of Vietnam: Fifteen years for reconciliation*. Hof van Sonoy, The Netherlands: International Fellowship of Reconciliation.

Gardiner, H. (1983). *Frames of mind: The theory of multiple intelligences*. New York: Basic Books.

Ghosananda, M. (1992). *Step by step: Meditations on wisdom and compassion*. Berkeley, CA: Parallax Press.

Gombrich, R. & Obeyesekere, G. (1988). *Buddhism transformed: Religious change in Sri Lanka*. Princeton, NJ: Princeton University Press.

Ikeda, D. (1999). The SGI's peace movement. In D. W. Chappell (Ed.), *Buddhist peacework: Creating cultures of peace* (pp. 129–138). Boston: Wisdom Publications.

Khongchinda, P. C. (1993). *The Buddha's socio-political ideas*. New Delhi: Navrang.

Lokamitra, D. (1999). The Dhamma revolution in India: Peacemaking begins with the eradication of the caste system. In D. W. Chappell (Ed.), *Buddhist peacework: Creating cultures of peace*. (pp. 29–38) Boston: Wisdom Publications.

McConnell, J. A. (1990). The Rohini conflict and the Buddha's intervention. In S. Sivaraksa et al, (Eds.), *Radical conservatism: Buddhism in the contemporary world* (pp. 200–208). Bangkok: Thai Inter-Religious Commission for Development.

Modsen, S. T. (1996). *State, society and human rights in South Asia.* New Delhi: Manohar.

Nhat Hanh, T. (1955). *Living Buddha, living Christ.* Berkeley, CA: Riverhead Books.

Payutto, P. (1993). Sangha: The ideal world community. In S. Sivaraksa et al. (Eds.), *Buddhist perception for desirable societies in the future* (pp. 274–285). Bangkok: Thai Inter-Religious Commission for Development.

Piburn, S. D. (Ed.). (1990). *The Dalai Lama, a policy of kindness: An anthology of writings by and about the Dalai Lama.* Ithaca, NY: Snow Lion.

Queen, C. S. & King, S. B. (Eds.) (1996). *Engaged Buddhism: Buddhist liberation movements in Asia.* Albany, NY: State University of New York Press.

Ray, R. (1994). *Buddhist saints in India.* New York: Oxford University Press.

Rummel, R. (1994). *Death by government.* New Brunswick, NJ: Transaction.

Schumann, H.W. (1989). *The Historical Buddha* (M. O'C. Walshe, Trans.) London: Penguin-Arkana.

Sharpe, E. (1975). The goals of inter-religious dialogue. In J. Hick (Ed.), *Truth and dialogue in world religions: Conflicting truth-claims* (pp. 77–95). Philadelphia: Westminster Press.

Sharpe, E. (1987). Dialogue of religions. In E. Mircea (Ed.), *The Encyclopedia of religion* (Vol. 4, pp. 344–348). New York: Macmillan.

Sivaraksa, S. (1999). Buddhism and a culture of peace. In D. W. Chappell (Ed.), *Buddhist peacework: Creating cultures of peace* (pp. 39–46). Boston: Wisdom Publications.

Vasak, K. (1982). *The international dimensions of human rights* (Volumes 1–2). Westport, CT: Greenwood.

Part IV

Future Directions

Global Impact

Chapter 13

On the Path to Peace and Wholeness

Conclusion to Psychology and Buddhism

G. Rita Dudley-Grant, C. Peter Bankart, and Kathleen H. Dockett

The completion of this book marks a tremendous effort over several years by the three editors and the many contributors. However, the timing of it's completion, in the aftermath of the tragic events of September 11, 2001 suggests that the "karma" of this effort, our collective energies and causes, determined that it would be completed at the time of greatest benefit to our audience. There are several sub-themes which have emerged from the chapters, including the alleviation of suffering at the individual, community, and global levels, the theory of dependent origination, empowerment at individual and societal levels, and the understanding of Buddhism as an engaged as well as individualistic practice, to name but a few. However, the overarching theme that speaks to this defining moment in our lives, is the commitment to peace and our ability as psychologists, Buddhists, or thoughtful human beings to bring about peaceful solutions to the terror, fear, and ethnic warfare that has been recognized as one of the greatest challenges to freedom in the twenty-first century (Chirot & Seligman, 2001; Ikeda, 2001; Payutto, 1996).

Buddhism as a religion has been recognized as a vehicle for peace. Indeed, Ikeda (2001) argues that "a religion that does not help people, that is not devoted to peace is not a proper religion... at its essence, religion is commitment – commitment to saving people from suffering. True religion strives to instill that commitment in peoples lives" (p. 1).

Jason and Moritsugu speak to this issue in their chapter, linking the Buddhist goal of reducing violence and conflict in the world to this shared goal within the discipline of community psychology. Thich Nhat Hanh (1993) has said "To preserve peace, our hearts must be at peace with the world, with our brothers and sisters" (p. 73). This point is well developed in the Dockett and North Schulte chapter on "Transcending Difference" which identifies as a root cause of ethnic conflict the failure to understand the nature of our existence and our interdependent relationships.

One could question the role of psychology in what appears to be a priori a political battle. What if any, is the role of the psychologist in the peace process? While Buddhism has established itself as a means of alleviating discord, promoting peace, and reducing suffering on the societal as well as the individual level, psychology, particularly as it is practiced in the West, has established itself as a "scientific" profession determinedly apolitical. As such, it consistently has sought to remove itself from the "subjectivity" inherent in human experience, which has plagued the discipline's early development, and elevate itself to the lofty "objectivity" associated with the physical sciences such as physics and chemistry. Indeed, "evidence-based practice" (Barlow, 2000) has been touted as the most positive redeeming value of the managed care era. However, Polly Young-Eisendrath has argued that we seek such scientific purity to our detriment in the sense of "biologizing" our behavior in the extreme. Her contention is that emphasis on the biological bases of behavior, in particular those that lead to suffering, undermines the ability to make significant behavior change. Practicing psychologists can also be seen as purveyors of the ultimate "coping mechanism," whether on the individual or community level, helping people to manage their individual stress and promoting resilient communities.

As psychologists addressing this tragedy, on the scene and around the world with our clients, and in our communities, we have addressed the issues of stress and helped our clients whether individually or at the societal level to come to terms with what some have called the "new reality." However, it has been the intent of this book to generate insight, thought, and action that goes beyond mere coping and stress management, although these are extremely worthwhile goals. Buddhism charges us to recognize that we are one with our environment, and that we have a responsibility to take action, as the external world is ultimately a reflection of our individual and collective reality. Thich Nhat Hanh has coined the term, "engaged Buddhism." This term was developed during the time of the Vietnam war when the Vietnamese Buddhist leaders took an active role in attempting to bring about a peaceful solution to the conflict that was devastating their country and destroying communities and their people.

We would posit that we must also recognize our responsibility as "engaged psychologists" playing a major role as social interventionists who can help our fellow human beings and ourselves to recognize our responsibility in creating peace in this world.

Alleviation of Suffering at the Individual, Community, and Global Levels

Buddhism is a pacifist religion as violence and war are seen as the result of misguided perceptions and reactions, resulting in suffering on all levels. Buddhist psychology has recognized its responsibility for assisting in the creation of peace. Throughout its entire several thousand year history creating peace has been an essential element of the reduction of suffering through the increase of wisdom.

> The idea of transforming consciousness and gaining wisdom is central to Buddhist psychology and perhaps represents Buddhism's most direct contribution to the idea of self-empowerment .... The delusion that the reified alaya [eighth] consciousness is one's true self is identified with fundamental ignorance, a turning away from the truth of the interconnectedness of all beings. It is this sense of one's self as separate and isolated from others that gives rise to discrimination against others, to destructive arrogance and acquisitiveness. (Kawada, 2001, p. 20)

We would add that this delusion of separateness allows us to visit the worst atrocities on each other in the name of the loftiest values such as purity, peace, and freedom. War and peace begins in the mind and heart of each individual. Our responsibility as psychologists, Buddhists, and mindful individuals must be to continue our development of empowerment and deepen our wisdom to create right actions that will ultimately lead to the elevation of the human spirit. As such, our attitudes toward war and peace, the consciousness of which has been brought on by these great events, must be examined and purified in such a way as to enable us to promote peaceful solutions to these problems that threaten our very existence. The contributors to this book have provided thoughtful and helpful insights into ways of thinking about these issues on individual as well as global levels, and it is hoped that the resulting stimulation of thoughts and ideas will move each reader to a greater level of empowerment and engagement in the processes of development of the human spirit.

The book has tried to address some of the causes of suffering from psychological and Buddhist perspectives that continue to lead us to human tragedy. It is safe to say that while parts of the world that have been disenfranchised politically, socially, economically or environmentally have been suffering for some time, we are all now feeling the effects of devastating loss, helplessness, and the fear of terrorist attacks from sources known and unknown. The Buddhist term for suffering is "dukkha". Young-Eisendrath defines it as "a state of being in which we are out of kilter because of a subjective disturbance that may be as mild as a momentary frustration or as severe as a depressive or psychotic state" (pp. XX). In these most difficult of times, when America is engaged in warfare, which is predicted to be longer and of a magnitude previously inexperienced, we can see intense emotional suffering stemming from being forced to come to grips with a new definition of the world and issues of safety and security. Young-Eisendrath posits that we have undermined our ability to adequately address this suffering by too great a reliance on what she terms the "biobabble" of scientific determinism. Bankart, in his chapter on five manifestations of the Buddha has also commented on the lost opportunities that western psychology has had to integrate and utilize Buddhist teachings into the theory and practice of Western psychotherapy. He attributes this loss primarily to what he calls "Orientalism," the ethnocentric tendency of Western Psychology to subjugate and arrogantly discredit Eastern theory, through what can now be seen as unfortunate misunderstandings of the processes and goals of meditation, mindfulness, and other practices. At the same time, he reviews the current primacy that Eastern techniques, particularly meditation and other mindfulness practices, have taken within the therapeutic and "new age" genres. He cautions that inappropriate use of these powerful techniques can be severely psychiatrically debilitating to individuals with a fragile psyche. He issues an even greater caution against "Western Buddhists [who] may, in fact, be in danger of the greatest act of Orientalism yet committed against the ancient teachings; turning it into a massive carnival of self-glorifying power-seeking materialistic narcissism" (p. 66).

Dudley-Grant has focused on the alleviation of suffering that results from addictive processes. She suggests that lessons learned from an integration of the twelve steps into Buddhist theory can strengthen the individual not only by taking responsibility for their actions, but also strengthening their commitment to the group. It is this recognition of self in relationship to others that is the necessary insight that can lead to the alleviation of suffering. Shantideva (of Tibetan Buddhism) states the concept well.

> What need is there to say more?
> The childish work for their own benefit,
> The buddhas work for the benefit of others,
> Just look at the difference between them.
>
> If I do not exchange my happiness
> For the suffering of others,
> I shall not attain the state of Buddhahood
> And even in samsara I shall *have no real joy*
> (as cited in Rinpoche, 1995, November 2)

This saying well encapsulates the mission of the bodhisattva, which is the highest state of life for humanity.

Dependent Origination

In addition to the theme of suffering addressed in many of the chapters, is the theme of our interconnectedness embodied in the doctrine of dependent origination. This doctrine originates in the Mahayana teachings, and speaks cogently to our mutual interdependence. To simplify a very intricate and complex theoretical formulation, the doctrine explains that we can only exist in relation to everything else. We retain our unique qualities but are dependent on other aspects of reality to form the whole that we define as "reality". In other words, reality is not some objective entity that we live in or observe, but rather is the subjective interconnectedness of all things, including our perceptions and interactions with them. Ultimately, we are connected at the deepest levels to all others as well as to our eternal selves.

In terms of the doctrine of dependent origination, a consistent theme through most of the chapters is the need to be more rather than less aware of ourselves in relation to each other and the world. Belinda Sieu Luan Khong exemplifies this quite well in her chapter on Daseinanalysis and Buddhism. In a subsequent presentation on the same subject, she made the following point:

> Mindfulness practice does not require us to empty our minds, to set out aside or suppress intellectualism. Rather it permits us to be constantly aware of the workings and the contents of the mind so as not to allow them to interfere with our ability to listen quietly. The Buddha encourages people to experience for themselves how one thing leads to another. Understanding this cycle, the person has the choice and the responsibility to interrupt this process so that things can be otherwise. By paying bare attention, we learn to separate our responses from the situation itself, and to respond appropriately. (Khong, 2001, p. 6)

Khong is encouraging us to understand and come to terms with our ability and responsibility regarding our behavior and its consequences. Shuichi Yamamoto further explains that our individual and collective desires have a direct impact, both positive and negative on our environment.

> As mentioned earlier, the Consciousness-Only doctrine holds that whatever is manifested in the environment and what kind of environment is created reflect the "common karma". In other words, what is internal in humans, such as desires, transform themselves into components of the external environment. (p. 251)

Thus the world, and every aspect of it, can be seen ultimately as the manifestation of our inner life (Erricker, 1995).

Empowerment at Individual and Societal Levels

This concept of the interconnectedness of self and environment can be overwhelming, however it can also be freeing and ultimately empowering. Indeed, empowerment of the individual to deal with suffering has been seen as a major goal of Shakyamuni Buddha and Buddhist psychology. Kawada (2001) has stated,

> Later practitioners [of Buddhism] would refer to the cosmic life force to which Shakyamuni awakened as the Buddha nature. They would explore means and methods of practice by which all people can manifest the vast energy, dignity, and wisdom of this life state; methods, in other words, of self-empowerment. (p. 19)

Empowerment at all levels is a key theme in this book, as the entire third section is devoted to empowerment and responsibility on the societal level. However, empowerment is a theme that is addressed on the individual level as well. Richard Hayes explicates that the goal of therapy is the development of a healthy mind. From the Buddhist perspective, this means the avoidance of excesses, both positive and negative, while emphasizing the importance of continued connectedness to family and community.

In some instances, the contributors have offered interventions that can aid the therapist to effectively assist their client. Thus, Ragsdale states:

> I believe that the invariant relation between meaning and value is implicit in Buddhist teaching. Its ultimate goal of enlightenment entails a transformation in the sphere of value, which is possible only through an awakening to the authentic meanings of self and world. (Consider here the Buddha's Four Noble Truths, which recognize ignorance as the cause of suffering.) These authentic meanings, freed of ignorance, consciously bear the insight of emptiness and dependent-arising. This entails – as though by definition – a full appreciation of the role of context in the relational determination of meaning, for context is the realm in which relationships arise. It moreover suggests a full conscious access to, and tolerance of, those contexts in unfolding experience. Liberation [or empowerment] is relational determination made fully accessible to consciousness. (p. 95)

The therapist working from a Gestalt perspective seeks to assist his patient to overcome their suffering through a deep understanding of their role in defining their life experience and response to it.

As psychologists, we are ethically mandated to respond to the emotional pain at all levels of human experience. Buddhist psychology can inform and offer avenues to develop the human psyche and the human spirit. This development is essential as true societal change can only be effected through change within the individual. Ikeda has said that a change within a single individual can bring about a change within the entire world. In other words that the "… inner determination of an individual can transform everything" (Ikeda, Saito, Endo, & Suda, 2000, p. 7). Conversely, we as human beings have developed our technology, but neglected our psychology. As Payutto (1996) states,

> Peace and happiness are on the wane, while troubles and misery grow … Why has this been so? … Because the individual human being has not been developed. Truly

> we have developed all kinds of things in the name of civilization, including science and technology, but we have paid too little attention to the development of ourselves. We think of ourselves as enjoyers of developments, not as objects of development. Our problems are much the same now as they were before, this year as three or ten thousand years ago, and our motives for action are of the same nature, even though they may take different forms. (p. 41)

Thus, Buddhist psychology, developed so many thousands of years ago remains quite relevant in the present day. The opening chapter, written by the editors, provides an excellent summary of the development of Buddhism with an overview of the Buddhist psychological theory.

Engaged Buddhism

In this time of turmoil, our authors have offered solutions predicated on our willingness to recognize and accept our societal responsibility and take action accordingly. In his chapter on Buddhist Social Principles, Chappell indicates that while mindfulness practice has traditionally been a mode of achieving inner peace, the Buddha proposed that dialogue, frequent and open, aspiring to consensus would lead to social harmony. Chappell proposed three crucial factors necessary to achieving that social well-being.

> First is constant mindfulness of the interdependent and impermanent factors in one's own consciousness that leads to nonattachment to any inner agenda; second is an appreciation of the factors in the lives of others that are similarly interdependent and impermanent; and third is a sense of compassion for others and moral commitment to social harmony. (p. 267)

He identifies several Buddhist leaders, among them Thich Nhat Hanh, the Dalai Lama, Daisaku Ikeda, and A. T. Ariyaratne, among others who share this same commitment to dialogue as a means of bridging the gaps not only between religions but also between peoples of all kinds.

Jason and Moritsugu also offer the use of Buddhist values and practices, as an effective means of enhancing community psychology practices. They suggest that it is the lack of a "road map," or adequate underpinning of values, which may render community psychological interventions less than effective. They state "Even though the elimination of deplorable environmental conditions are laudable goals, it is the thesis of this chapter that only a transformation of our values such as by embracing Buddhist principles will provide us the template to successfully work on the forces that cause unequal distribution of the worlds resources" (p. 199). The unequal distribution is seen as a major causative factor in the myriad social ills that plague our society. Dockett indicates that a major contribution of community psychology and Buddhist psychology is the notion of empowering organizations and communities that can inspire and promote positive behavior change and growth individually and collectively. Using Maton and Salem's (1995) construct of empowering organizations to analyze her twelve year longitudinal study of Nichiren Buddhism and the Soka Gakkai International-USA, Dockett details how its practices and philosophy teach a belief system that is "growth-inspiring, strengths-based, and beyond self... [It is an organization] established... for the purpose of enabling people to actualize the innate potentialities for value within their own lies and to create value within society" (p. 186). Thus, community psychology is seen as playing a crucial role in integration with Buddhist psychology in the peace process.

Recommendations

Anthony Marsella (1998; 2000a,b) has charged psychology with expanding its horizons to meet the emerging political, environmental, social, and cultural challenges of the twenty-first century. He states:

> If psychology is to survive and grow as a profession and academic discipline, it is essential for it to be responsive to the changing world in which we live. Unlike the world of the last few decades, today's world requires psychology to acknowledge the global context of our times, including the increased interdependency of our individual and collective lives. Today, events and forces in distant lands and cultures – once considered inconsequential and unimportant – have a daily impact upon our lives. Under these circumstances, psychology needs both to reconsider its training and research priorities, assumptions, methods, and ethics with a new vision, vigor, and commitment, and to respond to the emerging international challenges of over-population, poverty, environmental desecration, cultural disintegration, ethnopolitical warfare, and urbanization....
>
> I see internationalizing the psychology curriculum as a potent first step toward resolving the challenges facing the world because so many of these are rooted within political ideologies and economic systems that are culturally and nationally contextualized and generated. I propose that internationalizing the psychology curriculum begin with a recognition of the competencies that are needed by psychologists to function successfully (validly) in today's world. The things we do as psychologists – teaching, conceptualizing, researching, consulting, assessing, evaluating, intervening, preventing – must be considered within the range of levels in which we can demonstrate our competencies and participate in international and cultural activity arenas. We can be aware of cultural differences, share knowledge of these differences, consult across cultures, or actively participate in bringing about cultural changes....
>
> I would like to see our new psychology curriculum incorporate greater attention to indigenous psychologies, the non-western psychologies of such great cultural traditions as China, Islam, India, and the American Indians.... In brief,

> I call upon psychologists throughout the world to dialogue, to exchange views and actual positions, to learn the challenges facing our world, and in the process, to create a new professional and global consciousness that can advance our field, resolve problems, and restore dignity. It is within our capability to do so! It is our responsibility to do so! (2000b, p. 1)

Marsella views Buddhist psychology as a vehicle to inform and provide useful pathways for theoretical and research-based practical approaches to enhancing psychology's actions on the world stage. We, the editors and authors of this book, believe that Buddhism and psychology can forge a bond that can be mutually enhancing for the benefit of our society. Buddhism's rich, 3000-year history has only begun to be analyzed from the perspective of psychology. There is yet much to be learned. The practitioner, the scholar, the researcher, and the individual desirous of knowledge and growth can use the theses and findings of these chapters to further their thinking and their practice, and we hope improve their participation in this grand drama that is our universal life. We sincerely hope that as "engaged" individuals, we will also take full responsibility for creating the lasting peace that can ensure our human as well as technological development, long into the future, for ourselves and for humanity.

> After centuries of divorce between the spiritual and the worldly life, *the increasingly desperate situation of a planet that human beings are rapidly destroying cries out for a new kind of psychological integration*, which has only rarely existed before. Namely an integration between liberation – the capacity to step beyond the individual psyche into the larger, non-personal space of pure awareness – and personal transformation – the capacity to bring that larger awareness to bear on all one's conditioned psychological structures, so that they become fully metabolized, freeing the energy and the intelligence frozen inside them, thereby fuelling the development of a fuller, richer human presence that could fulfill the still unrealized potential of life on this earth. (Wellwood, 2000, p. 141)

References

Barlow, D. H. (2000). Evidence-based practice: A world view. *Clinical Psychology: Science and Practice, 7*, 241–242.

Chirot, D. & Seligman, M. E. P. (Eds.). (2001). *Ethnopolitical warfare: Causes, consequences, and possible solutions*. Washington, DC: American Psychological Association.

Erricker, C. (1995). *World faiths: Buddhism*. Chicago, IL: NTC/Contemporary Publishing.

Ikeda, D. (2001, June 22). True religion means commitment for peace. *World Tribune*, p. 1.

Ikeda, D., Saito, K., Endo, T., & Suda, H. (2000). *The wisdom of the Lotus Sutra: A discussion*. Santa Monica, CA: World Tribune Press.

Kawada, Y. (2001). Nichiren Buddhism and empowerment. *Living Buddhism, 5*(9), 18–23.

Khong, B. S. L. (2001, August). The Buddha's influence in the therapy room. In G. R. Dudley-Grant, (Chair), *Psychology and Buddhism*. Symposium conducted at the annual meeting of the American Psychological Association, San Francisco, CA.

Marsella, A. J. (1998). Toward a global-community psychology: Meeting the needs of a changing world. *American Psychologist, 53*, 1282–1291.

Marsella, A. J. (2000a, August). Psychology and global problems: Meeting the challenges of a new century. In T. Sasao (Chair), *Global challenges to social and community issues – Theory and practice*. Symposium conducted at the meeting of the American Psychological Association, Washington, DC.

Marsella, A. J. (2000b, Winter). Internationalizing the Psychology Curriculum, *International Psychology Reporter, 4*(3), 1–3.

Maton, K. I. & Salem, D.A. (1995). Organizational characteristics of empowering community settings: A multiple case study approach. *American Journal of community psychology, 23*, 631–656.

Nhat Hanh, T. (1993). *Love in action: Writings on nonviolent social change*. Berkeley, CA.: Parallax Press.

Payutto, P. A. (1996). *Buddhist solutions for the twenty-first century* (B. Evans, Trans.). Bangkok, Thailand: Buddhadhamma Foundation.

Rinpoche, S. (1995). *Glimpse after glimpse: Daily reflections on living and dying*. New York: HarperCollins.

Wellwood, J. (2000). Realization and embodiment: Psychological work in the service of spiritual development. In G. Watson, S. Batchelor, & G. Claxton (Eds), *The Psychology of Awakening* (pp. 137–166). York Beach, ME: Samuel Weiser.

About the Editors

C. Peter Bankart, Ph.D., is professor of psychology and director of the Student Counseling Service at Wabash College in Crawfordsville, Indiana. He is author of *Talking Cures: A History of Western and Eastern Psychotherapies* (1997), and numerous publications that explore the integration of Eastern thought with Western psychotherapeutics. He has taught on the faculty of the International Division of Waseda University in Tokyo.

Kathleen H. Dockett, Ed.D., is professor of psychology and former Chairperson of the Department of Psychology and Counseling at the University of the District of Columbia. She is author of *Resources for Stress Resistance: Parallels in Psychology and Buddhism* (1993). A community psychologist, her research and numerous presentations focus on Buddhism as a resource for the promotion of personal and societal well-being, and it's application to diversity and ethnic conflict.

G. Rita Dudley-Grant, Ph.D., MPH, ABPP, is a licensed clinical psychologist and director of program development at the Virgin Islands Behavioral Services in St. Croix. She is an APA Fellow, a member of the Board of Professional Affairs, past chair of the Committee on International Psychology, and past president of the Virgin Islands Psychological Association. She has presented on and been instrumental in a series of American Psychological Association programs examining the intersection of Buddhism and psychology.

Author Index

Subject Index